Donato F. Altomare, Filippo Pucciani (*Eds*)

Rectal Prolapse

Diagnosis and Clinical Management

Springer

Editors

Donato F. Altomare
Department of Emergency and Organ Transplantation
General Surgery and Liver
Transplantation Unit
University of Bari
Bari, Italy

Filippo Pucciani
Department of Medical and Surgical Critical Care
University of Florence
Florence, Italy

Library of Congress Control Number: 2007933189

ISBN 978-88-470-0683-6 Springer Milan Berlin Heidelberg New York
e-ISBN 978-88-470-0684-3

Springer is part of Springer Science+Business Media
springer.com

Cover layout: Simona Colombo, Milan, Italy
Typesetting: Compostudio, Cernusco s/N (Milan), Italy
Printing: Arti Grafiche Nidasio, Assago, Italy

Printed in Italy
Springer-Verlag Italia S.r.l., Via Decembrio 28, I-20137 Milan, Italy

Foreword

by John Nicholls

Rectal Prolapse: Diagnosis and Clinical Management is a unique publication. It is a multiauthor work edited by experts who have drawn together opinions by professionals highly recognised in the field. The book deals with a common condition in all its aspects – from aetiology and pathophysiology to treatment by the numerous available methods. The incidence of rectal prolapse will increase with the ageing population. In the young, functional defecation disorders sometimes associated with prolapse are frequently seen in colorectal practice and are an important cause of morbidity. For these reasons, the wide-ranging and detailed account of the subject contained within its pages makes the book particularly valuable. The contents give extensive information on the causes of prolapse and its investigation and treatment. In doing so, the editors have included contributors from home and abroad who have national and international standing. The concentrated experience that this offers is of the highest order.

The book deals comprehensively with the various forms of prolapse, including external prolapse, rectal intussusception and genital prolapse. Our understanding of the pathophysiology of rectal prolapse has advanced in the last 10–20 years due to the application of more sophisticated methods of neurophysiological assessment and of technical developments in imaging. The chapters on aetiology and investigation set out in detail the present position regarding the value of these advancements in clinical practice. The interface between rectal and genital prolapse is dealt with, as is the relationship of rectal prolapse to other anorectal symptoms such as incontinence and evacuation difficulty. The various abdominal and perineal procedures, including laparoscopic rectopexy, are described in separate chapters. Besides the classic operations, new treatments such as the STARR and EXPRESS procedures are dealt with, and their indications are considered in relation to the clinical presentation and the various other options. There is discussion on the relative merits of abdominal and perineal surgical approaches. Function following surgery receives considerable attention, and the difficult problems that may be posed by recurrence after surgery are dealt with. Nonsurgical treatment and rehabilitation are also described. There are chapters outlining best practice and a treatment algorithm that, being evidence based, set a standard of management guiding the reader through the decision-making process.

The book is beautifully laid out. The illustrations are exceptional. They include high-quality operative colour photographs and line drawings that demonstrate clearly the relevant stages of the procedure in question.

Rectal Prolapse: Diagnosis and Clinical Management gives a detailed and authoritative statement of current best practice through a wide-ranging account of all aspects of the condition. There is no other book on the subject that does so in such depth. The extensive bibliography will be a valuable resource to all practitioners involved in managing rectal prolapse, as well as to research workers in the field of functional bowel disease. The book should appeal not only to surgeons but also to gastroenterologists, physiologists and radiologists – whether in training or in established consultant practice.

London, September 2007

Prof. John Nicholls, MD
Emeritus Consultant Surgeon
St. Mark's Hospital
Professor of Colorectal Surgery
Imperial College, London

Foreword

by Floriano Marchetti
Stanley M. Goldberg

The treatment of rectal prolapse encompasses hundreds of different operations, and despite being known and studied for millennia, the subject still creates controversy. Never, since its first recorded description in the Eber papyrus of 1500 BC has so much attention and research, so much passion and discussion, been focused on this problem. Yet, the pathophysiologic bases of this condition remain elusive; the superiority of one technique over another unclear.

The surgical landscape for rectal prolapse has recently expanded to include new treatments such as the STARR and EXPRESS procedures. The apparent effectiveness of these new techniques has allowed greater insight into the understanding of the role of intussusception in the development of rectal procidentia. Conversely, these procedures have raised new questions and stirred an ongoing global controversy. If these operations are as effective as claimed, should we then operate on all patients presenting with obstructed defecation and internal intussusception? Will this prevent the development of rectal procidentia? Will the resulting rearranged pelvic anatomy prevent prolapse recurrence? Alternatively, will the same pathophysiologic mechanism that generated the prolapse in the first place, and which may not have been addressed, lead to recurrence? The answers are clearly not yet available, and long-term follow-up will hopefully assist us in the near future to attain those answers.

Furthermore, technical details, indications, and outcomes of these new techniques are not widely understood. Clearly, no significant comparison can be made if uniformity of indications, techniques, and goals is missing. No publication so far has extensively treated these issues; therefore, the majority of surgeons and almost all nonsurgical physicians involved in the treatment of rectal prolapse have no comprehensive and effective knowledge of the new operations. The richness and variety of choices for treating rectal prolapse may become confusing, and controversy may be paralyzing when dealing with a problem about which our understanding remains somewhat obscure.

These are some reasons many surgeons felt the need for one articulate and comprehensive volume that presented an all-inclusive understanding of the pathophysiology of rectal prolapse and state-of-the-art surgical treatment for it. There is, in fact, the obvious necessity to understand new techniques and perhaps the need to weed out old procedures that offer nothing other than a historical perspective in the understanding and treatment of this condition.

This daunting task was taken up by the editors and contributing authors of this book and implemented in an authoritative and concise fashion. *Rectal Prolapse: Diagnosis and Clinical Management* offers a body of information encompassing any aspect of pathophysiology, diagnosis, and treatment of rectal prolapse. It is a meticulous, exhaustive review of what is established, what is new, and what we should know about rectal prolapse and its treatment.

Rectal prolapse is routinely treated in colorectal surgery textbooks as a separate entity without any deep, comprehensive discussion of the pathophysiologic antecedents that lead to its development. This book details the current understanding of prolapse mechanisms as well as the long process of anatomic and physiologic changes and symptoms that lead to rectal procidentia and fecal incontinence. Several different treatment procedures – surgical and nonsurgical – are listed and technically described, as are their results. Each procedure is treated in separate, logically laid-out chapters, with constant reference to the pathophysiological processes of rectal prolapse.

Rarely, if ever, in a textbook have obstructed defecation, intussusception, and rectal prolapse been addressed together in a comprehensive and coordinated fashion in the attempt to understand the interrelations that tie these three entities together. The editors and authors of this book have successfully achieved that goal and provided this missing link. The layout is beautiful, and the illustrations are precise to the smallest detail. The pool of contributors includes some of the most authoritative experts on the subject in the world, and whereas colorectal surgeons everywhere will benefit the most from this book, it is a valuable resource to all health care professionals who deal with such patients.

Miami, October 2007

Prof. Floriano Marchetti MD
Assistant Professor of Clinical Surgery
Division of Colon and Rectal Surgery
DeWitt Daughtry Family Department of Surgery
Miller School of Medicine
University of Miami
Miami, FL, USA

Prof. Stanley M. Goldberg MD, FACS
Clinical Professor of Surgery
Division of Colon and Rectal Surgery
Department of Surgery
University of Minnesota
Minneapolis, MN, USA

Contents

Contributors

Donato F. Altomare
Department of Emergency and
Organ Transplantation
University of Bari
Bari, Italy

Luca Amadio
Department of Surgery
University of Padua
Padua, Italy

David C.C. Bartolo
Western General Hospital
Edinburgh, United Kingdom

Alberto Bazzocchi
Department of Radiology
Pelvic Floor Imaging Centre
Radiologia Golfieri
Malpighi-S-Orsola Hospital
Bologna, Italy

Roberto Bellomo
Department of Surgery
Civil Hospital
San Vito al Tagliamento (PN), Italy

Roberto Bergamaschi
Department of Surgery
Lehigh Valley Hospital
Penn State University Campus
Allentown, PA, USA

Francesco Bianco
Department of Surgery I
"S.G. Moscati" Hospital
Avellino, Italy

Gian Andrea Binda
Department of Surgery
Galliera Hospital
Genoa, Italy

Luisa Caggiano
Department of Surgery I
"S.G. Moscati" Hospital
Avellino, Italy

Mauro Cervigni
Department of Urogynecology
S. Carlo - IDI Hospital
Rome, Italy

Gianluca Colucci
Department of Surgery and Gastroenterology
University of Verona
Verona, Italy

Gian Gaetano Delaini
Department of Surgery and Gastroenterology
University of Verona
Verona, Italy

Raffaele De Caro
Department of Human Anatomy and Physiology
School of Medicine
University of Padua
Padua, Italy

Domenico Del Ciampo
Department of Surgery
Civil Hospital
San Vito al Tagliamento (PN), Italy

Giuseppe Dodi
Department of Surgery
University of Padua
Padua, Italy

Andre D'Hoore
Department of Abdominal Surgery
University Hospital Gasthuisberg
Leuven, Belgium

Michael Fealk
Department of Surgery
Lehigh Valley Hospital
Allentown, PA, USA

Ezio Ganio
Colorectal Eporediensis Centre
Department of Colorectal Surgery
Monza, Italy

Iacopo Giani
Department of Medical and Surgical Care
University of Florence
Florence, Italy

Pasquale Giordano
Department of Surgery
Whipps Cross University Hospital
London, United Kingdom

Rita Golfieri
Department of Radiology
Pelvic Floor Imaging Centre
Radiologia Golfieri
Malpighi-S-Orsola Hospital
Bologna, Italy

Aldo Infantino
Department of Surgery
Civil Hospital
San Vito al Tagliamento (PN), Italy

Urban Karlbom
Department of Surgery
University Hospital
Uppsala, Sweden

Amit Khanna
Department of Colorectal Surgery
Cleveland Clinic Florida
Weston, FL, USA

Marco La Torre
Department of Digestive and Endocrine Surgery
Hôtel-Dieu
University Hospital of Nantes
Nantes, France

Paul-Antoine Lehur
Department of Digestive and Endocrine Surgery
Hôtel-Dieu
University Hospital of Nantes
Nantes, France

Veronica Macchi
Department of Human Anatomy and Physiology
School of Medicine
University of Padua
Padua, Italy

Robert D. Madoff
Department of Surgery
Division of Colon and Rectal Surgery
University of Minnesota
Minneapolis, MN,USA

Anders Mellgren
Division of Colon and Rectal Surgery
University of Minnesota
Minneapolis, MN, USA

Dan R. Metcalf
Spectrum Health
Ferguson Clinic
Grand Rapids, MI, USA

Guillaume Meurette
Department of Digestive and Endocrine Surgery
Hôtel-Dieu
University Hospital of Nantes
Nantes, France

Pier Carlo Muzzio
IRCCS-Istituto Oncologico Veneto and
Department of Medical Diagnostic Sciences and
Special Therapies, Radiology
University Hospital
Padua, Italy

Franca Natale
Department of Urogynecology
S. Carlo - IDI Hospital
Rome, Italy

Hung Nguyen
Department of Surgery
Launceston General Hospital
Launceston, TAS, Australia

James W. Ogilvie Jr.
Department of Surgery
Division of Colon and Rectal Surgery
University of Minnesota
Minneapolis, MN,USA

Anna Padoa
Department of Obstetrics and Gynecology
Assaf Harofe Medical Center
Zrifin, Israel

Lars Påhlman
Department of Surgery
University Hospital
Uppsala, Sweden

Hugh M. Paterson
Department of Colorectal Surgery
Western General Hospital
Edinburgh, United Kingdom

Freddy Penninckx
Department of Abdominal Surgery
University Hospital Gasthuisberg
Leuven, Belgium

Vittorio L. Piloni
Department of Radiology
Pelvic Floor Imaging Centre
Radiologia Golfieri
Malpighi-S-Orsola Hospital
Bologna, Italy

Fabio Pomerri
Department of Medical Diagnostic Sciences and
Special Therapies, Radiology
University Hospital
Padua, Italy

Andrea Porzionato
Department of Human Anatomy and Physiology
School of Medicine
University of Padua
Padua, Italy

Filippo Pucciani
Department of Medical and Surgical Critical Care
University of Florence
Florence, Italy

Carlo Ratto
Department of Surgical Sciences
Division of Digestive Surgery
Catholic University
Rome, Italy

Marcella Rinaldi
Department of Emergency and
Organ Transplantation
University of Bari
Bari, Italy

Giovanni Romano
Department of Surgery I
"S.G. Moscati" Hospital
Avellino, Italy

Anthony J. Senagore
Spectrum Health
Ferguson Clinic
Grand Rapids, MI, USA

Alberto Serventi
Department of Surgery
Galliera Hospital
Genoa, Italy

Vance Sohn
Department of Surgery
Madigan Army Medical Center
Tacoma, WA, USA

Scott R. Steele
Department of Surgery
Madigan Army Medical Center
Tacoma, WA, USA

Steven D. Wexner
Department of Colorectal Surgery
Ohio State University and
Department of Surgery
University of South Florida College of Medicine
Cleveland Clinic Florida
Weston, FL, USA

Norman S. Williams
Centre for Academic Surgery
The Royal London Hospital
London, United Kingdom

Andrew P. Zbar
School of Clinical of Human Life Sciences
University of Tasmania
Launceston, TAS, Australia

SECTION I
Rectal Prolapse: Anatomy, Pathophysiology and Imaging

1 Perineum: Functional Anatomy

Raffaele De Caro, Andrea Porzionato, Veronica Macchi

Introduction

The perineum is the complex of tissues between the peritoneum and the skin that closes the pelvis inferiorly. The surface projection of the perineum and the form of the skin covering vary considerably depending on the position of the thighs: they are reduced when the tighs are adducted, whereas they widen when the tighs are flexed and abducted. The perineum is diamond-shaped, bounded by four lines: two from the pubic symphysis to the ischial tuberosities, and two from the ischial tuberosities to the coccyx. In the female, it is crossed anteriorly by the urethra and the vagina and posteriorly by the rectum; in the male, it is crossed anteriorly by the urethra and posteriorly by the rectum. Thus, in the female, the skin of the perineum is reduced compared with that in the male. Anatomical structures between the perineum and skin are constituted by muscles and fasciae, which are located in three planes: (1) the pelvic diaphragm, (2) the urogenital diaphragm, and (3) the superficial plane of the perineum.

Pelvic Diaphragm

The pelvic diaphragm is constituted by two laminar muscles, the levator ani and ischiococcygeus muscles, which – arising from the pelvic walls – are attached to the opposite pelvic walls (Figs. 1 and 2). Their fibres are primarily directed backwards to the coccyx and the rectum. The fasciae investing the muscles are the superior and inferior fasciae of the pelvic diaphragm. The two levator ani are similar to a funnel shape with the apex at the level of the puborectal sling. Each muscle attaches to the bone on the pubis anteriorly and the ischiatic spine posteriorly. Between these two bone attachments, the muscle is linked through a tendineus arcade to the fascia of the muscle obturator internus. From this line of attachments, the muscle fibres are directed backwards, medially and downwards, to attach to the perineal body on the posterior wall of the anorectal junction and on the anococcygeal raphe. The muscle is subdivided into portions that are named according to their attachments and the pelvic viscera to which they are related: (1) pubococcygeus muscle (supe-

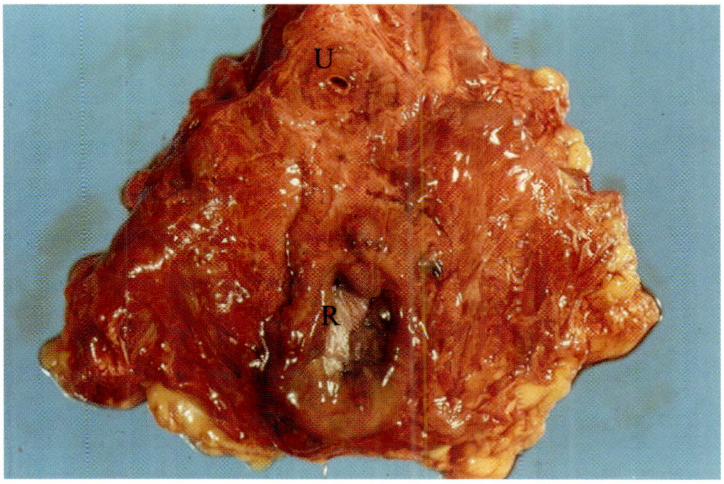

Fig. 1
Pelvic view of a male pelvic block (*R* rectum, *U* urethra)

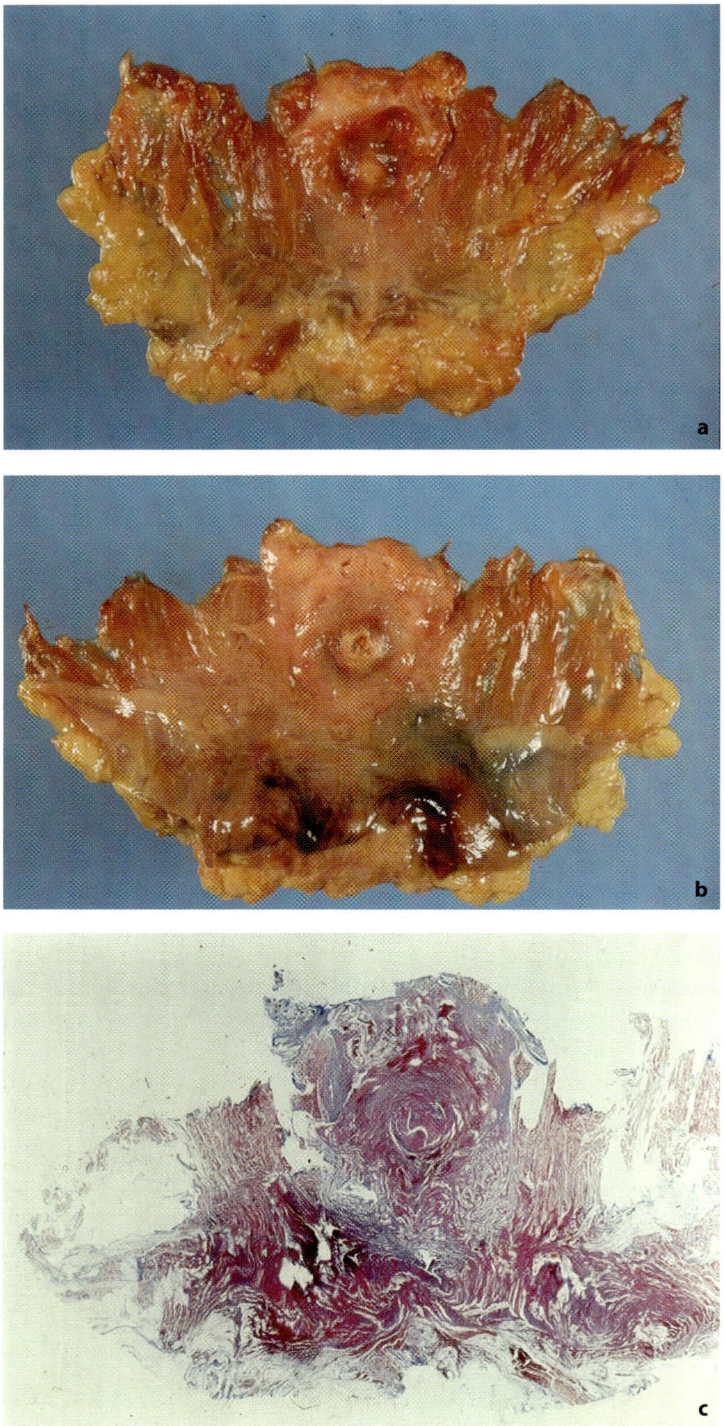

Fig. 2a-c
Perineal (**a**) and pelvic (**b**) aspects of the levator ani muscle isolated from the sample of Figure 1. Histological macrosection of the levator ani (**c**) (azan-Mallory stain)

rior level), (2) iliococcygeus muscle (intermediate level) and (3) puborectal muscle (inferior level). The levator ani muscles with their attachments to the perineal body separate the anterior urogenital hiatus and the posterior anal hiatus. The ischiococcygeus muscle arises from the tip of the ischial spine and is attached to the lateral margins of the coccyx and the fifth sacral vertebra. The consistency of the levator ani and the course of its fibres are variable, and in particular, the ischiococcygeus muscle may be nearly completely tendinous rather than muscular.

Urogenital Diaphragm

The urogenital diaphragm is a muscular-fascial sheet triangular in shape (urogenital triangle), anteriorly and laterally bound deeply by the pubic symphysis and ischiopubic rami. In males, it is crossed by the urethra and in females by the urethra and the vagina. It includes two muscles that lie between the superior and deep fascia of the urogenital diaphragm. The *deep transverse perinei* is attached to the medial aspects of the ischiopubic rami; posteriorly, it is attached to the perineal body where its fibres decussate with those of the opposite side. Together with the superficial transverse perinei, the muscles may help support the visceral canals that pass through them.

The compressor urethra is recognisable in females, and its fibres arise from the ischiopubic rami, pass anteriorly, and fuse with the contralateral fibres, lying anterior to the urethra *below sphincter urethrae*. However, the urethral sphincter mechanism is constituted by intrinsic striated and smooth muscle of the urethra and by fibres of the pubourethralis component of the levator ani, surrounding the membranous urethra in the male and the middle and lower thirds of the urethra in the female.

Superficial Plane of the Perineum

The superficial plane of the perineum contains superficial muscles, some placed around the terminal portion of the genital system (bulbospongiosus, ischiocavernosus and the *superficial transverse perinei muscles*) and others placed around the anal canal (external anal sphincter). This plane is limited superficially by the superficial perineal fascia.

Perineal Body

The perineal body is a poorly defined aggregation of fibromuscular tissue located between the rectum and urogenital triangles. It is attached to muscles and fasciae.

Rectum

The rectum (Fig. 3) is part of the large bowel and is about 12-cm long. It can be subdivided into superior and inferior parts. It is continuous with the sigmoid colon at the level of the third sacral vertebra. It descends in two curves on the sagittal plane: the sacral flexure of the rectum, along the sacrococcygeal concavity; and the perineal flexure, where it crosses the pelvic diaphragm. The passage through the pelvic diaphragm corresponds to the anorectal junction, and the angle it forms with the upper anal canal is termed the anorectal angle, 2–3 cm in front of and slightly below the tip of the coccyx. On the frontal plane, the rectum deviates in three lateral curves: the upper and lower are convex to the right; the middle bulges to the left. The taeniae blend above the rectosigmoid junction forming two wide muscular bands on the anterior and posterior aspects of the rectal wall. The upper third of the rectum is covered by the peritoneum on its anterior and lateral aspects; the middle third of the rectum is covered by the peritoneum only on the anterior aspect. The peritoneum is reflected superiorly onto the urinary bladder in males, to form the rectovesical pouch, or onto the posterior vaginal wall in females, to form the rectouterine pouch (pouch of Douglas). The peritoneum is loosely attached by fatty connective tissue to the muscular tunica, allowing for considerable expansion of the upper half of the rectum. In the internal surface of the rectum, some permanent semilunar transverse or horizontal folds are recognisable, consisting of the mucosa, the submucosa and the muscularis. The most superior fold, at the beginning of the rectum, and the middle fold, immediately above the rectal ampulla, are quite constant.

Anal Canal

The anal canal, 4-cm long, begins at the anorectal junction and is directed downwards and backwards. It is located between the perineal body an-

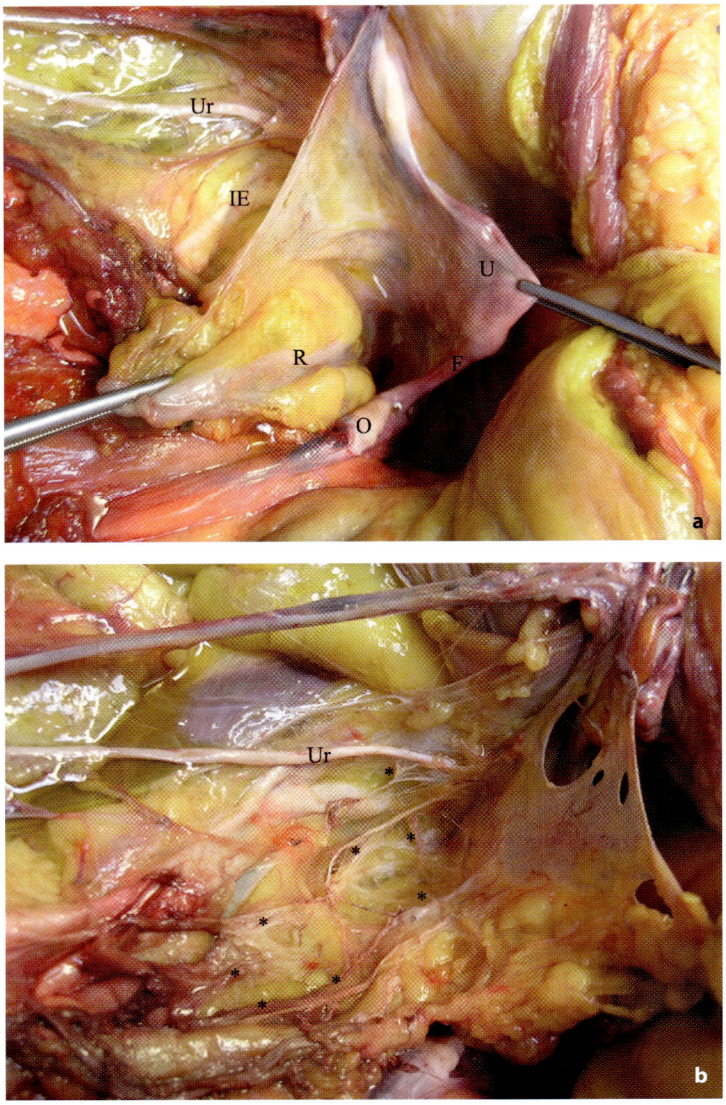

Fig. 3a,b

Aspect of the female pelvic viscera during anatomical dissection (**a**). The forceps grasp the uterus (*U*) and the rectum (*R*) showing the rectouterine pouch (*D*). After removal of the peritoneum laterally to the cervix (**b**), dissection shows the inferior hypogastric plexus (*asterisks*). *F* fallopian tube, *O* ovary, *IE* external iliac artery, *Ur* ureter

teriorly, the anococcygeal ligament posteriorly and the ischiorectal fossae laterally. Sphincteric muscles surround the rectum along its course, and at rest they cause an oval slit in the anteroposterior plane rather than a circular canal. Three portions can be subdivided as follows:

1. The first portion, 15-mm long, beginning at the anorectal junction and ending at the dentate line, presents mucosa with a stratified cubic epithelium. There are six to ten vertical folds, the anal columns, which contain a terminal radicle of the superior rectal vessels. The lower ends of the columns are joined by mucosal folds, the anal valves, between which lie small recesses referred to as anal sinuses. In the embryonic period, the dentate line is the site of the anal membrane, appearing at the junction between the entodermic portion of the anal canal, derived from the cloacae, and the ectodermic portion, derived from the proctodeum.
2. The second portion, 15-mm long, is the transition zone, or pecten. It is nonkeratinised, stratified, squamous epithelium that lacks sweat and sebaceous glands and hair follicles but contains numerous somatic nerve endings. It extends from the dentate line to the white line of Hilton, corresponding to the intersphincteric anal groove (boundary between the lower border of the internal sphincter and the sub-

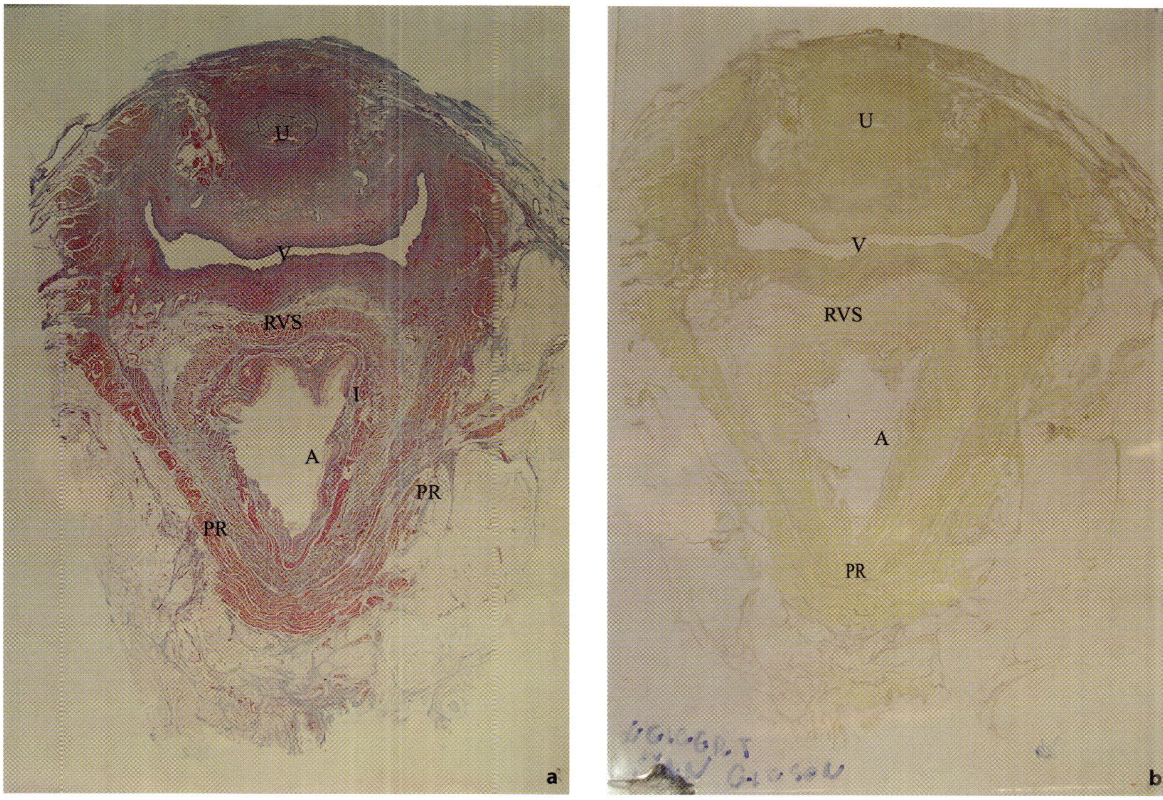

Fig. 4a,b
Transverse sections of the female pelvic viscera with azan-Mallory (**a**) and Weigert-van Gieson (**b**) stains showing topography and histological characteristics of puborectal sling (*PR*), rectovaginal septum (*RVS*) and internal anal sphincter (*I*). *U* urethra, *V* vagina, *A* anal canal

cutaneous portion of the external sphincter).

3. The third part, 10-mm long, is located inferiorly to the white line of Hilton and is continuous with the skin.

The walls of the anal canal are surrounded by the sphincteric complex, the puborectal muscle and the internal and external anal sphincters.

Puborectal Muscle

The puborectal muscle is the caudal and most medial portion of the levator ani and is constituted by a superior and inferior lamina (Fig. 4). The inferior lamina progresses backwards from the insertion on the pubis to join the contralateral muscle behind the anorectal junction. In this way, it forms a sling, anchoring the junction to the pubis and determining perineal flexure. Posteriorly, the anococcygeal ligament anchors the junction to the coccyx. The muscle's lateral fibres show anteroposterior direction, and the medial fibres show a descending longitudinal course and juxtapose with the smooth longitudinal musculature of the anal wall, interposing between the internal and the external sphincters. The most superficial anterior fibres of the puborectal muscle insert in front of the rectum and contribute to formation of the levator muscle of the prostate gland in the male and the pubovaginal muscle in the female. Their margins delimit the urogenital hiatus.

Internal Anal Sphincter

The internal anal sphincter (Fig. 4) is constituted by a thickening of the circular layer of the smooth muscle of the anal canal. It is 5- to 8-mm thick and surrounds the superior three fourths of the anal canal and ends at the level of the linea alba.

External Anal Sphincter

The external anal sphincter is a striated muscle surrounding the anal canal for its entire length and is formed by three parts: subcutaneous, superficial and deep. The first (subcutaneous) and the third (deep) parts of the muscle are ring-like and do not insert on the coccygeus, whereas the second part is oval and inserts on the coccygeus. The subcutaneous part is a flat band 15-mm wide surrounding the inferior part of the anal canal beneath the inferior margin of the internal sphincter. Anteriorly, some bundles insert onto the tendineus centre and mix with bundles from the superficial transverse muscles, whereas posteriorly they insert on the anococcygeal ligament. The superficial part arises from the posterior surface of the most caudal coccygeal vertebra and from the anococcygeal raphe. The muscle bundles are directed anteriorly to form two bands surrounding the inferior half of the internal sphincter and insert into the tendineus centre. This is the only part of the muscle that is anchored to the bone. It is interposed between the subcutaneous and deep part. The deep part is ring-like and surrounds the superior part of the internal sphincter. Posteriorly, it inserts on the anococcygeal ligament; anteriorly, some bundles continue with the bundles of superficial transverse muscle. Cranial bundles are not separable from the puborectal muscle. Besides these muscles, at the level of the anal canal, there are two other muscular formations without strict sphincterial functions: the muscle wrinkler of the anal skin and the muscularis mucosae.

Corrugator Cutis Ani

The corrugator cutis ani corresponds to the common longitudinal muscular layer, interposed between the internal and the external sphincters, arising from the anorectal junction. It juxtaposes the longitudinal bundles of the intrinsic muscle layer of the anal wall. Distally, this muscle lamina becomes fibroelastic and divides into about ten fibroelastic septa irradiating and crossing the subcutaneous part of the external sphincter to insert into the derm of the perianal skin. One of these septa passes between the inferior margin of the internal sphincter and the external sphincter and is called the intermuscular anal septum. It is responsible of the intersphincteric anal groove.

Muscularis Mucosa

The muscularis mucosa is constituted by longitudinal and circular bundles of smooth muscular fibres located between the mucosal and submucosal layers.

Innervation of the anal sphincters derives from:

1. The orthosympathetic nerve fibres: these arise from the lateral column of myelomeres T-11, T-12, L-1 and L-2 and run through the inferior hypogastric plexus to inhibit the musculature of the rectal ampulla and excite the musculature of the internal sphincter.
2. The parasympathetic nerve fibres: these arise from the sacral myelomeres S-2, S-3 and run through the pelvic splanchnic nerves (erigentes nerves) to excite the musculature of the rectal ampulla and to inhibit the internal sphincter.
3. The pudendal nerve: this runs through the inferior rectal branch arising from myelomeres S-2, S-3 and the perineal branch of S-4 to excite the musculature of the external sphincter and the puborectal muscle.

Personal Contributions

Subperitoneal Connective Tissue in the Female Pelvis

Traditionally, a system of ligamentous suspensory structures (the sacropubic laminae of Farabeuf and the cardinal ligaments of Mackenrodt) is described in the female pelvis. According to some authors, the so-called visceral pelvic fascia (endopelvic fascia) includes a fibrous connective system that forms two paired ligaments [1]. The first ligament constitutes the sacropubic laminae of Farabeuf, which have an anteroposterior course and may be subdivided into four segments: sacrorectal, rectouterine, uterovesical and pubovesical. The second suspensory mechanism is constituted by the cardinal ligaments of Mackenrodt, which run transverse from the pelvic wall to the uterine cervix. These structures should sustain the pelvic organs, particularly the cervix, together with the connective condensations forming visceral fascias (rectal, cervicovaginal and vesical fascia, respectively). The spaces among them are filled with fibroadipose tissue that, according to anatomical literature, has no active role in supporting the intrapelvic organs. In De Caro et al. [2], the subperitoneal connective tissue was studied with histological and morphometric techniques and plastination. The subperitoneal connective tissue of the female pelvis consists of varying amounts of adipose tissue divided into small lobules by thin connective laminae. These laminae are connected to the visceral and parietal layers of the pelvic fascia and are closely connected to the vascular and nervous bundle sheaths crossing the pelvis. At the level of the so called sacrouterine and cardinal ligaments, we were unable to find connective ligamentous structures, and they correspond respectively to the inferior hypogastric plexus and uterine vessels, around which there is areolar adipose tissue with smooth muscle cells. In the absence of real connective ligaments, the subperitoneal connective tissue forms a three-dimensional network of thin connective laminae that are connected to the visceral adventitia, parietal layer of the pelvic fascia and neurovascular bundles crossing the pelvis. These connective laminae surround the adipose lobules of different sizes (smaller near the viscera; larger at the periphery). The subperitoneal connective tissue constitutes an anatomical structure that, beyond the functional limits of any individual ligament, may have "active" supporting properties.

Rectourethralis Muscle

The rectourethralis muscle has been described in different ways in the literature. Henle [3], in his first description of the "prerectal" muscle, did not define its attachments. In the work by Roux [4], muscle fibres were described as deriving, to a minor extent, from the dorsal aspect of the inferior half of the prostatic urethra and, to major extent, from the membranous urethra. Both bundles were described as travelling obliquely backwards and upwards to the anterior rectal wall and passing through the longitudinal and circular muscular layers, ending in the submucosa. For Poirier [5] the rectourethralis muscle represented a reinforcement of the rectal musculature in the male. In his description, muscle fibres attached to the urogenital diaphragm, the urethral musculature and the prostate and went towards the anterior rectal wall. Some fibres travelled upwards, attaching to the inferior aspect of the peritoneum of the cul-de-sac of Douglas, whereas other more numerous fibres attached to the rectal wall, travelling upwards and downwards and continuing with the longitudinal and circular muscular layers. According to Wesson [6], the rectourethralis muscle attached posteriorly to the anterior longitudinal layer of the rectum, at the level of the verum montanum and coursed forwards to attach anteriorly to the posterior raphe of the external urethral sphincter. This muscle would be responsible for the perineal flexure of the rectum and its close approach to the prostate apex. Myers et al. [7] confirmed the presence of muscular bands attaching anteriorly into the perineal body and posteriorly to the anal canal (anoperineal bands) and to the anterior surface of the rectum (rectoperineal bands). Brooks et al. [8] described it as arising as two lateral arms from the smooth muscle of the anterior rectal wall, fusing in the midline and attaching to the perineal body. In addition, Matsubara et al. [9] found that at the interface between the rectourethralis muscle and the rectum, there was an intermingling of fibres with the outer layer of the longitudinal smooth muscle of the rectum.

The analysis by our group [10] showed that the fibres of the rectourethralis muscle attached to the longitudinal muscular layer of the rectum and of the anal canal. In no histological sections were fibres seen extending to the circular layer or to the submucosa, as formerly stated by Roux and Poirier [4, 5]. We also confirmed the presence of the two components of the muscle, i.e., the rectoperinealis and the anoperinealis muscles. Concerning the anterior portion of the muscle, both sagittal and transverse sections showed clear separation of its smooth fibres from the prostatic and membranous urethra and their attachment to the perineal body. The rectourethralis muscle, being separated from the prostatic and membranous urethra by the septum rectovesicale, is located in the caudal portion of the prerectal space. This location and, in particular, the absence of attachment to the prostatic or membranous urethra make the original term "prerectal" as used by Henle more correct than the term "rectourethralis". The latter term, in fact, was introduced by authors who considered the muscle to directly attach to the urethra.

Rectovaginal Septum

The rectovaginal septum (RVS) (Fig. 4) is commonly described as a strong connective tissue between the rectum and the vagina. Through an histological, plastination and morphometric study [11], the RVS has been evaluated on transverse sections collected at the cranial and caudal levels of the middle third (level II) and inferior third (level III) of the vagina. The RVS is located in an oblique coronal plane, close to the posterior vaginal wall, and is formed by a network of collagen, elastic fibres, smooth muscle cells with nerve fibres emerging from the autonomic inferior hypogastric plexus and variable numbers of small vessels. The RVS is thicker at cranial levels II and III with respect to caudal level II, both in the midline (1.75 and 1.70 vs. 0.2 mm, $p < 0.05$) and lateral portions of the septum (2.67 and 2.64 vs. 0.17 mm, $p < 0.05$). At the caudal level II, there are no statistically significant differences between the thicknesses of the lateral portions and the midline (0.17 vs. 0.2 mm, $p > 0.05$). The RVS resembles an hourglass shape, with a flattened central portion in the frontal plane. Given its position in the centre of the pelvis, the RVS plays a connecting role between the perineal body and the overlying portions of the endopelvic fascia. It may also play an active role in modulating pelvic-wall musculature tone during variations in endorectal pressure.

Longitudinal Anal Muscle

The longitudinal anal muscle (LAM) has been described as a layer of muscular tissue interposed between the external and internal anal sphincter [12], but there is no general agreement in the literature as to its attachments and constitution. Lesshaft [13] stated that the posterior part of the levator ani from the sacrococcygeal column travelled down to the posterior part of the perineal portion of the rectum. The external fibres inserted in the pelvic aponeurosis (tensor fasciae pelvis), and the internal fibres inserted in the context of the internal sphincter and the deep part of the anal skin. Cruveilhier [14] described the levator ani contributing with some fibres towards augmenting the outer muscle coat to form the conjoint longitudinal muscle of the anus. Milligan and Morgan [15] attributed the contribution to the LAM to the puborectalis posteriorly and the deep external anal sphincter anteriorly, whereas Courtney [16] described the LAM as a vertically oriented, striated muscle that received contributions from the puborectalis, pubococcygeus and ileococcygeus muscles. Shafik [17] subdivided the LAM into three layers (medial, intermediate, lateral), separated by four fascial septa, which split and decussate below the lower end of the longitudinal muscle to form the "central tendon". In their review, Lunniss and Phillips [18] reported that the LAM consisted of a muscular part formed by the fusion of striated muscle fibres from the puboanalis, the innermost part of the puborectalis, with smooth tissue from the longitudinal muscle of the rectum. The layer then becomes completely fibroelastic and splits into septa, running between bundles of the subcutaneous external sphincter, to terminate in the perianal skin. More recently, Petros [19] described the contribution to the LAM by the levator ani plate, the lateral part of the pubococcygeus muscle and the puborectalis muscles. The LAM partly surrounds the rectum posteriorly but is not inserted into it and runs inferiorly into both the deep and superficial external anal sphincter. Its topography and histologic characteristics were studied by our group [20]. We found that the LAM appears as a layer of muscular tissue interposed between the internal and external anal sphincters. From the anorectal junction, it extends along the anal canal, receives fibres from the puborectalis and medial part of the pubococcygeus muscles and terminates with fibroelastic septa (7–9), which penetrate the external anal sphincter, reaching the deep part of the dermis. In the transverse plane, the mean thickness of the LAM is 1.63 ± 0.44 mm. Immunohistochemical staining showed that the LAM consists predominantly of striated muscle fibres with scarce smooth muscle fibres. Due to its attachments, the LAM may play a role in supporting and binding together the internal and external sphincter complex.

References

1. Staskin DR, Hadley HR, Leach GE et al (1986) Anatomy for vaginal surgery. Sem Urol 4:2
2. De Caro R, Aragona F, Herms A et al (1998) Morphometric analysis of the fibroadipose tissue of the female pelvis. J Urol 160:707–713
3. Henle J (1873) Handbuch der systematischen Anatomie des Menschen. Braunschweig, F. Vieweg u. Sohn, pp 533–910
4. Roux C (1881) Beitrage zur Kenntniss der Aftermuskulatur des Menschen. Archiv fur Mikroskop Anat 19:721–733
5. Poirier P (1895) Traite d'anatomie humain, vol. 4. L Battaille, Paris, pp 80–82
6. Wesson MB (1922) The development, and surgical importance of the rectourethralis muscle and Denonvilliers' fascia. J Urol 8:339–359
7. Myers RP, Cahill DR, Devine RM, King BF (1998) Anatomy of radical prostatectomy as defined by magnetic resonance imaging. J Urol 159:2148–2158
8. Brooks JD, Eggener SE, Chao WM (2002) Anatomy of the rectourethralis muscle. Eur Urol 41:94–100
9. Matsubara A, Murakami G, Arakawa T et al (2003) Topographic anatomy of the male perineal structures with special reference to perineal approaches for radical prostatectomy. Int J Urol 10:141–148
10. Porzionato A, Macchi V, Gardi M et al (2005) Histotopographic study of the rectourethralis muscle. Clin Anat 18:510–517
11. Stecco C, Macchi V, Porzionato A et al (2005) Histotopographic study of the rectovaginal septum. Ital J Anat Embryol 110:247–254
12. Standring S, Ellis H, Healy JC et al (eds) (2005) Gray's Anatomy, 39th edn. Churchill Livingstone, London, p 1199
13. Lesshaft P (1892) Grundlagen der theoretichen Anatomie. Mason, Leipzig
14. Cruveilhier H (1852) Traite d'Anatomie Descripitve. Labe, Paris
15. Milligan E, Morgan CN (1934) Surgical anatomy of the anal canal with special reference to anorectal fistulae. Lancet 224:1150–1156; 1213–1217
16. Courtney H (1950) Anatomy of the pelvic diaphragm and anorectal musculature as related to sphincter preservation in anorectal surgery. Am J Surg 79:155–173
17. Shafik A (1976) A new concept of the anatomy of the anal sphincter mechanism and the physiology of defecation. III. The longitudinal anal muscle: anatomy and role in anal sphincter mechanism. Invest Urol 13:271–277
18. Lunniss and Phillips (1992) Anatomy and function of the anal longitudinal muscle. Br J Surg 79:882–884
19. Petros PE (2004) The female pelvic floor. Springer, Heidelberg, pp 18–20; 43–45
20. Macchi V, Porzionato A, Stecco C et al (2007) Histotopographic study of the longitudinal anal muscle. Pelvi-Perineology 26:30–32

2 Rectal Prolapse: Pathophysiology

Filippo Pucciani

Introduction

Rectal prolapse, procidentia, "complete" prolapse or "first-degree" prolapse, is defined as a circumferential, full-thickness intussusception of the rectal wall with protrusion beyond the anal canal [1]. This definition emphasises two important points: (1) rectal prolapse is the expression of a full-thickness intussusception, and (2) protrusion is outside the anus. The cause of rectal prolapse is still not completely understood. It is likely the result of a multifactorial aetiology, and any single standard theory would be improbable and imprecise. This implies that each patient potentially has his or her own specific pathogenetic profile, which is the result of a mix of several aetiological factors. A great division has developed between supporters of the "sliding hernia" and those who support the rectal intussusception theory. Rectal prolapse has been related to either a form of sliding hernia, as most patients have a redundant sigmoid colon, deep pelvic-peritoneal cul-de-sac, diastasis of the levator ani muscles, loss of posterior rectal fixation and loss of the usual anorectal angle; or to the final stages of a progressively worsening intussusception, as similarities in manometric findings can be found among patients with rectal prolapse, rectoanal intussusception and solitary rectal ulcer syndrome. In contrast with this dichotomous illustration of the facts, there are many other important factors that can play a role in the pathophysiology of rectal prolapse. In an attempt to find a common thread, a few questions should be answered:

- Why is rectal prolapse uncommon in men?
- How and why does a full-thickness intussusception of the rectum occur?
- How and why does external protrusion of the rectum occur?
- What is the role of the pelvic floor muscles (PFM), pelvic fascia and connective tissue, which together are designed to hold the internal organs within the pelvic cavity?
- How and why does rectal prolapse occur alone or in combination with other pelvic organ prolapses?
- What is the multidirectional relationship among rectal prolapse, defecation and faecal continence?
- What happens to colonic motility in rectal prolapse?
- What is the relationship between rectal prolapse and solitary rectal ulcer syndrome?

Rectal Prolapse in Men

Epidemiological aspects emphasise the low incidence of rectal prolapse in men ($\approx$10%) vs. women ($\approx$90%) [2]. Differently from women, the incidence of rectal prolapse in men does not increase with age and remains constant throughout life. The topic has yet to be studied extensively, and there is no clear explanation for this epidemiological phenomenon. We deduce that the structure of the male pelvic floor, which is strongly supported by the prostate, and the low incidence of obstructed defecation compared with women may be two significant factors that may help explain the different incidence between the sexes. The prostate is a powerful anchorage for all pelvic organs, which, for example, provides an insurmountable impediment to sliding: indeed, a descending perineum is very rare in men [3], and rectal prolapse is usually related to a defective pelvic floor [4]. Similarly, obstructed defecation created by pelvic floor dyssynergia is more frequent in women [5], and the same demography is present in patients affected by rectoanal intussusception [6], which is considered to be a sort of preprolapse state [7, 8]. However, it remains to be ascertained why some men have rectal prolapse. At present, the problem seems inexplicable.

Full-thickness Intussusception of the Rectum

Rectal prolapse may be the end point of a full-thickness circumferential intussusception that began as a rectorectal intussusception at ≈8 cm from the anal verge, evolved into a rectoanal intussusception and finally everted outside the perineum [7–9]. The main criticism against this theory is that, to date, it has not been possible to significantly prove the entire pathogenetic evolution during the life of the single patient. Indeed, the time spectrum of intussusception is quite broad, lasting many years. The spectrum begins in middle age (median age 44 years) [10] as a rectorectal intussusception, with chronic straining and symptoms and signs of obstructed defecation, which is related to pelvic floor dyssynergia. Over the years, intussusception develops into a rectoanal intussusception, which is often related to descending perineum syndrome (DPS), expecially in patients with minor grades of faecal incontinence that overlap obstructed defecation [11]. Finally, rectal prolapse occurs late in life, peaking (43% of cases) at between 70 and 89 years of age [12].

At defecography, the site of the "on-off" point for rectorectal intussusception appears during evacuation about 5.5 cm from the anorectal junction anteriorly. This anatomical point corresponds to the distal limit of the peritoneum within the pouch of Douglas [8]. Impaired evacuation, as a consequence of pelvic floor dyssynergia, gives rise to chronic straining, with vector-force lines and high intra-abdominal pressures canalised into the Douglas cul-de-sac. At this weak point, the anterior rectal wall is forced into intussusception, and the process begins. Intussusception thickness at proctography can be just over 3 mm [13], but sometimes, the thickness can increase more than 8 mm; in these patients, a suspected anterior enterocele and/or an enlarged posterior mesorectum may explain the grossly thickened measurements [10]. Rectoanal intussusception appears at defecography as a "funnel-shaped infolding", occurring during evacuation. Patients with an infolding depth >10 mm (≈27% of all patients with rectoanal intussusception) have lower anal pressures than patients with infolding depth <10 mm. This last report suggests that faecal incontinence could develop in patients with a deeper and larger intussusception [14].

Nevertheless, the risk of full-thickness rectal prolapse developing in patients medically treated for large intussusception (infolding depth >10 mm) is very small (3.8%) [6]. Among the many patients affected by obstructed defecation, even if rectal intussusception can be identified in ≈39% of patients who undergo investigation for rectal evacuatory symptoms [10], only a small number will develop a late rectal prolapse [15]. This also implies that other pathogenetic factors, beyond rectoanal intussusception, are involved in inducing the occurrence of rectal prolapse.

External Protrusion of the Rectum

Ageing, an impaired perineum and structural changes of the rectum play additional roles in the pathophysiology of the external protrusion of the rectum. In the literature, the anatomy and function of the perineum has received less attention than the pelvic floor. The perineum is the part of the trunk that lies caudal to the pelvic floor; it contains the perineal body (central perineal tendon) and the deep and superficial transverse perineal muscles. Anatomical findings prove that the perineal body is the site along which the tendineus fibres from the two sides of the perineal muscles decussate each other across the midline [16]. This anatomical arrangement permits simultaneous contraction of the muscles on both sides, with the presumable effects of shortening and broadening the central perineal tendon, leading to stretching and elevation of perineal muscles. During an increase in intra-abdominal pressure, the perineal muscles contract reflexively ("straining-perineal reflex") and act as a perineal support against the increased pressure [17]. These anatomical and functional data therefore support the hypothesis that perineal muscles most likely prevent perineal descent and prolapse through the perineum [18]. Widening of the levator hiatus could expose the perineal muscles to the direct effects of chronic intra-abdominal pressures, weakening these muscles and promoting perineal descent [18].

Ageing becomes an important additional factor. In asymptomatic women, anorectal sensorimotor function (anal resting and squeeze pressures, rectal compliance, rectal sensation) and perineal function both decline with ageing: the perineum is lower, at rest and during defecatory manoeuvres, in older than in younger women and has some grade of laxity [19]. Therefore, ageing and impairment of the levator ani and transverse perineal muscles may be important cofactors that create an environment predisposing to DPS [17]. Moreover, a significant relationship ($p<0.003$) has been detected between the length of rectal intussusception and the extent of perineal descent during straining [20]. These signs seem to converge on a common report of a flabby perineum, which is age related and independent from pudendum neuropathy, in patients affected by rectal prolapse. It is easy, then, to understand how chronic straining efforts may push the rectum out through a flabby perineum that is devoid of restraining anatomical support.

Structural changes of the rectum have also been detected in patients with rectal prolapse. A lack of fixation of the rectum to the sacrum is a common anatomical report, and it can be observed at the time of both laparoscopy and defecography. It is not clear whether fixation loss is primary or secondary to external migration of the rectum, but whatever the aetiology, the result is lengthening of the mesorectum. Likewise, rectal wall displacement takes place anteriorly; rectal prolapse associated with posterior enterocele may occur via sliding on/along the rectovaginal septum in women with a deep congenital rectovaginal pouch [21]. Finally, the conjoined longitudinal muscle layer of the rectum (or septum of the anal canal), where the levator ani muscle joins the anorectum [22], can be considered reasonably altered when dealing with a widened levator hiatus with thin pubovisceral muscles [23], such as the case in external protrusion of the rectum.

Pelvic Floor Muscles, Pelvic Fascia, Connective Tissue

The support of pelvic viscera is multistructural, and according to the integral theory, PFM, pelvic fascia, ligaments and connective tissue interact with each other in order to sustain the viscera [24]. PFM are composed of the portions of the levator ani muscle and the muscles of the cavernous organs [25]. Experimental and clinical evidence suggests that damaged PFM play a role in the pathophysiology of rectal prolapse.

It has been reported that a transgenic mouse strain deficient in a urokinase-type plasminogen activator (uPA-/-), derived from the wild C57B16 strain, develops a high incidence of rectal prolapse [26]. The study of the PFM of uPA-/- mice with rectal prolapse provided interesting data regarding the effects of chronic muscular stretching on PFM in the same way that the levator ani muscle could be stretched in humans, with severe pelvic prolapse [27]. Histological analysis showed that the lesion was mainly myopathic in origin ("centronucleated myofibres") and lacking in any denervation features. This experimental report suggests that whatever the primary cause of pelvic prolapse in humans (obstetrical trauma, pelvic surgery, ageing, chronic straining), continuous stretching of the PFM could cause supplementary myopathic injury.

Pelvic floor myopathic changes have also been documented in young Egyptian men affected by rectal prolapse when associated with schistosomiasis [28]. Histopathological, ultrastructural and immunohistochemical studies on biopsies taken from the PFM of these patients during surgery for rectal prolapse suggest an immunological mechanism [cytoplasmic staining with anti-immunoglobulin (Ig)G and anti-IgM schistosomiasis antibodies] for some myopathic changes (loss of striation, distortion of myofibrillar pattern, irregularity in the sarcomere), evidencing an aetiological relationship between schistosomiasis, PFM and rectal prolapse.

Further clinical evidence supports the hypothesis of pelvic muscle involvement in the physiopathology of rectal prolapse. Pelvic floor weakness is the hallmark of DPS. The defecographic image of rectoanal intussusception as a funnel-shaped folding, considered a possible rectal pre-prolapse state, is often present in women affected by DPS [11]. Dynamic magnetic resonance imaging (MRI), very helpful in evaluating defects in the pelvic floor associated with posterior compartment and rectum, detected a levator ani hernia in 75% of women with DPS [29].

Paediatric-age rectal prolapse may also be related to functional disorders of the PFM. A small number of patients with paraplegia or cauda equine lesions may be affected by rectal prolapse, and pelvic floor weakness is considered the main pathogenetic factor [30]. Malnutrition, congenital hypothyroidism, Ehlers-Danlos syndrome and cystic fibrosis also show some incidence of rectal prolapse, probably related to a pelvic floor disorder: varying from case to case, pelviperineal muscles, connective and adipose tissue and components of the pelvic fascia may be involved. Last but not least, rectal prolapse is a known postoperative problem in children with anorectal malformations, and the incidence of prolapse in patients with a low muscle-quality score has been shown to be significantly increased [31].

A defective pelvic floor, independent of the neuropathic or myopathic origin of muscle impairment, offers the anatomical basis through which the rectum could extend forward to the point of external protrusion. A deep, adynamic pelvic cul-de-sac, formed in patients who excessively strain to defecate, could be the *locus minoris resistentiae* for rectal herniation, as could happen in a sliding hernia [4]. Through a defect in the pelvic diaphragm, the anterior wall of the rectum could produce an intussusception within the rectal and anal canals, extending beyond the anal verge [12].

In truth, rectal prolapse surgery, which has been used primarily to eliminate the pouch of Douglas, has been associated with high recurrence rate, thus suggesting a more complex pathogenetic mechanism than the simple "sliding factor" [32]. Nevertheless, association of the Altemeier procedure with levatorplasty has a lower recurrence rate of rectal prolapse than the same surgical procedure without levatorplasty [33].

Pelvic Organ Prolapse and Rectal Prolapse

Pelvic organ prolapse and rectal prolapse may occur together. A gynaecological series reports a 6.1% incidence of rectal prolapse among women with genital prolapse [34]; a coloproctological series reports that 48% of patients with rectal prolapse suffer from genital prolapse [35]. The sagittal sequences of MRI display the pelvic floor and the various pelvic compartments: anterior urinary, middle genital, posterior anorectal and the fourth peritoneal. Therefore, MRI permits a multicompartment pelvic approach [36]. In the posterior component of women with pelvic organ prolapse, there is a large cross-section area of the levator hiatus [23]. This is a morphological sign of levator ani defects and suggests that a lesion to the pelvic floor support could occur in women with both pelvic organ and rectal prolapses. Birth injury could be a contributing factor, but denervation of the PFM is present in patients with both rectal and genital prolapses, and it may likely be the common a etiological denominator [34]. Nevertheless, it is impossible to determine whether rectal prolapse brings on vaginal eversion or whether the two prolapses occur simultaneously. It is likely that rectal intussusception may mechanically distort the rectovaginal septum and may be capable of creating permanent injury to the vaginal support structure. Indeed, failure to preoperatively recognise rectal intussusception is a common cause of failure of a vaginal vault suspension procedure [34]. A final reflection is that several combined (gynaecological and rectal) surgical procedures may be used to treat both rectal and pelvic organ prolapse via the perineal and/or abdominal approach, but whichever the procedure chosen, it must be able to correct pelvic floor support defects.

Rectal Prolapse, Defecation, Faecal Continence

Patients affected by rectal prolapse have several long-lasting signs and symptoms of change in bowel habits. Dyschezia and chronic constipation may be the earliest symptoms, which begin many years before the appearance of prolapse; over the course of time, the rectal prolapse extends outside the anus during bowel movements. Initially, it is self-reducing at the end of defecation, but it later requires hand-assisted manoeuvres. Later, faecal incontinence may occur, especially when the prolapse becomes irreducible. The anal sphincter is dilated and a patulous anus is often observed. Several aetiological factors, anatomical and functional, have been identified in patients with rectal prolapse and faecal incontinence. Rectal prolapse may itself cause reversible rectoanal inhibition, which would account for the low anal pressures found in incontinent patients. Rectoanal inhibition (due to inhibition of the electromyographic activity of the internal anal sphincter) is associated with high-pressure rectal waves, which, disappearing after successful resection rectopexy, seem to be caused by the intussusception entering the rectum [37].

The report that rectal prolapse in patients with faecal incontinence is associated with an increased anal pressure asymmetry index in the absence of the anal sphincter defect at ultrasonography is also very interesting [38]. This could be explained by the wide opening effects of the walls prolapsing into the anal canal. Nevertheless, the pathophysiology of faecal incontinence is strongly related to the stretching of pudendal nerves. The injury to these nerves could be due to repeated defecatory stretching of the pelvic floor. In fact, electrophysiological investigation and anorectal manometric findings show that pelvic floor denervation with severe abnormalities in anal function is present in patients with rectal prolapse and faecal incontinence but not in those with rectal prolapse without incontinence [39]. Pudendal neuropathy is more common, severe and often bilateral in women with rectal prolapse and faecal incontinence than in continent patients with rectal prolapse [40]. Moreover, histological studies of the external anal sphincter and the puborectalis muscle in patients with faecal incontinence and rectal prolapse have shown features typical of denervation [41]. Nevertheless, the permanent external protrusion of the rectum may induce faecal soiling arriving at true faecal incontinence simply because it is outside the perineum.

Last but not least, resting motor activity in the sigmoid colon could be abnormal. The motility index in patients with rectal prolapse, faecal incontinence and intermittent diarrhoea is significantly greater than in controls [42]. Thus, the relationship between rectal prolapse and impairment of faecal continence is not linear and, at this time, the pathogenetic pathway of incontinence is not well defined. However, one unforeseen therapeutic result is that incontinence may improve following most surgical procedures for rectal prolapse.

Colonic Motility

Constipation may occur after operative procedures for rectal prolapse, but the cause is unknown. For example, anorectal obstruction or impaired colonic state is considered, by turns, the causes of constipation after rectopexy [43–45]. In patients affected by rectal prolapse and chronic constipation, the preoperative evaluation of colonic motility, by means of transit-time studies and colonic manometry, seems to be able to identify those with slow transit constipation [42]. In fact, reduced high-amplitude propagated contractions (HAPCs) and prolonged colonic transit have been detected in patients with rectal prolapse and constipation. Therefore, in these patients, rectopexy failed to restore HAPCs, improve colonic transit or reduce constipation [46]. This is probably the group of patients with rectal prolapse who would experience slow transit constipation anyway, regardless of whether they received surgical treatment for prolapse or not.

The problem is different when patients develop postoperative constipation when constipation was absent prior to surgery. Constipation has been attributed to postoperative autonomic neuropathy (a consequence of rectal lateral ligament division) and/or to the presence of a redundant sigmoid loop (kinking and mechanical obstruction) [47]. Sigmoid colon resection can be added to rectopexy in order to reduce the incidence of postoperative constipation [48], and a few prospective randomised studies confirm that the best results are obtained using rectopexy with sigmoidectomy than for rectopexy alone [49, 50]. Probably, resection of the sigmoid colon removes the segment of bowel that could subsequently become neuropathic as a consequence of rectal dissection and/or division of the lateral ligaments [51].

In conclusion, before choosing the surgical option, it is advisable to study colonic motility behaviour in the patient affected by both rectal prolapse and chronic constipation.

Rectal Prolapse and Solitary Rectal Ulcer Syndrome

Proctoscopic findings, which can be either a typical ulcer with hyperaemic edges and surrounding induration or an exophytic polypoid lesion seen on the anterior rectal wall usually 6–8 cm from the anal verge, define the pathology of solitary rectal ulcer syndrome (SRUS). Although the hypothesis of repeated mucosal trauma and ischaemia is generally accepted, SRUS is a complex syndrome, as it can occur in patients suffering from outlet obstruction and in those with overt rectal prolapse. Anorectal physiological reports differ between patients with and without rectal prolapse [52, 53]. SRUS patients without a prolapse have high anal pressures, which increase with straining, and a paradoxical puborectalis contraction occurs more frequently than in SRUS patients with a prolapse. These reports agree with transrectal ultrasound data. In patients without prolapse, the rectal wall is thicker, and enlargement of the muscularis propria indicates a rectal wall that is chronically overloaded by motor activity working against a nonrelaxing puborectalis muscle [54]. However, the mucosal changes in patients with prolapse might be related, instead, to the mechanical trauma of mucosa during the eversion through the anus. Moreover, low anal pressures and the absence of paradoxical puborectalis contraction are the usual manometric reports [50].

Conclusion

It is difficult to find guidelines to better understand the pathophysiology of rectal prolapse. Many varying factors are present, each differing from patient to patient. The aetiology of this disorder is multifactorial: impaired anorectal motility, anatomical pelviperineal changes, concomitance of pelvic organ prolapses, altered colonic motility, all together contribute to the multifaceted aspect of rectal prolapse. Nevertheless, it is important for the practitioner to be aware of all the possible aetiological factors in order to design and execute the appropriate therapy.

References

1. Lowry AC, Simmang CL, Boulos P et al (2001) Consensus statement of definitions for anorectal physiology and rectal cancer, Washington, D.C., May 1, 1999. Dis Colon Rectum 44:915–919
2. Kairaluoma MV, Kellokumpu IH (2005) Epidemiologic aspects of complete rectal prolapse. Scand J Surg 94:207–210
3. Harewood JC, Coulie B, Camilleri M et al (1999) Descending perineum syndrome: audit of clinical and laboratory features and outcome of pelvic floor retraining. Am J Gastroenterol 94:126–130
4. Moschcowitz AV (1912) The pathogenesis, anatomy and cure of prolapse of the rectum. Surg Gynecol Obstet 15:7–21
5. Rao SS, Tutya AK, Vellema T et al (2004) Dyssynergic defecation: demographies, symptoms, stool patterns and quality of life. J Clin Gastroenterol 38:680–685
6. Choi GS, Hwang YH, Salum MR et al (2001) Outcome and management of patients with large rectoanal intussusception. Am J Gastroenterol 96:740–744
7. Devadhar DS (1965) A new concept of mechanism and treatment of rectal procidentia. Dis Colon Rectum 8:75
8. Broden B, Snellman B (1968) Procidentia of the rectum studied with cineradiography. Dis Colon Rectum 11:330–347
9. Mackle EJ, Parks TG (1986) The pathogenesis and pathophysiology of rectal prolapse and solitary rectal ulcer syndrome. Clin Gastroenterol 15:985–1002
10. Dvorkin LS, Gladman MA, Epstein J et al (2005) Rectal intussusception in symptomatic patients is different from that in asymptomatic volunteers. Br J Surg 92:866–872
11. Pucciani F, Boni D, Perna F et al (2005) Descending perineum syndrome: are abdominal hysterectomy and bowel habits linked? Dis Colon Rectum 48:2094–2099
12. Altemeier WA, Culbertson WR, Schowengerdt C, Hunt J (1971) Nineteen years experience with the one-stage perineal repair of rectal prolapse. Ann Surg 173:993–1001
13. Shorvon PJ, McHugh S, Diamant NE et al (1989) Defecography in normal volunteers: results and implications. Gut 30:1737–1749
14. Choi GS, Salum MR, Moreira H et al (2000). Physiologic and clinical assessment of patients with rectoanal intussusception. Tech Coloproctol 4:29–33
15. Mellgren A, Schultz I, Johansson C et al (1997) Internal rectal intussusception seldom develops into total rectal prolapse. Dis Colon Rectum 40:817–820
16. Shafik A, Ahmed I, Shafik AA et al (2005) Surgical anatomy of the perineal muscles and their role in perineal disorders. Anat Sci Int 80:167–171
17. Shafik A, El-Sibai O, Shafik AA, Ahmed I (2003) Effect of straining on perineal muscles and their role in perineal support: identification of the straining-perineal reflex. J Surg Res 112:162–167
18. Shafik A, Shafik AA, Shafik I, El-Sibai O (2006) Study of the role of the transverse perineal muscles during rectal filling. Int J Colorectal Dis 21:698–704
19. Fox JC, Fletcher JG, Zinsmeister AR et al (2006) Effect of aging on anorectal and pelvic floor functions in females. Dis Colon Rectum 49:1726–1735
20. Tsiaoussis J, Chrysos E, Athanasakis E et al (2005) Rectoanal intussusception: presentation of the disorder and late results of resection rectopexy. Dis Colon Rectum 48:838–844

21. Baessler K, Schuessler B (2005) Anatomy of the sigmoid colon, rectum, and the rectovaginal pouch in women with enterocele and anterior rectal wall procidentia. Clin Anat 19:125–129
22. Arakawa T, Muratami G, Nakajima F et al (2004) Morphologies of the interfaces between the levator ani muscle and pelvic viscera, with special reference to muscle insertion into the anorectum in elderly Japanese. Anat Sci Int 79:72–81
23. Hsu Y, Chen L, Huebner M et al (2006) Quantification of levator ani cross-sectional area differences between women with and those without prolapse. Obstet Gynecol 108:879–883
24. Petros PE (2004) The female pelvic floor function, dysfunction and management according to the integral theory. Springer, Heidelberg, pp 180–190
25. Fritsch H, Lienemann A, Brenner E, Ludwikowski B (2004) Clinical anatomy of the pelvic floor. Adv Anat Embryol Cell Biol 175:1–64
26. Carmeliet P, Schoonjans L, Kieckens L et al (1994) Physiological consequences of loss of plasminogen activator gene function in mice. Nature 368:419–424
27. Yiou R, Delmas V, Carmeliet P et al (2001) The pathophysiology of pelvic floor disorders: evidence from a histomorphologic study of the perineum and a mouse model of rectal prolapse. J Anat 199:599–607
28. Hussein AM, Helal SF (2000) Schistosomal pelvic floor myopathy contributes to the pathogenesis of rectal prolapse in young males. Dis Colon Rectum 43:644–649
29. Gearhart SL, Pannu HK, Cundiff GW et al (2004) Perineal descent and levator ani hernia: a dynamic magnetic resonance imaging study. Dis Colon Rectum 47:1298–1304
30. Nash DF (1972) Bowel management in spina bifida patients. Proc R Soc Med 65:70–71
31. Belizon A, Levitt M, Shoshany J et al (2005) Rectal prolapse following posterior sagittal anorectoplasty for anorectal malformations. J Ped Surg 40:192–196
32. Gourgiotis S, Baratsis S (2007) Rectal prolapse. Int J Colorect Dis 22:231–243
33. Boccasanta P, Venturi M, Barbieri S, Roviaro G (2006) Impact of new technologies on the clinical and functional outcome of Altemeier's procedure. A randomized controlled study. Dis Colon Rectum 49:652–660
34. Peters WA, Smith RM, Drescher CW (2001) Rectal prolapse in women with other defects of pelvic floor support. Am J Obstet Gynecol 184:1488–1495
35. Altman D, Zetterstrom J, Schultz I et al (2006) Pelvic organ prolapse and urinary incontinence in women with surgically managed rectal prolapse: a population-based case-control study. Dis Colon Rectum 49:28–35
36. Maubon A, Aubard Y, Berkane V et al (2003) Magnetic resonance imaging of the pelvic floor. Abdom Imaging 28:217–225
37. Farouk R, Duthie GS, MacGreor AB, Bartolo DCC (1994) Rectoanal inhibition and incontinence in patients with rectal prolapse. Br J Surg 81:743–746
38. Damon H, Henry L, Roman S et al (2003) Influence of rectal prolapse on the asymmetry of the anal sphincter in patients with anal incontinence. BMC Gastroenterol 3:23
39. Neill ME, Parks AG, Swash M (1981) Physiological studies of the anal sphincter musculature in faecal incontinence and rectal prolapse. Br J Surg 68:531–536
40. Roiq JV, Buch E, Solana A et al (1998) Anorectal function in patients with complete rectal prolapse. Differences between continent and incontinent individuals. Rev Esp Enfferm Dig 90:794–805
41. Parks AG, Swash M, Urich H (1977) Sphincter denervation in anorectal incontinence and rectal prolapse. Gut 18:656–665
42. Keighley MRB, Shouler PJ (1984) Abnormalities of colonic function in patients with rectal prolapse and faecal incontinence. Br J Surg 71:892–895
43. Dolk A, Broden G, Holstrom B et al (1990) Slow transit of the colon associated with severe constipation after the Ripstein operation. A clinical and physiologic study. Dis Colon Rectum 33:786–790
44. Siproudis L, Robert A, Gosselin A et al (1993) Constipation after rectopexy for rectal prolapse. Where is the obstruction? Dig Dis Sci 38:1801–1808
45. Kellokumpu IH, Vironen J, Scheinin T (2000) Laparoscopic repair of rectal prolapse. A prospective study evaluating surgical outcome and changes in symptoms and bowel function. Surg Endosc 14:634–640
46. Brown AJ, Nicol L, Anderson JH et al (2005) Prospective study of the effect of rectopexy on colonic motility in patients with rectal prolapse. Br J Surg 92:1417–1422
47. Brown AJ, Anderson JH, McKee RF, Finlay IJ (2004) Strategy for selection of type of operation for rectal prolapse based on clinical criteria. Dis Colon Rectum 47:103–107
48. Frykman HM, Goldberg SM (1969) The surgical treatment of rectal procidentia. Surg Gynecol Obstet 129:1225–1230
49. McKee RF, Lauder JC, Poon FW (1992) A prospective randomized study of abdominal rectopexy with and without sigmoidectomy in rectal prolapse. Surg Gynecol Obstet 174:145–148
50. Luukkonen P, Mikkonen J, Järvinen H (1992) Abdominal rectopexy with sigmoidectomy vs rectopexy alone for rectal prolapse: a prospective randomized study. Int J Colorectal Dis 7:219–222
51. Speakman CTM, Madden DV, Nicholls RJ, Kamm MA (1991) Lateral ligament division during rectopexy causes constipation but prevents recurrence: results of a prospective randomized study. Br J Surg 78:1431–1433
52. Kang YS, Kamm MA, Nicholls RJ (1995) Solitary rectal ulcer and complete rectal prolapse: one condition or two? Int J Colorectal Dis 10:87–90
53. Morio O, Meurette G, Desfourneaux V et al (2005) Anorectal physiology in solitary ulcer syndrome: a case matched series. Dis Colon Rectum 48:1917–1922
54. Van Outryve MJ, Pelckmans PA, Fierens H, Van Maercke YM (1993) Transrectal ultrasound study of the pathogenesis of solitary rectal ulcer syndrome. Gut 34:1422–1426

3 Functional Imaging in Rectal Prolapse

Vittorio Luigi Piloni, Alberto Bazzocchi, Rita Golfieri

Introduction

Imaging data has gained great relevance in the preoperative assessment of severe pelvic organ prolapse, including vaginal vault descent, enterocele, rectocele and cystocele. This is at least partly due to inaccurate characterisation and failure to identify all of the involved sites when using physical examination alone, leading to incomplete surgical repair with subsequent persistence or recurrence of the prolapse. Despite their potential advantages in determining which organs are involved, however, available imaging procedures, i.e. contrast radiography, ultrasonography and, more recently, dynamic magnetic resonance imaging (MRI), still share some important limitations, such as lack of standardisation, validation and availability. In fact, existing methods of performing examinations and measurements of individual parameters vary greatly among researchers, making comparison of study results difficult. In addition, significant differences still exist in the definition and terminology of the most common pelvic descent processes as well as in the classification and quantification systems adopted.

This report represents an attempt to provide the clinician (surgeon) with a sort of "nautical chart" to sail with caution around the world of existing imaging studies, which will help him or her reach the "harbour" of pelvic prolapse surgical repair. In particular, the reader will be offered a concise description of the fundamentals, technical strengths and limitations of each of the three methods mentioned above in order to understand the optimal indications for their application. The intention of the authors was to produce a document to be circulated to members of the Italian Society of Colorectal Surgery (SICCR)'s coloproctological society involved in rectal prolapse management for a 1-year review and trial before establishing its clinical utility.

Description of Pelvic Organ Prolapse

Definition of the most common abnormalities should conform to the standards recommended by the international committee on pelvic organ prolapse and pelvic floor dysfunctions [1]. The clinical description of pelvic floor anatomy, however, differs significantly from that depicted by imaging techniques, because the former is determined during the physical examination of the external genitalia and vaginal canal (female), and the specific site of vaginal bulge usually replaces such terms as cystocele, enterocele and rectocele, regardless of which structure will most likely be found on the other side of vaginal protrusion. Traditionally, visceral prolapse during physical examination is evaluated relative to the hymen ring, which provides a precisely identifiable landmark. For measurements, the anatomic position of six defined points (two on the anterior vaginal wall, two in the superior vagina and two on the posterior vaginal wall) is usually given in centimetres above (proximal) or below (distal) the hymen and expressed by negative or positive numbers, respectively. Conversely, despite no universally accepted imaging system for describing the anatomic position of pelvic organs, the key feature of bladder, rectal and genital prolapse seen on imaging techniques lies in their low position, either at rest or on straining, relative to the pubococcygeal line. This is defined as a line joining the inferior border of the symphysis pubis to the last sacrococcygeal joint and has been chosen because it represents the line of attachment of the muscular and ligamentous components of the pelvic floor [2]. In addition, with the exception of perineal sonography, the pubococcygeal line can easily be traced, allowing comparable measurement of pelvic organ descent by imaging techniques.

Technical Aspects and Image Analysis

Contrast Radiography

Traditionally, fluoroscopic cystocolpoproctography, i.e. evacuation proctography combined with opacification of the pelvic viscera [3–7], is considered the imaging technique of choice for investigating pelvic floor prolapse affecting the bladder (cystocele), vagina (vaginal vault prolapse), small bowel (enterocele) and rectum (rectocele). Preparation for the fluoroscopic examination requires that, at the arrival of the patient at the X-ray department, a standard dose of 120 ml of liquid barium suspension (Pronto Bario HD 68% wt/vol, Bracco, Milan, Italy) is given orally to opacify the small-bowel loops, which usually are visualised in the lower pelvis 2–3 h later. After small-bowel opacification, the patient's bladder is catheterised, and 100 ml of 60% diatrizoate sodium solution (Opacist, Bracco) are introduced. Then, with the patient still lying supine on the X-ray table, the vagina is also opacified, with 5 ml of a thick barium paste (Pronto Bario OE 113% wt/vol, Bracco). Usually, this small dose of contrast prevents the loss of barium through the introitus when tilting the patient upright. Finally, after vaginal opacification, the patient is asked to turn 90° on her left side to assume the Sims position, and the rectum is filled with 200 ml of the same thick barium paste. The entire procedure lasts no more than 10 min. At this point, with the patient seated on a specially designed commode, intermittent fluoroscopy is used for proper centring the region of interest, and lateral radiographs are obtained at rest, on squeeze and during coughing, straining, voiding and evacuation. After the emptying phase, two more series of images are taken with the patient straining maximally. Digital images are postprocessed at the same console after having dismissed the patient. Measurements of the distances of pelvic organs from anatomic landmarks and angles are made possible by incorporating a radiopaque centimetre ruler within the field of view. According to the literature, standard measurements include: (1) the position of the bladder base, vaginal vault and anorectal junction calculated at 90° to the pubococcygeal line, (2) the anorectal angle, defined as the angle between the longitudinal axis of the anal canal and the posterior rectal wall, measured at rest, squeeze, strain and emptying and (3) the anorectal junction (defined as the junction of the rectal ampulla and anal canal) whose descent is considered excessive if seen projecting more than 2.5 cm below the pubococcygeal line at rest or if more than 3 cm on minimum strain. Images are also evaluated for any other structural abnormality, such as enterocele, defined as small bowel within the rectovaginal septum reaching or crossing the upper one third and distal two thirds of vagina; and rectocele, defined as an anterior rectal wall bulge exceeding 2 cm.

Ultrasonography

In the early 1980s, transperineal sonography was developed for the dynamic investigation of stress urinary incontinence as an alternative to videocystography [8–13]. Many contributions followed in the subsequent years, which highlighted the potential of this noninvasive technique in a number of clinical applications, including nongynaecological, inflammatory [14] and, more recently, coloproctological diseases [15–22]. Despite considerable variation among centres, the procedure today is quite easy to perform and relatively easy to interpret. Currently, ultrasonography of the pelvic floor has assumed a central role in the diagnostic workup and has been proposed as the first imaging approach for proper diagnosis and management of pelvic prolapse syndromes, as it helps discriminate those patients with anatomical abnormalities who are likely to undergo elective treatment from those requiring conservative treatment.

The procedure we follow is a modification and a synthesis of that described originally by Rubens et al. [15] and that by Sandridge and Thorp [17]. More particularly, the patient is asked to reach the imaging department with her bladder half filled by natural urine. Then, she is placed in the Sims position, and 60 ml of hypoechoic contrast (the same as that used for evacuation proctography) are administered through a rectal tube to enhance rectal visualisation, as described by us in previous reports [21, 23]. Thereafter, the patient is turned supine with her knees bent and feet flat on the table and is asked to place a finger into the vagina (self-digitation) to allow penetration and subsequent trapping of air bubbles within the lumen in order to improve identification of both anterior and posterior vaginal walls. Although transducers with frequencies in the 3- to 5-MHz range positioned at the interlabial region producing a pie-shaped field of view have commonly been described for transperineal sonography, we prefer using a 5- to- 7.5-MHz endocavitary probe for the following two reasons: (1) the head of the transducer can be placed closer to the region of interest so as to provide superior axial and lateral resolution of the pelvic anatomy, and (2) with the head of the transducer placed at the introital region, scanning through an arc of 195° is possible in the sagittal plane so that the entire pelvic floor is depicted, including the lower border of the symphysis pubis (anteriorly) and the coccyx (posteriorly). The only drawback when using the endocavitary probe is represented by a greater distortion of image anatomy. On the other hand, the obtained sonographic image compares more favourably with that from both contrast radiography and MRI. Whatever the probe employed, transducers are connected to an ultrasound scanner equipped with advanced software, freeze-frame and post-processing facilities (MyLab5, Esaote, Genoa, Italy).

Prevention of cross-contamination between patients is achieved by adopting a disposable cover (latex condom or the finger of a surgical glove) over the tip of the probe. Examination of the region of interest includes the systematic combination of longitudinal with transversely oriented scans in order to localise the anatomical structures accurately and provide three-dimensional (3D) measurements during rest, squeeze and straining manoeuvres by the patient before emptying the bladder and rectum.

In order to obtain quantitative sonogram data, the following anatomic landmarks and measurements are noted:

1. Bladder-neck position: With the inferior border of the symphysis as the reference point, the x-axis is constructed by drawing a line between the superior and inferior border of the symphysis (central line). The position of the anterior margin of the bladder neck with respect to the x-axis is noted at rest and on straining. Its minimal distance from the reference line is calculated in millimetres and expressed as a number preceded by – (above) or + (below).
2. Posterior urethrovesical (β) angle: According to Schaer et al. [12], it is defined as the angle formed between a line drawn tangent to the proximal half of the urethra and a line drawn tangent to the lowermost back aspect of the bladder base.
3. Anterior urethral (α) angle: This refers to the slope of the proximal half of the urethral axis with respect to the x-axis of the pubic bone. Values are expressed in degrees and range from 60° to 110° in control groups.
4. Urethral sphincter width and thickness: These measurements are only performed when an endoprobe operating at 6.5 MHz frequency is available. A mean width of 17.33 mm (range 15–20 mm), thickness of 9.3 mm (range 8–10 mm), smooth sphincter length of 15.1 mm (range 13–19 mm) and striated sphincter length of 7 mm (3–11 mm) are reported.
5. Bladder-wall thickness: According to Khullar et al. [13], this is measured, when the urinary residual volume is ≤20 ml, perpendicular to the bladder lining at the thickest part of its four walls. A mean wall thickness of <5 mm is seen in over 85% of patients with no evidence of detrusor instability.
6. Anal length: According to Sandridge and Thorp [17], this is measured on sagittal scans with calliper placed at the anal verge and anorectal junction. The latter is assumed to be located where the gut lumen turns down over the puborectalis muscle. The same anatomical landmark is used to measure the diameter of the anus from the outside borders of the muscularis propria.
7. Internal and external anal sphincters: These are measured in their short axis at either the 3, 6 or 9 o'clock position from the cross section of the anal canal at a point where it is seen to assume a perfect ring shape. The reported mean thickness is 5 ± 1.3 mm, range 3–7 mm (external sphincter) and 3 ± 0.9 mm, range 2–5 mm (internal sphincter).
8. Thickness of the puborectalis muscle: This is measured on axial scans at the midpoint of its lateral portion, where the muscle diverges from the anal canal. The same anatomic landmark is also used to draw a line tangent to the lateral aspect of the muscle on both sides to al-

Table 1. Cross-sectional area of anal canal at sonography in women with (n=20) and without (n=10) rectal prolapse

Parameter	Control			Prolapse		
	Outer		Inner	Outer		Inner
Average area and SD (cm²)						
Rest	2.30 (0.43)		1.09 (0.24)	2.61 (0.84)		1.23 (0.37)
Strain	2.21 (0.48)		1.08 (0.25)	3.83 (1.12)		3.02 (0.73)
Inner-to-outer ratio (%)						
Rest		47.4 (5.11)			48.1 (6.3)	
Strain		49.6 (8.2)			81.3 (2.9)*	
Increase on straining (Δ)						
Outer		-0.082			+0.38*	
Inner		-0.007			+0.42*	

SD standard deviation
*$p < 0.01$

low measurement of the angle formed in between, which is referred to as the puborectalis angle. Mean values reported are 5 ± 1.04 mm, range 2.5–7 mm (thickness) and 40 ± 8.8° (angle).

9. Cervix descent: The lowermost dislocation on straining is measured relative to a line drawn tangent to the central axis (x-axis) of the symphysis pubis.
10. The anal cross-sectional area is calculated at rest and on straining by outlining the inner and outer margins of the smooth internal sphincter muscle and measuring the included area at the level of the middle anal canal in the axial plane. Average values in control groups and patients with rectal prolapse are listed in Table 1.

Magnetic Resonance Imaging

MRI has been used since 1991 [24] to evaluate pelvic floor movement in order to provide a global view of the pelvic viscera and pelvic floor musculature. Thanks to the rapid advances in technology during the last decade [25, 26] and no use of ionising radiation, MRI is considered, especially in young female patients, the single imaging modality capable of providing both superior anatomic details and complete depiction of bladder and rectal emptying in a safe and noninvasive manner.

Due to the limited availability of vertically oriented systems throughout the world, MRI of the pelvic floor is usually performed with the patient supine. This has been claimed to affect the detection rate of some abnormalities, such as mucosal prolapse, rectal intussusception, rectocele less than 2 cm in depth and external rectal prolapse, highlighting the effect gravity has on depiction of these findings. This was not our experience, however. At our department, static and dynamic MRI of the pelvis is performed using a 1.5-T superconducting conventional (horizontal) magnet system (Signa, General Electric Medical System, Milwaukee, WI, USA) equipped with high-speed gradients and surface phased-array coils wrapped around the patient's pelvis. Following bladder emptying via catheterisation and refilling with 100 ml of sterile water solution mixed with 1.5 ml of gadopentetate dimeglumine, a soft rubber tube is placed in the rectum to act as a luminal marker and for subsequent contrast administration without interruption during scanning or patient movement. Static T2-weighted images with an empty rectum are obtained, first to provide complete anatomic evaluation at rest in the axial, coronal and sagittal planes using fast recovery spin echo pulse sequence (TR/TE, 3,400/85 ms; field of view, 32 cm; slice thickness, 5 mm; interslice gap, 1 mm; matrix size, 320 × 224 zipped to 512; BW, 31.25; and four excitations). Then, following administration of 120 ml of ultrasound gel mixed with 1.5 ml of gadopentetate dimeglumine via the previously positioned rectal tube, dynamic images are obtained during rest, squeezing and straining in the midsagittal plane using a T1-weighted fast spoiled gradient recalled acquisition pulse sequence (flip angle, 60°; TR/TE, minimum; field of view, 32 cm; section thickness, 20 cm; BW, 62.5; matrix size, 256 × 160; and one excitation). After this, the bladder voiding and rectal emptying phases are imaged after the patient is instructed to start the movement at will and just make notice of it by intercom to allow contemporary acquisition of images by the examiner. Finally, the urogenital hiatus is imaged again in the axial plane using a T2-weighted fast spin echo pulse sequence while the patient is straining maximally.

Quantification of pelvic floor relaxation and visceral prolapse on sagittal images is performed according to Comiter et al. [27] using the HMO classification system, where the "H-line" (levator hiatus) measures the distance from the pubis to the posterior margin of the external anal orifice, the "M-line" (muscular pelvic floor relaxation) measures the descent of the levator plate from the pubococcygeal line and the "O" classification (organ prolapse) characterises the degree of sacral prolapse beyond the H-line. Moreover, according to Kelvin et al. [28], a cystocele is defined as descent of the bladder base below the reference line. It is graded as small if the bladder base extends less than 3 cm below this line, moderate if this extension measures from 3 to 6 cm and large if it extends 6 cm or more below this line. Vaginal vault prolapse is defined as descent of the vaginal vault or any part of the remaining cervix below the pubococcygeal line. The degree of vaginal vault prolapse is graded as small if the vaginal vault or cervix extends less than 3 cm below this line, moderate if the extension measures from 3 to 6 cm below this line and large if it extends 6 cm or more below this line. An enterocele or sigmoidocele is defined as descent of the small bowel or sigmoid colon below the pubococcygeal line. Enterocele and sigmoidocele are graded as small if they extend less than 3 cm below the pubococcygeal line, moderate if they extend from 3 to 6 cm below this line and large if they extend 6 cm or more below this line. A peritoneocele is defined as herniation of the peritoneal cul-de-sac with or without contained small bowel or sigmoid colon and is measured in the same manner as enterocele and sigmoidocele.

In addition, the axial images are used to calculate the pelvic floor hiatal area and the perimeter at rest and during maximum strain, which are measured at the level of the most inferior point of the symphysis pubis. The anterior–posterior diameter corresponds to the distance from the pubic symphysis to the ventral margin of the puborectalis muscle sling; the transverse diameter is the distance between the medial borders of the levator ani muscle. The area of the hiatus is estimated by using these two diameters (A and B) to calculate the area of an oval ($A \cdot B \cdot \pi$) and is expressed in square centimetres. In women with normal support and without prior surgery, the reported hiatus area is 5.4 cm^2 ± 1.71 standard deviation (SD), whereas in women with uncorrected grade 2–3 prolapse, the figure increases to 9.6 cm^2 ± 3.97 SD and remains larger (13.3 cm^2 ± 3.86 SD) in women with recurrent prolapse [29].

Image Display

In order to reduce difficulties in interpretation and eliminate discrepancies between radiographs, sonograms and MRI sagittal images of the pelvis with regard to the side of the pictures, the documentation is standardised to display the caudal side of the patient's body at the lower edge of the screen, the cranial at the top, the dorsal on the right and the ventral on the left. To obtain this, when performing transperineal sonography, the upside-down facility is activated so that the transducer is seen at the bottom and the image is always generated from below upwards. On all other planes, i.e. axial and coronal, the right and left sides are designated following the convention used for routine imaging, where the left side of the monitor corresponds to the right side of the patient and vice versa.

With regard to bony landmarks, the lower edge of the symphysis pubis has been given high priority to allow comparison among contrast radiography, sonography and MRI. Other anatomic landmarks (where possible) include the tip of coccyx, the ischial spine and tuberosity and the promontory of the sacrum.

Appearances of Rectal Prolapse

When scrutinised for evidence of rectal prolapse, conventional radiographic contrast-enhanced studies, ultrasonography and MRI offer comparable, even though peculiar, appearances (Fig. 1); thus, image findings should be integrated as follows:

Contrast Radiography

Mucous prolapse is seen as a rectal wall infolding of <3 mm in thickness confined to the anterior or posterior margin that does not show a tendency to migrate distally on straining or during evacuation. Conversely, a circumferential infolding of the

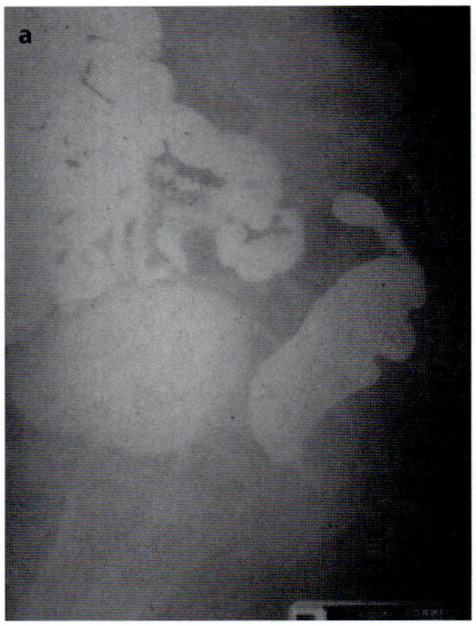

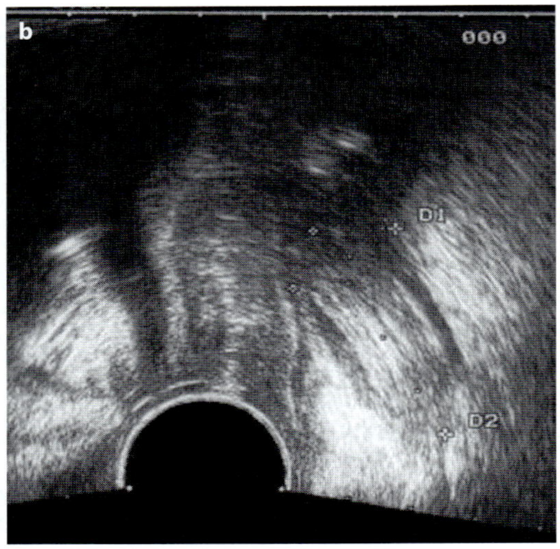

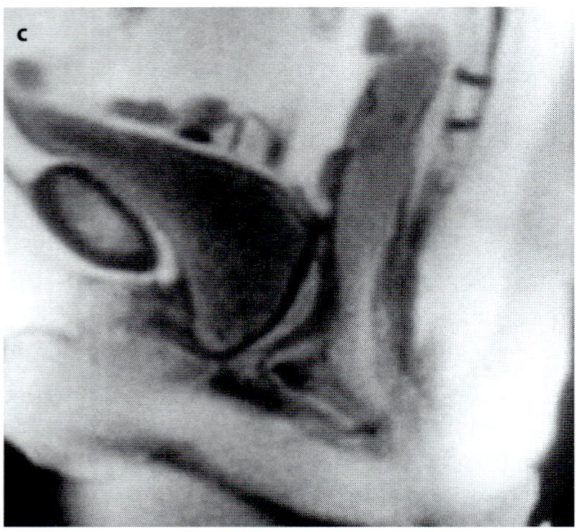

Fig. 1a-c
Pelvic floor imaging by three different methods, each with its own strengths and limitations: Enterocystoproctography (**a**) offers real-time depiction of visceral relationship and movement; sonography (**b**) shows at best extraluminal anatomy of the urethra, vaginal canal and anal canal; magnetic resonance imaging defecography (**c**) allows noninvasive evidence of contemporary intra-anal intussusception and cystocele

rectal wall ≥3 mm that descends towards the anal canal is defined as intussusception. It is termed intrarectal when it remains within the rectum and intra-anal if its apex penetrates the anal canal. Traditionally, morphological features of the intussusception that are determined include thickness, depth of descent and the point of inversion from the anal verge. In addition, intussusception can be graded by using a three-point scale depending on the involved rectal wall appearance at the end of evacuation, as follows: grade 1 intussusception is a 3- to 5-mm-thick intraluminal filling defect that presumably has a mucosal component only; grade 2 intussusception is 5- to 10-mm thick and includes both the mucosal and mural components; a grade 3 or full-thickness intussusception is assumed if the prolapsed folds are thicker than 10 mm, penetrate the anal canal and appear to impede the expulsion of rectal content. We recently developed a standardised classification system for evaluating rectal intussusception, which consists of four grades (Fig. 2) and deals not only with the demonstration of the size of intraluminal filling defect but relates in particular to the level reached by the head of intussuscipiens within the lumen of the anal canal. In grade 1 intussusception, the head of intussuscipiens does not overcome the upper one third of the anal canal; in grade 2, it reaches the proximal two thirds; in grade 3, it is seen to impinge down on the distal one third; in grade 4, it overcomes the anal verge. A complete external rectal prolapse is diagnosed when the entire thickness of the rectal wall is extruded through the anal canal, is termed reducible when it disappears at the end of the evacuation spontaneously or by effect of voluntary squeezing of the pelvic floor musculature, and termed unreducible if it can be reduced only by hand. Finally, a recto-

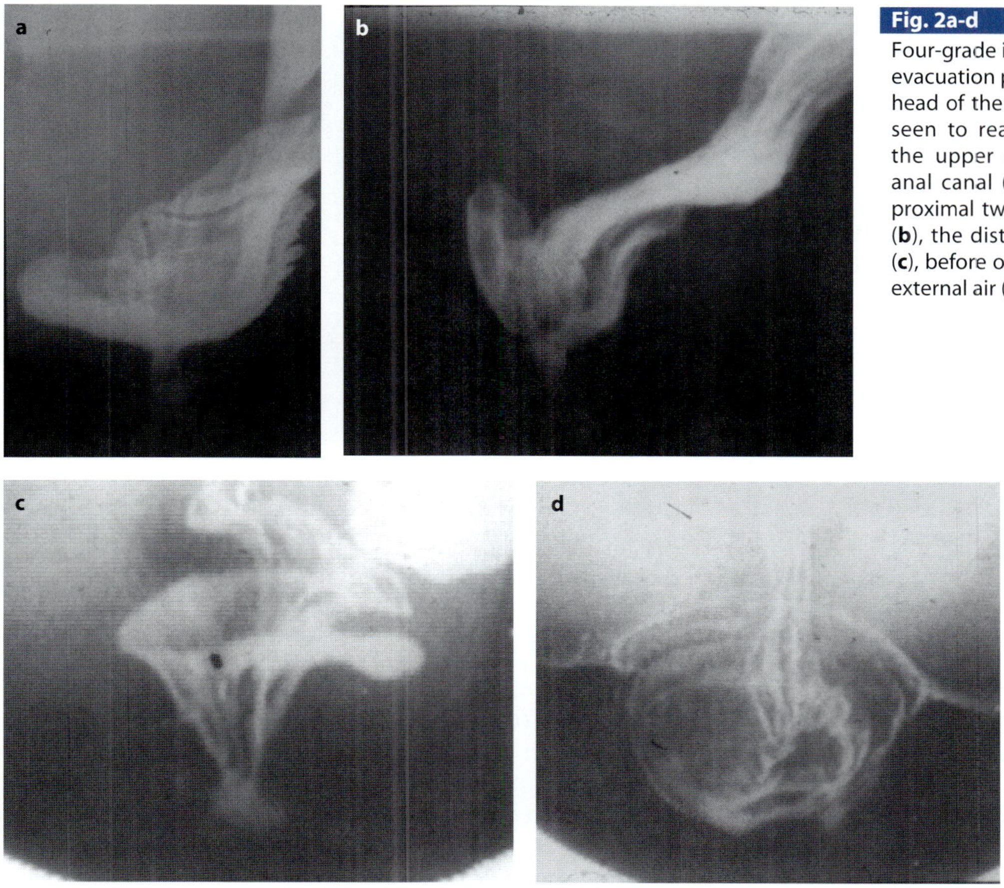

Fig. 2a-d

Four-grade intussusception at evacuation proctography: The head of the intussuscipiens is seen to reach progressively the upper extremity of the anal canal (grade 1) (**a**), the proximal two thirds (grade 2) (**b**), the distal third (grade 3) (**c**), before opening out to the external air (grade 4) (**d**)

cele appears as any rectal protrusion anterior to a line extended upwards through the anal canal. Its depth, either at rest or on straining, should be measured as the shortest distance from the deepest margin of the actually reached anterior rectal wall and the expected line mentioned above. Rectocele is graded as small if it measures less than 2 cm in depth, moderate if it measures from 2 to 4 cm and large if it measures 4 cm or more.

Sonography

A distinct advantage of perineal sonography over contrast radiography is its ability to depict the cross-sectional anatomy of the anal canal in fine detail, including that of the mucosa–submucosa complex and the internal and external anal sphincters. Obtaining information on both these structures is unanimously considered an essential part of the anorectal prolapse syndrome, with important therapeutical implications. Via the transperineal or the transvaginal route, the undisturbed anatomy of the anal canal is always displayed (identification rate, 100%) as follows: The virtual lumen of the anal canal is wrapped up by the hypoechoic mucosa that reproduce the "X-like" shape of a clover. Directly outside the mucosa, two to three triangular-shaped images of intermediate echogenicity, which represent the submucosa, are found. The internal anal sphincter is the innermost muscular structure, which is the continuation of the circular part of the rectal mucosa wall. It is clearly seen as a symmetric, 3-mm-thick hypoechoic ring completely encircling the submucosa. Outside the internal sphincter is the mixed echogenic intersphincteric space. Within this space is the relatively hypoechoic longitudinal muscle, which is a continuation of the longitudinal part of the rectal muscular wall. The intersphincteric space is bordered by the relatively echoic external sphincter. The intensively hyperechoic puborectal muscle is the most peripheral structure of the upper part of the sphincter. The

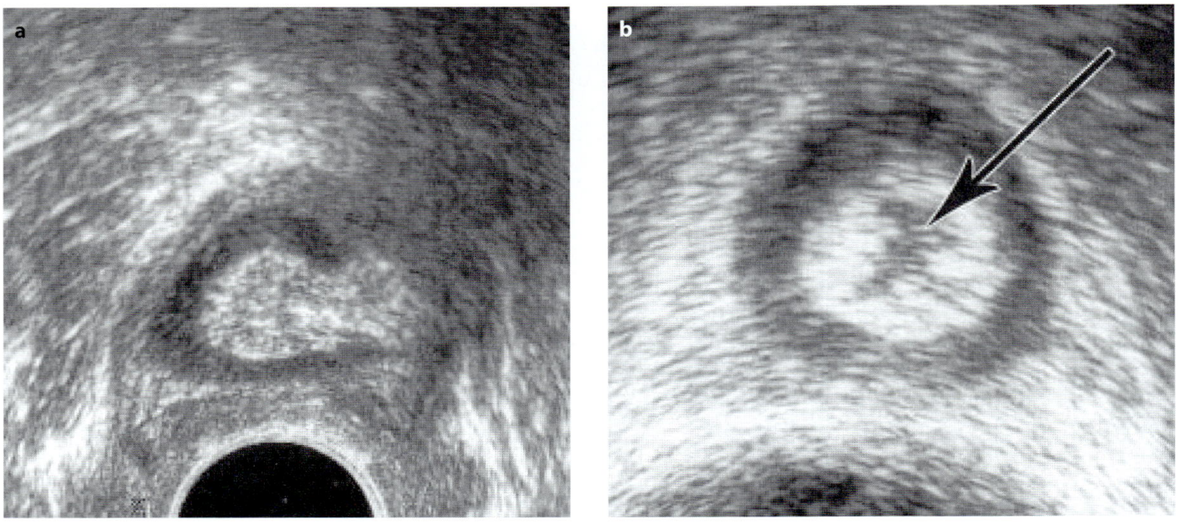

Fig. 3a, b

Axial view of mucous prolapse (**a**) at sonography in comparison with normal pattern (**b**). The X-shaped hypoechoic image (*arrow*) represents the mucosa

upper part of the anal sphincter complex is connected to the levator ani muscle. In case of mucous prolapse, a focal deformity becomes visible on axial scans, which affects one or more of the arms of the X-shaped hypoechoic mucosa, leading to the appearance of a cudgel (Fig. 3). This finding presumably corresponds to the intraluminal filling defect of contrast radiography described as grade 1 intussusception, which has a mucosal component only. On the other hand, a circumferential infolding of the rectal wall that descends and penetrates the anal canal with its apex (intra-anal intussusception) will determine a different pattern, as follows: taking the hypoechoic internal sphincter as reference, the cross-sectional area of the anal canal measured on straining from the inner border of the sphincter is seen to enlarge until it overcomes the one measured from its outer border by 50%. When present, a full-thickness prolapse involving both the mucosal and mural components can also be assumed (which corresponds to grades 2 and 3 intussusception at radiography), which is seen to impinge on the anal lumen and to obstruct defecation. Conversely, a complete external rectal prolapse with associated faecal incontinence is diagnosed when the entire thickness of the rectal wall is extruded through the anal canal and appears encircled by concentric rings of an attenuated or disrupted internal anal sphincter (Fig. 4). The issue of this discriminating capability by sonography is highly suggestive and encourages further investigation when considering that for patients with rectal prolapse and obstructed defecation as their primary symptom, only approximately 40% improve following surgery, whereas continence improves to some degree in up to 75% for those with incontinence as their main symptom.

More fundamental, when compared with contrast radiography, is the limitation of sonographic evacuation series. In fact, it has been argued that just stressing the perineum gives useful information. However, most important, abnormalities of pelvic floor function in the posterior compartment, such as trapping in a rectocele and enterocele, occur only when the rectum is stressed maximally by evacuation. Thus, transperineal sonography may have to include rectal voiding to become a valuable study in coloproctology. Not by chance, a special technique has been developed by us that is capable of providing details of the anorectal anatomy during evacuation of semisolid barium sulphate suspension. Characteristically, this substance appears radiopaque at contrast radiography and – unlike acoustic gel, hydrogen peroxide or tap water – is homogeneously anechoic at sonography, thus enhancing optimal visualisation of inner anorectal layers. For the emptying phase, patients are scanned in the squatting position with their knees flexed and thighs ab-

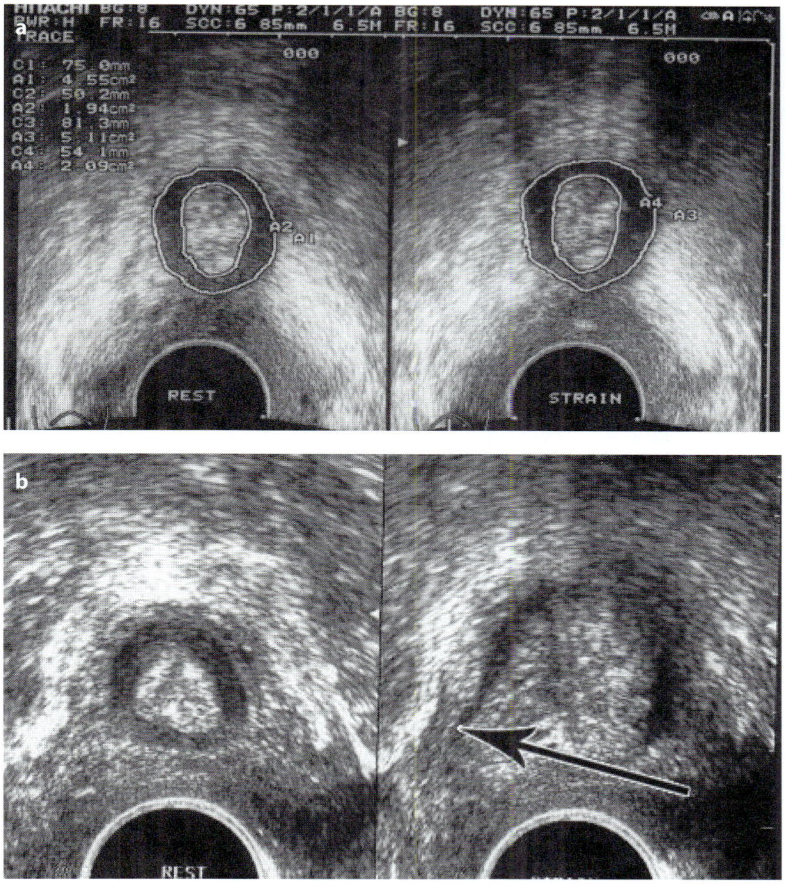

Fig. 4a, b
Cross-sectional measurement from the inner and outer margins of the internal anal sphincter (*tracing*) by sonography of an asymptomatic woman (**a**). Note the significant (>50%) increase of the internal area occurring in a different patient (**b**) with external prolapse, episodes of faecal incontinence and internal sphincter derangement (*arrow*)

ducted sufficiently to allow placement of the transducer in a sagittal orientation between the labia majora after having positioned a pad on the floor of the diagnostic room. Major drawbacks of this technique are: (1) it is somewhat difficult for the sonographer, who sits in front of the patient, to keep the probe fixed in place during the process of evacuation and (2) the potential risk of wrong assessment due to shift of the anatomic plane during straining, resulting in measurements of sections different from those intended. Consequently, determination of the rectal base position with respect to the reference line by evacuation sonography has not been proved sufficiently accurate and reproducible to match dynamic contrast radiography in case of rectal prolapse. On the other hand, it is capable of showing soft tissue details not seen on defecographic sequences, including a curvilinear hyperechoic structure that extends from the posterior border of the gut lumen to the anterior anorectal junction on sagittal dynamic images, which has been suggested to represent the locked-valve mechanism initially proposed by Phillips and Edwards [30]. This structure, which becomes visible only at sonography – thanks to the anechoic contrast medium injected intrarectally – lies as a flap over the upper end of the anal canal, effectively occluding it. At the beginning of defecation, a downwards bulge is seen to occur in the linear stripe, which is followed by opening of the anorectum into a funnel shape. It is possible to suggest that any impairment in the mechanism for breaking the seal of the valve may lead to outlet obstruction, strain defecation and eventually to rectal prolapse.

Magnetic Resonance Imaging

With the exception of lower accuracy by MRI in diagnosing external rectal prolapse in comparison with evacuation proctography, probably because patients are investigated supine, the two methods exhibit similar sensitivity. Thus, the po-

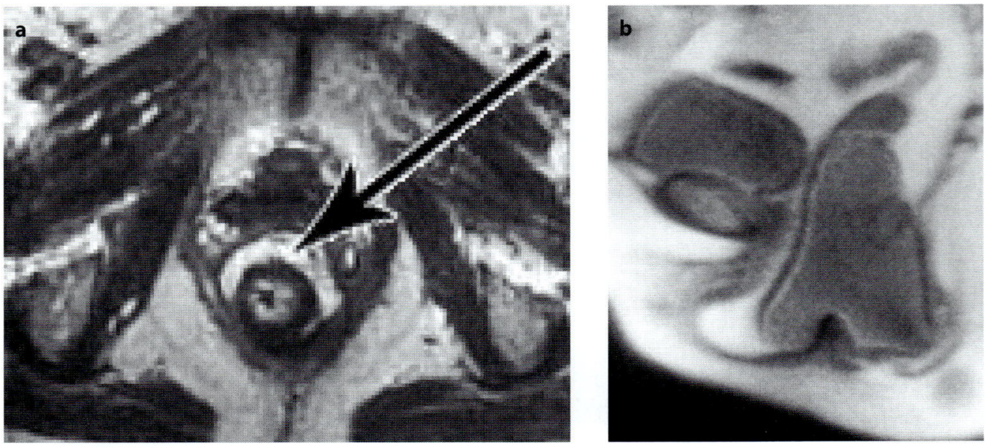

Fig. 5a, b

Axial T2-weighted magnetic resonance imaging of levator hiatus showing complete detachment (*arrow*) of rectovaginal fascia (**a**) leading to a low-type anterior rectocele (**b**)

tential use of MRI in place of X-ray contrast studies in proctology is highly suggestive. On the other hand, in view of the limited value of dynamic conventional radiography in demonstrating the presence and extent of anatomic derangements of adjacent structures, in particular those responsible for hiatus closure, MRI is mandatory for evaluating fat recesses, muscles and fascia [31–35]. Concepts of defects in the rectovaginal septum and its connections to the pelvic wall and perineal body that give rise to rectocele and rectal prolapse have undergone significant revision in recent years. An excellent discussion of current concepts of these common conditions can be found in the classical papers of DeLancey [36]. According to him, evaluation by MRI in living women – thanks to its multiplanar capability and high tissue contrast – can display specific sites of damage occurring in each component (i.e. pubovisceral and iliococcygeal) of the levator ani muscle or fascia and further clarify the relationships among the appearance of rectal descent, symptoms and the underlying anatomic defects present. Therefore, MRI is particularly indicated for cases of overt complexity when more precise surgical planning is necessary. In fact, the need for individually designed treatment has also been emphasised by observation of different types of rectocele and rectal prolapse as follows: Defects occurring in the middle of the vagina (high type) with an intact perineal body leading to rectocele should be addressed by plicating the rectovaginal fascia. Conversely, reuniting the fibres of the perineal body that have been separated from level II support is mandatory in case of a perineal rectocele (low type) occurring below this region (Fig. 5). Thus, the goal of MRI pelvic floor investigation in rectal prolapse and rectocele should focus on demonstrating the presence and extent of soft tissue deformations and focal defects of the muscular and fascial components. In particular, as demonstrated by Chou and Delancey [34], the importance of not seeing a structure in a given location, referred to as "the missing sign", is considered a distinct levator ani defect and helps separate anatomic variation from anatomic abnormalities.

On axial T2-weighted MRI sections through the arch of the pubic bone, midurethra and urogenital hiatus, special attention is given to the following:

1. Identification of vaginal shape, distance between the lateral vaginal wall and the pubic bone or levator ani muscle and lateral displacement of the vagina into the area normally occupied by the muscle as an indication of paravaginal tears and pelvic floor relaxation; abnormal vaginal shapes include concave anterior, flat and asymmetric.
2. Focal attenuation or defects in the pubovisceral and iliococcygeal muscles, along with loss of part of them, detachment from the endopelvic fascia or any signal intensity or thickness asymmetry due to fatty degeneration occurring in all sequences and scan planes.
3. Integrity of fascial condensations of the en-

dopelvic fascia called ligaments, parametria (cardinal and uterosacral ligaments), and paracolpia (condensations arising from the lateral aspect of the vagina).

4. Increased width of the levator hiatus (> 5 cm^2); any unilateral or bilateral discontinuity, focal thinning, ballooning or outward bulging in the puborectalis muscle with fat, fluid or pelvic viscera protruding out through the defect (perineal hernia).

Criteria that have been proposed for diagnosing rectal prolapse on sagittal MRI include:

1. Anterior displacement of the rectum with folding upon itself due to poor posterior mesorectal fixation.
2. Anterior, posterior or lateral bulging (rectocele).
3. Stretching and attenuation of the perineal body.
4. Descent of the anorectal junction relative to the pubococcygeal line greater than 2 cm.
5. Descent and caudal angulation of the levator plate such that its anterior projection does not cross the pubic bone.

Finally, coronal sections are ideal for displaying the pubovisceral part of the levator ani muscle where it is seen to fuse with the smooth muscle layer of the vaginal wall. On the more posterior images, the iliococcygeal part, with its typical convex configuration, and the puborectalis sling are depicted on either side of the rectum. The plane of section in this orientation is also suitable to display the fibres of paracolpium and parametrium connecting the vagina to the pelvic side wall.

Conclusion

Rectal prolapse is common in middle-aged and elderly women and is often associated with constipation, obstructed defecation and stress urinary incontinence. In such patients with symptoms of multicompartment defects, diagnostic imaging can be a useful preoperative planning tool. The imaging techniques involved include cystocolpoproctography, perineal sonography and dynamic MRI, the criteria for diagnosing rectocele and rectal prolapse derived from proctographic examinations being generally applicable to either ultrasonography or MRI.

In summary, contrast radiography provides a baseline to which other modalities can be compared in order to assess the presence and extent of rectal prolapse and to investigate all three pelvic compartments, but their drawbacks include high exposure to ionising radiation and absence of information on surrounding soft tissue. Perineal sonography, on the other hand, is safe, inexpensive and well tolerated by the patient, but has limited value during the emptying phase and is highly operator dependent. Its main value consists of allowing quick and easy investigation of relationships between pelvic organs and giving objective evidence of concomitant anal sphincter derangements. MRI is increasingly being used to image global pelvic floor dynamics and is especially useful for imaging anatomic structures not otherwise visible, such as muscles, fascia and fat recesses. Consequently, the major role of MRI is to provide images of loss of integrity of muscular and fascial supports. The advantages of MRI are nonexposure to ionising radiation and high soft tissue contrast for assessing pelvic floor morphology. The technique is suitable for optimal standardisation, and its only drawback is the limited local availability and cost. Hopefully, a combination of all three imaging modalities in rectal prolapse will lead to a better understanding of the precise nature of anatomic changes associated with symptoms and better treatment selection and prevention.

Aknowledgements

The authors are especially indebted to Dr. Ebe Tartufo for her assistance in formatting the manuscript.

References

1. Bump RC, Mattiasson A, Bo K et al (1996) The standardization of terminology of female pelvic organ prolapse and pelvic floor dysfunction. Am J Obstet Gynecol 175(1):10–17
2. Ekberg O, Mahieu PHG, Bartram CI et al (1990) Defecography: dynamic radiological imaging in proctology. Gastroenterol Int 3:63–69
3. Kelvin FM, Maglinte DDT, Benson JT (1994) Evacua-

tion proctography (defecography): an aid to the investigation of pelvic floor disorders. Obstet Gynecol 83:307–314
4. Hock D, Lombard R, Jehaes C et al (1993) Colpocystodefecography. Dis Colon Rectum 36:1015–1021
5. Kelvin FM, Maglinte DDT, Benson JT et al (1994) Dynamic cystoproctography: a technique for assessing disorders of the pelvic floor in women. AJR Am J Roentgenol 163:368–370
6. Maglinte DDT, Kelvin FM, Hale DS et l (1997) Dynamic cystoproctography: a unifying diagnostic approach to pelvic floor and anorectal dysfunction. AJR Am J Roentgenol 169:759–767
7. Maglinte DDT, Kelvin FM, Fitzgerald DSH et al (1999) Association of compartment defects in pelvic floor dysfunction. AJR Am J Roentgenol 172:439–444
8. Brown MC, Sutherst JR, Murray A et al (1985) Potential use of ultrasound in place of X-ray fluoroscopy in urodynamics Br J Urol 57:88–90
9. Kohorn EI, Sciascia AL, Jeanty P et al (1986) Ultrasound cystourethrography by perineal scanning for the assessment of female stress urinary incontinence. Obstet Gynecol 68:269–272
10. Quinn MJ, Beynon J, McC. Mortensen NJ et al (1988) Transvaginal endosonography: a new method to study the anatomy of the lower urinary tract in urinary stress incontinence. Br J Urology 62:103–105
11. Kolbl H, Bernaschek G, Wolf G (1988) A comparative study of perineal scan and urethrocystography in patients with genuine stress incontinence. Arch Gynecol Obstet 244:39–45
12. Schaer GN, Khoechli OR, Schuessler B et al (1995) Perineal ultrasound for evaluating the bladder neck in urinary stress incontinence. Obstet Gynecol 85:220–224
13. Khullar V, Cardozo L, Salvatore S et al (1996) Ultrasound: a noninvasive screening test for detrusor instability. Br J Obstet Gynecol 103:904–908
14. Chang TS, Bohm-Velez M, Mendelson EB (1993) Nongynecological applications of transvaginal sonography AJR Am J Roentgenol 160:87–93
15. Rubens DJ, Strang JG, Bogineni-Misra S et al (1988) Transperineal sonography of the rectum: anatomy and pathology revealed by sonography compared with CT and MR imaging. AJR Am J Roentgenol 170:637–642
16. Sultan AH, Loder PB, Bartram CI et al (1994) Vaginal endosonography: new approach to image the undisturbed anal sphincter. Dis Colon Rectum 37:1296–1299
17. Sandridge DA, Thorp JM (1995) Vaginal endosonography in the assessment of the anorectum. Obstet Gynecol 86:1007–1009
18. Halligan S, Northover J, Bartram CI (1996) Vaginal endosonography to diagnose enterocele. Br J Radiol 69:996–999
19. Peschers UM, DeLancey JO, Schaer GN et al (1997) Exoanal ultrasound of the anal sphincter: normal anatomy and sphincter defects. Br J Obstet Gynaecol 104 (9):999–1003
20. Alexander AA, Liu JB, Merton DA et al (1997) Fecal incontinence: transvaginal US evaluation of anatomic causes Radiology 199:529–532
21. Piloni V (2001) Dynamic imaging of pelvic floor with transperineal sonography. Tech Coloproctol 5:103–105
22. Beer-Gabel M, Zbar AP (2002) Dynamic transperineal ultrasound in patients presenting with obstructed evacuation Tech Coloproctol 6:141
23. Piloni V, Spazzafumo L (2005) Evacuation sonography. Tech Coloproctol 9:119–126
24. Yang A, Mostwin JL, Rosenhein NB et al (1991) Pelvic floor descent in women: dynamic evaluation with fast MR imaging and cinematic display. Radiology 179:25–33
25. Lienemann A, Anthuber C, Baron A et al (1997) Dynamic MR colpocystorectography assessing pelvic-floor descent. Eur Radiol 7(8):1309–1317
26. Fielding JR, Griffiths DJ, Versi E et al (1998) MR imaging of pelvic floor continence mechanisms in the supine and sitting positions. AJR Am J Roentgenol 171:1607–1610
27. Comiter CV, Vasavada SP, Barbaric ZL et al (1999) Grading pelvic prolapse and pelvic floor relaxation using dynamic magnetic resonance imaging. Urology 54(3):454–457
28. Kelvin FM. Maglinte DDT, Hale DS et al (2000) Female pelvic organ prolapse: a comparison of triphasic dynamic MR imaging and triphasic fluoroscopic cystocolpoproctography. AJR Am J Roentgenol 174:81–88
29. DeLancey JOL, Hurd WW (1998) Size of the urogenital hiatus in the levator ani muscles in normal women and women with pelvic organ prolapse. Obstet Gynecol 91:364–368
30. Phillips SF, Edwards DAW (1965) Some aspects of anal continence and defaecation. Gut 6:396–406
31. Healy JC, Halligan S, Reznek RH et al (1997) Patterns of prolapse in women with symptoms of pelvic floor weakness: assessment with MR imaging. Radiology 203:77–81
32. Pannu HK, Kaufman HS, Cundiff GW et al (2000) Dynamic MR imaging of pelvis organ prolapse: spectrum of abnormalities. Radiographics 20(6):1567–1582
33. Tunn R, DeLancey JOL, Quint EE (2001) Visibility of pelvic organ support system structures in magnetic resonance images without an endovaginal coil. Am J Obstet Gynecol 184:1156–1163
34. Chou Q, DeLancey JOL (2001) A structured system to evaluate urethral support anatomy in magnetic resonance images. Am J Obstet Gynecol 185:44–50
35. Tunn R, DeLancey JOL, Howard D et al (2003) Anatomic variation in the levator ani muscle, endopelvic fascia, and urethra in nulliparas evaluated by magnetic resonance. Am J Obstet Gynecol 188: 116–121
36. DeLancey JOL (1999) Structural anatomy of the posterior pelvic compartment as it relates to rectocele. Am J Obstet Gynecol 180:815–823

4 An Overview of Neurophysiologic Tests in Rectal Prolapse

Carlo Ratto

Introduction

Diagnostic assessment in patients with rectal prolapse is a debatable field due to the very different clinical presentation of this condition and different preferences towards the variety of available diagnostic tests. Only full-thickness protrusion of the entire rectal wall through the anal canal should fall under the definition of "rectal prolapse". However, internal rectal intussusception is very often included in this definition [1] because it is regarded as an early stage of overt rectal prolapse. In reality, rectal intussusception represents a wide variety of clinical and radiological conditions (schematically, rectoanal and rectorectal) with or without the association of other abnormalities (rectocele, sigmoidocele, enterocele, perineal descent, uterovaginal prolapse, cystocele), all of which contribute to obstructed defecation. Recently, the interpretation of intussusception has been challenged based on the high percentage of asymptomatic persons showing internal intussusception during defecography but which can disappear by the time of a follow-up defecography [2]. Moreover, whereas complete rectal prolapse is frequently associated with a weak pelvic floor, incomplete rectal intussusception may be associated with paradoxical pelvic floor contraction. Therefore, intussusception remains the most likely theory for the pathogenesis of rectal prolapse, whereas internal rectal intussusception is of uncertain pathogenetic and clinical relevance in this interpretation.

A multimodal diagnostic assessment should be regarded as the only way to obtain an accurate pathogenetic interpretation of rectal prolapse/intussusception. Complete evaluation of the patient's history and thorough examination are mandatory, followed by diagnostic tests that include the evaluation of both colonic and rectoanal functions. Bowel-transit studies, anorectal manometry, defecography (associated with dynamic radiological assessment of the anterior, central and posterior pelvic floor compartments) and endoanal ultrasound should contribute to precise identification of lesions and dysfunctions related to the prolapse.

With this in mind, neurophysiologic tests should play a central role. They have contributed to the interpretation of rectal prolapse pathophysiology, showing abnormalities in the pelvic floor muscles, including dysfunction of internal and external sphincters and levator ani, possibly related to pelvic floor stretching during pregnancy, labour or a long history of constipation. Relationship with the consequent pudendal neuropathy has been elucidated and pelvic floor weakness suspected as a predisposing condition to rectal protrusion through the anal hiatus. Moreover, neurophysiologic tests have been regarded as having a pivotal significance in selecting patients for treatment and predicting its outcome. However, the real role of such tests is still under debate.

Anorectal Neurophysiology Tests

These procedures include a few tests directed to patients already investigated with history and physical assessment and other procedures in whom pelvic muscular and/or nervous functions seem to be altered. The tests usually consist of electrical impulses and/or record electrical traces derived from myographic and nerve-conduction examinations. Evolution of instruments, examination techniques and indications has occurred over the last 20 years.

Anorectal Electrophysiology Technique

Electrophysiological studies are usually carried

out using a neuromyography system equipped with software dedicated to anorectal physiological evaluation. Examination includes tests evaluating electrical muscle activity and nerve functionality. In performing such tests, either a recording function or an electrostimulating function or both can be requested. The neuromyographic instrument needs to be connected to dedicated cables and electrodes. Before anorectal electrophysiology, an enema is usually required to clean the rectal ampulla. The most preferred patient position is the left lateral during this procedure. A ground electrode soaked in normal saline is placed around the thigh.

The purpose of *electromyography* (*EMG*) is to investigate the electrical activity of the external anal sphincter and the other striated pelvic floor muscles at rest and during squeezing and straining. Over time, four different types of electrodes have been developed: concentric needle, monopolar wire, single-fibre and surface. The concentric needle electrode consists of a thin needle (0.1 mm in diameter) covered by an insulating resin, which is able to uptake electrical activity of the small area into which it has been inserted. This needle is unable to record single muscle-fibre action potentials. Under the guidance of digital anal exploration, the needle must be inserted into the external sphincter or puborectalis muscle. Recordings from the four anal canal quadrants should be obtained. This procedure is quite uncomfortable for the patient. The electrode could slide in a different position during trace acquisition and, even if multiple recording samples are taken, the mapping obtained is far from being considered sufficient to delineate accurately the real area of normal and abnormal muscle. The monopolar wire should reduce the patient's discomfort and avoid the electrode sliding because it is kept in site by a small hook placed at the electrode tip. A single-fibre electrode is thinner than the monopolar wire and is able to record individual motor-unit potentials. Appropriate signal amplification recording is necessary. Also, fibre density can be calculated based on 20 different recordings from each anal hemisphere. Evaluation with the single-fibre electrode is more accurate than using the two electrodes previously described but remains uncomfortable. Surface electrodes, mounted on an endoanal plug or a small external adhesive plaque, are able to record gross muscle activity but unable to delimit areas of functional deficit. They are more useful to study paradoxical contraction of striated muscles than to evaluate eventual sphincter damage in incontinent patients.

Mucosal sensitivity can be evaluated with electrostimulation not only in the rectum (as does manometry) but also in the anal canal using a bipolar ring electrode (containing two platinum wires 1-cm apart) mounted on a Foley catheter. An appropriate setting of stimulus duration and rate must be done before starting examination. During this test, the electrode is inserted into the anus first. From zero, the current amplitude is slowly increased until the patient feels a buzzing or tingling sensation in the anus. At least three measurements need to be taken, choosing the lower threshold value for the report. A similar procedure is used for mucosal sensitivity analysis in the rectum. Rectal ampulla must be reached by the electrode. Under slowly increasing current (parameter setting is different than that used for anal sensitivity test), three values should be obtained, taking the lowest as the rectal threshold sensation to be reported.

Finally, *pudendal nerve terminal motor latency (PNTML)* is measured, allowing evaluation of the pelvic floor neuromuscular integrity. A disposable St. Mark's pudendal electrode is mounted onto the volar side of the examiner's gloved index finger. The index finger is inserted into the rectum, with the fingertip reaching the course of each pudendal nerve and the proximal finger phalanx sited within the anal canal. During this test, both electrostimulation and recording function need to be activated. Four cables run within the electrode, conveying stimuli from the machine to the fingertip (to the anode and cathode) in order to stimulate the pudendal nerve fibres, and from the finger tip to the machine to record the striated muscle response visualised on the screen. The latency (expressed in milliseconds) from stimulus onset to the first deflection of the response is calculated for each pudendal nerve.

Indications for Anorectal Electrophysiology and Findings

As mentioned above, indications for anorectal electrophysiology are usually decided upon on the basis of the patient's history and physical assessment if pelvic, muscular and/or nervous disorders are hypothesised. Moreover, data from other diagnostic procedures (mainly manometry and ultrasound) should confirm the decision to submit the patient to anorectal electrophysiology.

In constipated patients, EMG is used to demonstrate a paradoxical puborectalis contraction or lack of relaxation. In this condition, striated muscle activity recorded during straining is either increased or not changed when compared with at-rest activity. These findings could be related to a paradoxical increase or unchanging anal pressure during straining observed with manometry. In reality, EMG features of the pelvic floor in coordination are very frequently observed, even if a large number of false positive results have to be considered. Indeed, a significant number of patients with this EMG result do not refer relevant constipation, so that the test needs to be critically evaluated. In cases of constipation and EMG demonstration of anismus, cinedefecography could also be useful.

In patients with sphincter lesions, no electrical activity may be found in cases of wide, complete replacement of normal muscular tissue with scar or, more frequently, polyphasic potentials as signs of a reinnervation process. Polyphasic potentials do present multiple spikes of muscle activity, prolonged in duration, and an increased fibre density (FD). In evaluating sphincter injury, endoanal ultrasound has higher sensitivity and specificity than EMG in mapping the lesion; however, only EMG can assess neuromuscular integrity. In this regard, these two procedures are complementary to each other.

Evaluation of anal mucosal electrosensitivity could have clinical relevance in a few clinical conditions. Apart from the alterations registered in patients with prolapsing haemorrhoids (higher threshold levels), in neurogenic incontinence, a wide spectrum of findings can be observed, probably related to the degree of pudendal neuropathy.

Also, rectal sensation measurements by electrophysiological study are meaningful. In patients suffering from constipation, threshold levels are frequently higher than normal, even if this is not the rule. In incontinent patients with only sphincter lesion(s), mucosal electrosensitivity could be normal. In those with neurogenic incontinence, there could be a wide variability of findings; concerning manometric rectal sensation measurement, its meaning has to be intensively interpreted and correlated with results from other tests.

Alterations in PNTML are identified in relation to patient age, being more frequent in older patients. This is probably due to several causes, including chronic straining in constipated patients presenting perineal descent due to continuous stretching of pudendal nerves. However, this feature is not constant, and the direct relationship between pudendal neuropathy and constipation is not demonstrated. In a large number of patients with faecal incontinence (with or without urinary incontinence) and rectal prolapse, the PNTML is abnormally prolonged. PNTML levels are thought to have a predictive value in patients undergoing treatment, but this assumption remains controversial.

Discussion

Although neurophysiologic evaluation could be done using the variety of tests mentioned above, in the literature, there is a lack of reports concerning complete evaluation of patients with rectal prolapse or intussusception. In most series, the only electrophysiological procedure reported is the PNTML; only in a few studies has FD been evaluated. A wide debate still exits about the physiologic and clinical significance of PNTML, as well as its diagnostic and prognostic role. It should reflect a part of the functional neuromuscular integrity of the anorectum and, more largely, of all pelvic organs. The pudendal nerve is involved in both motor and sensory functions. Therefore, in patients affected by rectal prolapse, pudendal neuropathy should be frequently expected. However, a variety of alterations can be encountered. Schematically, patients suffering from rectal intussusception usually refer with outlet obstruction due to occult rectal invagination but could also have a pathophysiological basis for the incontinence in cases of large rectal infolding; patients with full-thickness prolapse can be incontinent (to different degrees) to faeces or they may be constipated.

Rectorectal or rectoanal intussusception (also called internal intussusception, internal rectal prolapse, intrarectal prolapse or internal procidentia) has been reported to occur in up to 50% of the normal population [3]. It has been regarded as a prestage of overt prolapse [4–6], and step-by-step development has been described. Fleshman et al. [7] classified the intussusception–prolapse sequence into five grades based on rectal motility, intussusception, and anal sphincter relaxation: grade I, nonrelaxation of the sphincter mechanism; grade II, mild intussusception or motility from the sacrum; grade III, moderate intussusception; grade IV, severe intussusception; grade V, rectal prolapse. However, it is controversial whether this sequence must be considered accurate. Mellgren et al. [2] followed up 38 untreated patients with defecographic diagnosis of rectal intussusception; only two (5.2%) had developed overt rectal prolapse by the time of the second defecography. Later, Choi et al. [8] found that only one out of 26 patients (3.8%) with untreated rectal intussusception had a full-thickness rectal prolapse.

Unfortunately, these is a lack of electrophysiological assessment of patients with rectal intussusception, and this condition frequently is integrated into series including pelvic outlet obstruction and/or perineal descent. The common denominator with these clinical conditions should be the possible pudendal denervation due to continuous straining and consequent nerve-fibre stretching. Vaccaro et al. [9] found an overall incidence of pudendal neuropathy of 23.6% when examining 161 patients with chronic constipation, it being unilateral in 11.2% and bilateral in 12.4%. It was significantly related to patient age, confirming other studies performed with single-fibre EMG [10, 11]. They also found a relationship between pudendal neuropathy and paradoxical puborectalis contraction, which was significant in patients with bilaterally prolonged PNTML. Finally, motor-unit-potential recruitment decreased in constipated patients with pudendal neuropathy [9]. One year later, the same group of researchers [12] reported cinedefecography and PNTML data in 147 patients with chronic constipation (91 with normal pattern of evacuation, 56 with pelvic outlet obstruction). Overall incidence of pudendal neuropathy was 23.8% (10.9% unilateral, 12.9% bilateral). There was no significant difference between subgroups of patients (unobstructed vs. obstructed) concerning pudendal neuropathy, which was only related to increased patient age [12]. Also, Jorge et al. [13] found no association between pudendal neuropathy and increased perineal descent (studied with cinedefecography) in 213 patients suffering from constipation, idiopathic faecal incontinence or chronic rectal pain. Their findings were in contrast with data from Ho and Goh [14], who demonstrated that PNTML was the only independent variable predicting perineal descent (measured with perineometry) in 141 patients with chronic constipation, neurogenic faecal incontinence, rectal mucosal prolapse or female urinary stress incontinence.

Alterations in neurophysiologic parameters in full-thickness rectal prolapse are very frequent. Pfeifer et al. [15] analysed 1,026 patients differentiated into four groups: faecal incontinence, chronic constipation, idiopathic rectal pain, and rectal prolapse. In prolapse patients, a higher rate (47.2%) was affected by pudendal neuropathy when compared with patients with incontinence (32%), constipation (27.8%) or rectal pain (23.1%). Abnormal PNTML was unilateral in 18% and bilateral in 20.2% of patients. The authors found a correlation between pudendal neuropathy and patient age. Neurophysiologic abnormalities in rectal prolapse can be dependent on whether patients present incontinence or constipation.

Incontinence occurs in 35–100% of patients with rectal prolapse [16–20]. This dysfunction has been attributed to abnormal relaxation of the internal anal sphincter (due to a continuously elicited rectoanal inhibitory reflex) and the consequent decrease of resting pressure and, subsequently, incontinence [21–25]. However, Neill et al. [26] reported decreased resting anal pressure in rectal prolapse patients irrespective of presence or absence of incontinence. On the contrary, others [27, 28] reported a higher resting tone in continent patients with prolapse. Also, a significant reduction of maximal squeeze pressure has been considered as an associated abnormality in patients with rectal prolapse and incontinence [21, 26, 27]; a denervation of anal striated muscles has been shown in these patients [27, 29]. The rectum of patients with prolapse has been found to be hypersensitive and hyperreactive, which promptly respond to minor organ distension [21], which, then, determines incontinence [30, 31]. These findings can also be associated with increased activity of the colon, and particularly the sigmoid colon, in rectal prolapse patients [32, 33], possibly resulting in protrusion of the intussuscepted rectum through the anus. Neill et al. [26] demonstrated that preoperative EMG was abnormal in patients with rectal prolapse and incontinence, whereas it was normal in rectal prolapse patients without incontinence. Osterberg et al. [34] studied 72 patients with faecal incontinence using anorectal manovolumetry, anal ultrasound, defecography and electrophysiological examination including PNTML and FD. They found an abnormal PNTML in 46% and an increased FD in 82% of patients; these features were most common in patients with rectal prolapse or intra-anal intussusception. PNTML did not correlate with either manometric parameters or severity of incontinence, whereas an increased FD was significantly associated with lower anal pressures and decreased rectal sensibility.

The significance of neurophysiologic parameters following treatment has also been questioned. Birnbaum et al. [35] analysed prospectively 24 patients with full-thickness rectal prolapse, finding faecal incontinence in 50%; all patients were operated on with low anterior resection or retrorectal sacral fixation. Anorectal manometry and PNTML were tested before and after surgery. Postoperatively, four out of 12 incontinent patients referred improvement of continence, whereas three out of 12 continent patients developed incontinence; therefore, the overall incidence of incontinence after surgery was 46% (11 out 24 patients). In 12 patients, PNTML was measured both pre- and postoperatively. Among nine patients with normal preoperative PNTML, only two remained that way, whereas the others developed prolonged latency (unilaterally in four, bilaterally in three), with faecal incontinence clinically evident in four. Among three patients with preoperatively prolonged PNTML (two unilateral, one bilateral), all developed incontinence after surgery. A total of 19 patients underwent PNTML measurement after operation; faecal incontinence incidence was higher in patients with postoperative bilateral prolonged PNTML (83%) than in those with unilateral prolonged PNTML (38%) or normal PNTML (20%). Whereas no correlation was found between PNTML and resting pressure, pudendal latency was related to a decreased squeeze pressure. Authors attributed the postoperative pudendal neuropathy to progressive ischaemic neurogenic injury not reversed by surgical correction of rectal anatomy only. In their opinion, persistency of straining to defecate due to poor rectal emptying could continue pudendal injury. More recently, Glasgow et al. [36] reported long-term results of 106 patients treated with perineal proctectomy with levatorplasty for rectal prolapse; 45 were studied pre- and postoperatively with anorectal manometry and PNTML. Normal manometry and normal PNTML were detected in only three patients. A prolonged PNTML was measured preoperatively in 55.6% of patients (60% with bilateral pudendal neuropathy). Both preoperative incontinence and constipation decreased significantly after surgery (from 77.8% to 35.6%, $p < 0.0001$; and from 33.3% to 6.7%, $p < 0.003$, respectively). Faecal continence was particularly improved in patients with preoperative squeeze pressure >60 mmHg. PNTML did not correlate with functional outcome after surgery.

In rectal prolapse, between 25% and 50% of patients present constipation [37–39], sometimes associated with slow-transit colon [26, 37]. However, the colon could have normal transit time but poor propulsive activity [40]. Others showed a frequent paradoxical activity of the external anal sphincter [39]. All these features could contribute to increased extrusion of the rectum under the associated straining.

Conclusion

Theoretically, neurophysiologic tests should provide unique and fundamental information concerning the pathophysiology of rectal prolapse and, consequently, could play a primary role in treatment planning and prevision of patient outcome. Unfortunately, the wide variety of cases included in every single series (intussusception and full-thickness prolapse, incontinent and constipated patients), the lack of numerous series of patients studied prospectively and with strict diagnostic criteria, the quite exclusive use of PNTML (accepted by some, criticised by others) and the lack of a complete electrophysiologic examination all contribute to the fact that the place of these tests in the diagnostic workup remains debatable. At this time, anorectal electrophysiology in rectal prolapse patients should be considered as complementary to other diagnostic procedures, namely, anorectal manometry, cinedefecography, colonic transit time test and endoanal ultrasound. Comprehensive results should give the best interpretation of the disease pathophysiology. This step is of primary importance in planning the most appropriate management, choosing between a conservative approach or surgery. However, specifically in relation to this, a prospectively designed diagnostic protocol could be worthwhile in the near future aimed at identifying subgroups of patients selectively chosen to one treatment or another. Interpretation of such data could be useful also to verify the functional impact of the treatment option adopted in relation to the neurophysiologic condition both pre- and posttreatment.

References

1. Jarrett MED (2007) Rectal prolapse. In: Ratto C, Doglietto GB (eds) Fecal incontinence. Diagnosis and treatment. Springer, Milan, pp 261–265
2. Mellgren A, Bremmer S, Johansson C et al (1994) Defecography – results of investigations in 2,816 patients. Dis Colon Rectum 37:1133–1141
3. Shorvon PJ, McHugh S, Diamant NE et al (1989) Defecography in normal volunteers: results and implications. Gut 30:1737–1749
4. Ihre T, Seligson U (1975) Intussusception of the rectum-internal procidentia: treatment and results in 90 patients. Dis Colon Rectum 18:391–396
5. Broden B, Snellman B (1968) Procidentia of the rectum studied with cinedefecography: a contribution to the discussion of causative mechanism. Dis Colon Rectum 11:330–347
6. Devadhar DS (1965) A new concept of mechanism and treatment of rectal procidentia. Dis Colon Rectum 8:75–77
7. Fleshman JW, Kodner IJ, Fry RD (1989) Internal intussusception of the rectum: A changing perspective. Neth J Surg 41:145–148
8. Choi JS, Hwang YH, Salum MR et al (2001) Outcome and management of patients with large rectoanal intussusception. Am J Gastroenterol 96:740–744
9. Vaccaro CA, Cheong DM, Wexner SD et al (1994) Role of pudendal nerve terminal motor latency assessment in constipated patients. Dis Colon Rectum 37:1250–1254
10. Percy JP, Neill ME, Kandiah TK, Swash M (1982) A neurogenic factor in faecal incontinence in the elderly. Age Ageing 11:175–179
11. Neill ME, Swash M (1980) Increased motor unit fiber density in the external anal sphincter muscle in anorectal incontinence: a single fiber EMG study. J Neurol Neurosurg Psychiatry 43:343–347
12. Vaccaro CA, Wexner SD, Teoh T-A et al (1995) Pudendal neuropathy is not related to physiologic pelvic outlet obstruction. Dis Colon Rectum 38:630–634
13. Jorge JMN, Wexner SD, Ehrenpreis ED et al (1993) Does perineal descent correlate with pudendal neuropathy? Dis Colon Rectum 36:475–483
14. Ho YH, Goh HS (1995) The neurophysiological significance of perineal descent. Int J Colorect Dis 10:107–111
15. Pfeifer J, Salanga VD, Agachan F et al (1997) Variation in pudendal nerve terminal motor latency according to disease. Dis Colon Rectum 40:79–83
16. Mortenson NJMcC, Vellacott KD, Wilson MG (1984) Lahaut's operation for rectal prolapse. Ann R Coll Surg Engl 66:17–18
17. Watts JD, Rothenberger DA, Buls JG et al (1985) The management of procidentia: 30 years experience. Dis Colon Rectum 28:96–102
18. Yoshioka K, Hyland G, Keighley MRB (1989) Anorectal function after abdominal rectopexy: parameters of predictive value in identifying return of continence. Br J Surg 76:64–68
19. Andrews NJ, Jones DJ (1992) Rectal prolapse and associated conditions. BMJ 305:243–245
20. Stenchever MA (1984) Management of genital prolapse in the geriatric patient. Geriatr Med Today 3:75–78
21. Sun WM, Read NW, Carmel T et al (1989) A common pathophysiology for full-thickness rectal prolapse, anterior mucosal prolapse and solitary rectal ulcer. Br J Surg 76:290–295
22. Farouk R, Duthie GS, MacGregor AB et al (1994) Rectoanal inhibition and incontinence in patients with rectal prolapse. Br J Surg 81:743–746
23. Spencer RJ (1984) Manometric studies in rectal prolapse. Dis Colon Rectum 27:523–525
24. Williams JG, Wong WD, Jensen L et al (1991) Incontinence in rectal prolapse: a prospective manometric study. Dis Colon Rectum 34:209–216
25. Farouk R, Duthie GS, Bartolo DCC et al (1992) Restoration of continence following rectopexy for rectal prolapse and recovery of the internal anal sphincter electromyogram. Br J Surg 79:439–440
26. Neill ME, Parks AG, Swash M (1981) Physiological studies of the anal sphincter musculature in fecal incontinence and rectal prolapse. Br J Surg 68:531–536
27. Mathenson DM, Keighley MRB (1981) Manometric evaluation of rectal prolapse and fecal incontinence. Gut 22:126–129
28. Santini L, Pezzullo L, Caraco C et al (1995) Fecal incontinence and rectal prolapse, clinicofunctional assessment. Minerva Chir 50:741–745
29. Parks AG, Swash M, Urich H (1977) Sphincter denervation in anorectal incontinence and rectal prolapse. Gut 18:656–665
30. Siproudhis L, Bellissant E, Jujuet F et al (1998) Rectal adaptation to distension in patients with overt rectal prolapse. Br J Surg 85:1527–1532
31. Tsiaoussis J Chrysos E, Glynos M et al (1998) Pathophysiology and treatment of anterior rectal mucosal prolapse syndrome. Br J Surg 85:1699–1702
32. Keighley MRB, Williams NS (1999) Rectal prolapse. In: Keighley MRB, Williams NS (eds) Surgery of the anus, rectum and colon, 2nd end. Saunders, London, pp 794–842
33. Keyghley MRB, Shouler PJ (1984) Abnormalities of colonic function in patients with rectal prolapse. Br J Surg 71:892–895

34. Osterberg A, Graf W, Eeg-Olofsson KE et al (2000) Results of neurophysiologic evaluation in fecal incontinence. Dis Colon Rectum 43:1256–1261
35. Birnbaum EH, Stamm L, Rafferty JF et al (1996) Pudendal nerve terminal motor latency influences surgical outcome in treatment of rectal prolapse. Dis Colon Rectum 39:1215–1221
36. Glasgow SC, Birnbaum EH, Kodner IJ et al (2006) Preoperative anal manometry predicts continence after perineal proctectomy for rectal prolapse. Dis Colon Rectum 49:1052–1058
37. Madoff RD (1992) Rectal prolapse and intussusception. In: Beck DE, Wexner SD (eds) Fundamentals in anorectal surgery. McGraw-Hill, New York, pp 89–103
38. Madoff RD, Williams JG, Wong WD et al (1992) Long-term functional results of colon resection and rectopexy for overt rectal prolapse. Am J Gastroenterol 87:101–104
39. Metcalf AM, Loening-Baucke V (1988) Anorectal function and defecation dynamics in patients with rectal prolapse. Am J Surg 155:206–210
40. Brown AG, Hogan AF, Anderson JH et al (1999) Colonic motility is abnormal before surgery for rectal prolapse. Br J Surg 86:263–266

5 Classification of Internal and External Rectal Prolapse

Fabio Pomerri, Pier Carlo Muzzio

Introduction

Physical examination has traditionally been, and continues to be, the mandatory initial step in the evaluation of patients with constipation or faecal incontinence. This is because the initial treatment decision and the necessity of further investigations of patients with pelvic floor dysfunction depend on primary clinical assessment of the patient [1]. Even if authors [2] found good correlation between clinical assessment and defecography in high-grade intussusceptions when studying subjects with defecatory difficulties, several reports in the nonradiologic literature have documented the relative insensitivity of the history and physical examination in diagnosing the cause of constipation and detecting pelvic organ prolapse [1, 3–6]. The common clinical physical examination tends to underestimate the degree of prolapse and may be able to diagnose only 30–40% of rectal prolapse [7]. Therefore, the precise preoperative diagnosis supplied by defecography can help in the selection of a rationale treatment programme, placing the patient into a treatment-defined group, determining the type of operation and giving objective evidence for the corrective scope and degree of operation. However, there are few guidelines for defining clinically significant rectoanal intussusception and prolapse. For example, the frequency of rectoanal intussusception has been reported to occur in up to 50% of the normal population [8]. The absence of specific criteria defining functional disorders and conflicting results of physiologic tests has made the understanding of anorectal disorders difficult.

Personal Experience

Clinical presentation and radiologic findings in 2,837 consecutive patients (430 men, 2,407 women; age range, 14–87 years; mean age, 56.5 years) with proctologic, micturitional or gynaecologic symptoms were reviewed and analysed. Patients underwent a total of 3,042 dynamic evacuation examinations: defecography was used for 548 examinations (18%), colpodefecography for 541 (17.8%), and cystocolpodefecography for 1,953 (64.2%). Most patients were referred for radiologic evaluation by coloproctologists over a 10-year period, and 249 (8.8%) were found to have rectal intussusception or prolapse. Defecography was also performed in 43 asymptomatic subjects (17 men, 26 women; age range, 45–78 years; mean age, 58.7 years), who were recruited by advertisement. All subjects gave their fully informed consent to take part in the study, which was approved by the local ethics committee [9].

Normal Study

Normal anorectal configuration at the end of the evacuation was defined based on the findings in a control group of 43 asymptomatic subjects who underwent defecographic examination, the subjects being examined in the lateral position [9]. As the rectum collapses, the side walls become apposed [10, 11], and the longitudinal rectal axis shortens. In the lateral view, the mucosa creates a slight indentation of the rectal outline as residual barium is compressed between the folds. Rectal mucosal folds of a few millimetres, mainly in the posterior wall of the rectum (Fig. 1), are common radiology findings during evacuation and reflect pleating of mucosa as the rectum collapses. In no case did the fully distended rectum show any such fold [11]. At maximal straining on completion of evacuation, the rectal outline guttering increases,

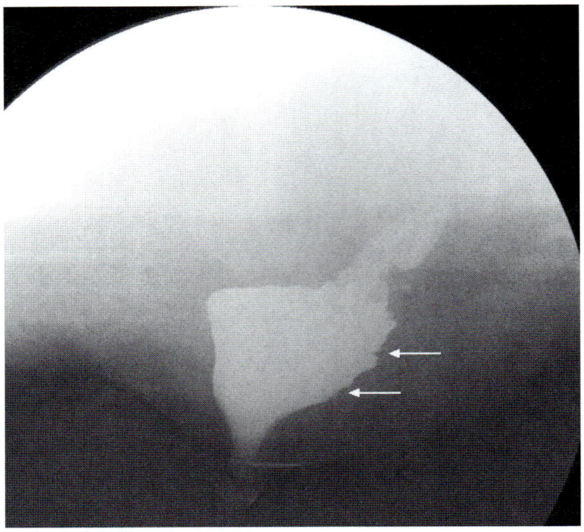

Fig. 1

Image at midevacuation. Thin rectal mucosal folds (*arrows*) in an asymptomatic 54-year-old man

representing mucosal folding up to 1 cm in width, and the gap between the folds becomes thinner.

Differing methodologies and imprecisely defined patterns make comparison and interpretation of many radiologic studies difficult. Much confusion arose over grading the development of mucosal folding, mucosal prolapse, and intussusception as a continuum. It was reported that circumferential invagination of the full thickness of the rectal wall is a common phenomenon in normal volunteers during straining [8]. Mucosal folding may occur only in one wall of the rectum or it may be circumferential. It can be difficult to distinguish normal rectal mucosal folds from rectal intussusception on the basis of morphological changes and subjective quantification of the thickness of rectal folding [12]. When normal rectal mucosal folding appears circumferential, rectal morphologic changes may mimic intussusception, which was observed in 13 (30%) of 43 asymptomatic subjects on completion of evacuation (Fig. 2). Rectal folding measured 8.7 ± 3.8 mm thick on the anterior aspect of the rectal wall and 7.3 ± 4.2 mm on the posterior aspect, all measurements being taken from images at maximum straining at the end of forced evacuation [9].

Appropriate assessment of dynamic patterns is crucial to the defecographic diagnosis of normal rectal folds. The motion recording of the examination should be analysed and an overall visual assessment of the anorectum made, which should be preliminary to any static radiographic measurement. Dynamic rectal outline changes are most easily appreciated from video recording during evacuation of a barium paste [10]. Some authors describe distal movement in the rectal mucosal folds [13]. Distal folding movement is related to rectal longitudinal axis shortening during evacuation, and we agree with other authors that the folds themselves should not show any distal descent [11]. According to the measurements and lack of abnormal distal excursion of mucosal folding with dynamic imaging involving video in asymptomatic subjects, we conclude that mucosal folding at the end of forced evacuation is neither mucosal prolapse nor low-grade rectal intussusception but a normal finding.

Pathologic Functional, Structural Findings and Grading

Rectal Prolapse

According to the criteria stated at the Tripartite Consensus Conference on Definitions for Anorectal Physiology and Rectal Cancer, *internal prolapse* (intussusception) is a full-thickness intussusception of the rectal wall without protrusion beyond the anal canal demonstrated on defecog-

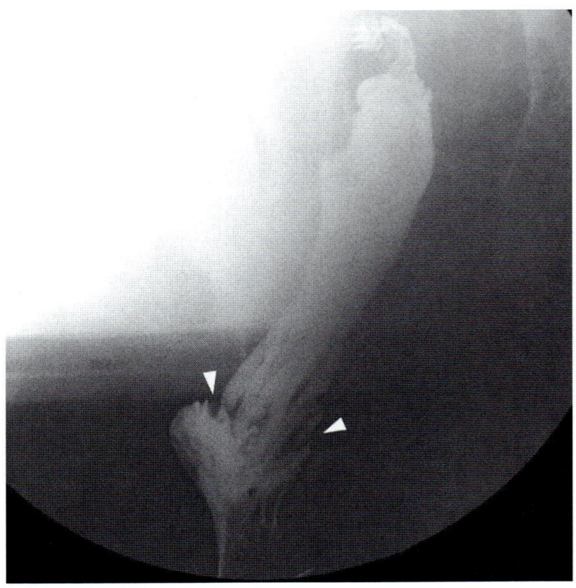

Fig. 2

An asymptomatic 71-year-old man. Mucosal folding up to 1 cm in width (*arrowheads*) mimicking intussusception on completion of forced evacuation raphy. *Rectal prolapse* is a circumferential, full-thickness intussusception of the rectal wall with protrusion beyond the anal canal [14]. Intussusception has also been labelled internal rectal intussusception, internal prolapse of the rectum, occult rectal prolapse, intrarectal prolapse and internal procidentia. Rectal intussusception may be defined as intrarectal or descent with all layers of the rectal wall, which does not emerge through the anal verge. Rectal prolapse contains all layers of the rectal wall emerging through the anal canal, resulting in part of it remaining outside intermittently or permanently.

Defecographic diagnosis of true rectal intussusception and prolapse should be based first on the rectal outline dynamics seen from video recording, mainly at maximum straining on completion of evacuation. Evacuation of barium paste leads to a ring-shaped or funnel-shaped rectal infolding of the midrectum into the adjacent lower rectum [15, 16]. Annular rectal infolding is seen associated with gradual or sudden abnormal descent by varying degrees. The rectal prolapse may remain intrarectal (hidden) (Fig. 3), extend into the anal canal (intra-anal) (Fig. 4), or pass through the anal canal and verge (external) (Fig. 5). Intussusception confined to the rectum is a little more frequent (98/2,837; 3.5%) defecographic finding

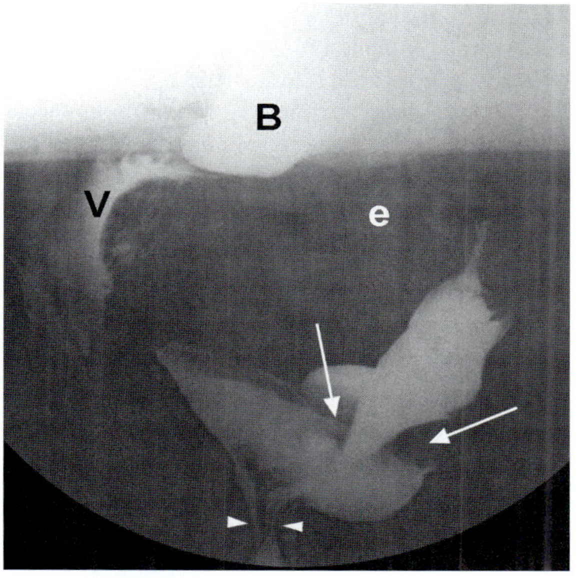

Fig. 3
Intrarectal intussusception (*arrows*) in a 76-year-old woman complaining of incomplete evacuation. The anal canal width (*arrowheads*) is normal, because the intussusception is confined to the rectum. The ratio between the intussuscipiens diameter and the intussusceptum lumen diameter is greater than 2.5. An enterocele (*e*) is also present. *V* vagina, *B* urinary bladder

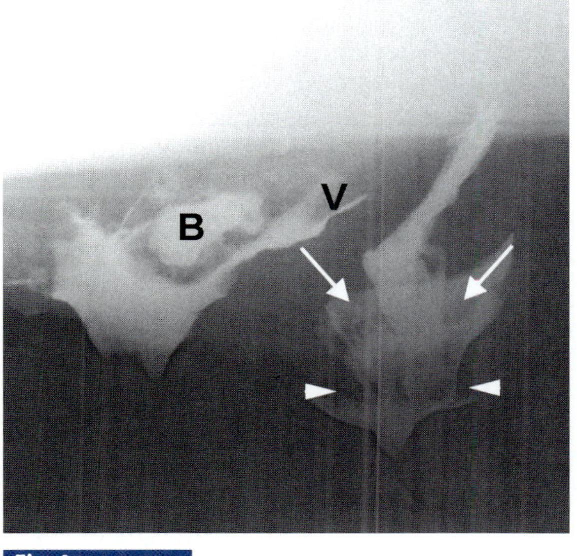

Fig. 4
Intra-anal intussusception (*arrows*) in an 84-year-old woman with feelings of incomplete rectal evacuation. The funnel-shaped infolding of the rectum enters the anal canal and reaches the anus (*arrowheads*). *V* vagina, *B* empty urinary bladder

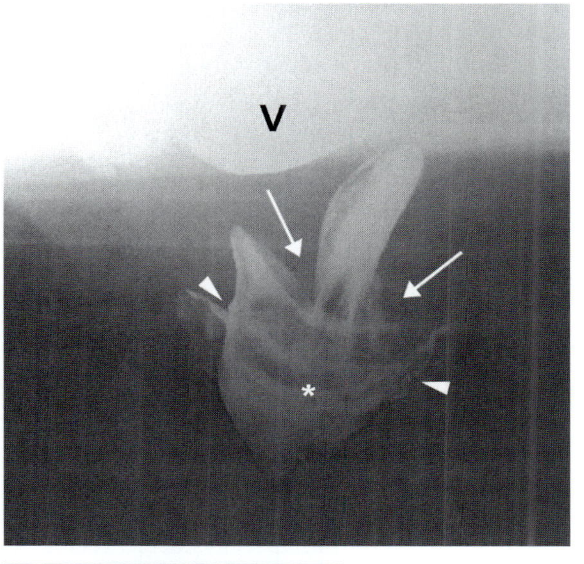

Fig. 5
Rectal prolapse (*arrows*) in a 69-year-old woman complaining of faecal incontinence. At the end of evacuation, the rectal wall (*asterisk*) protrudes through the anus (*arrowheads*). *V* vagina

than intra-anal intussusception (75/2,837; 2.6%) and rectal prolapse (76/2,837; 2.7%) in patients with disordered anorectal function.

The following morphological parameters were measured: anterior and posterior rectal fold thickness, intussuscipiens diameter, intussusceptum lumen diameter and ratio between the two diameters. All measurements were taken at the upper point of invagination and from the final images after forced evacuation, because the unemptied rectum may prevent rectal wall descent. Mean measurements for anterior and posterior rectal wall fold thickness were significantly greater than those in asymptomatic subjects, with rectal outline changes mimicking rectal intussusception [9]. Infolding in intussusception is thicker than in other conditions because it consists of two layers of the entire rectal wall. Anterior folding may be broader because it may contain a peritoneocele, with or without an enterocele, which was confirmed by both combined defecography and peritoneography [17] or open magnetic resonance defecography [18]. Mean intussuscipiens diameter measurement was greater and the mean intussusceptum lumen diameter measurement was lower in rectal intussusception and prolapse than in control subjects, these being linked to a thicker infolding in rectal intussusception and prolapse, which widens the intussuscipiens and narrows the intussusceptum lumen. The mean value of the ratio, with a cutoff of 2.5, was thus significantly higher in rectal intussusception and prolapse [9]. Defecography is usually indicated when rectal prolapse is suspected but not confirmed on physical examination. An external prolapse is not part of a diagnostic problem, but defecography will differentiate mucosal from full-thickness prolapse, show the degree of rectal prolapse and highlight combined pelvic anomalies.

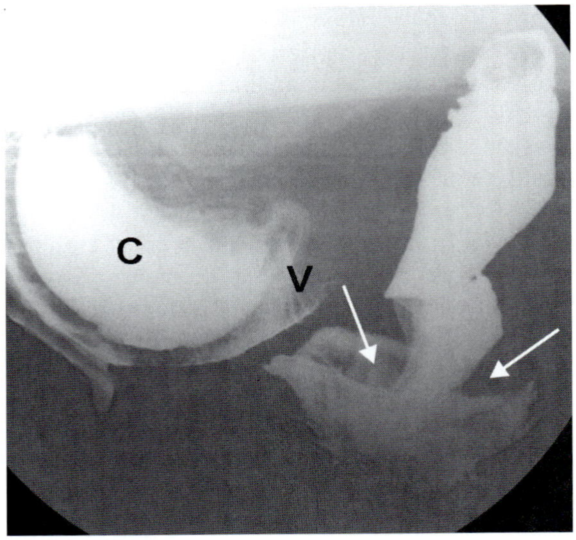

Fig. 6

Cystocolpodefecography of a 39-year-old woman with difficult evacuation and rectal pain. The lateral radiograph taken on completion of forced evacuation shows rectal prolapse (*arrows*) and cystocele (*C*). *V* vagina

Associated Defects

An isolated rectal prolapse is highly unusual. If prolapse is identified, one is tempted to attribute symptoms to the prolapse, but the prolapse may be secondary to an underlying functional disorder. Constipated patients who strain excessively may develop rectal prolapse, cystocele, rectocele, enterocele, sigmoidocele, uterine or vaginal vault prolapse or pelvic floor descent [19]. We concur with other investigators that the association of pelvic organ disorders involving the urinary, genital and anorectal systems is frequent in patients with rectal prolapse. In our experience, the frequency of combined defecographic anomalies including pelvic floor descent, rectocele, peritoneoenterocele or sigmoidocele, uterine or vaginal vault prolapse, cystocele and pelvic floor dyssynergia was 73.8%, 60.8%, 54.2%, 20.9%, 11.1% and 2.6%, respectively (Figs. 3–6). The predominant complaints were constipation including incomplete (64.2%) or difficult evacuation (46.8%), constipation combined with faecal incontinence (13.3%), faecal incontinence (22.5%) and other complaints including rectal pain (40.4%), bleeding (32.7%), urinary incontinence (35.7%) and mucous (36.2%).

Mucosal Prolapse

Mucosal prolapse is a protrusion of the rectal mucosa into or beyond the anal canal [14]. Prolapse limited to rectal mucosa is a common proctologic pattern presenting with complaints of incomplete (54.3%) or difficult (40.6%) evacuation, pain or tenesmus (37.9%), bleeding (37.1%), mucous (25.7%) and faecal incontinence (16.3%). The pathologic condition is characterised by prolapse of the mucosa though the anus, either spontaneously or during straining at defecation. The prolapse was permanently external in some cases, whereas it could be reduced manually or dimi-

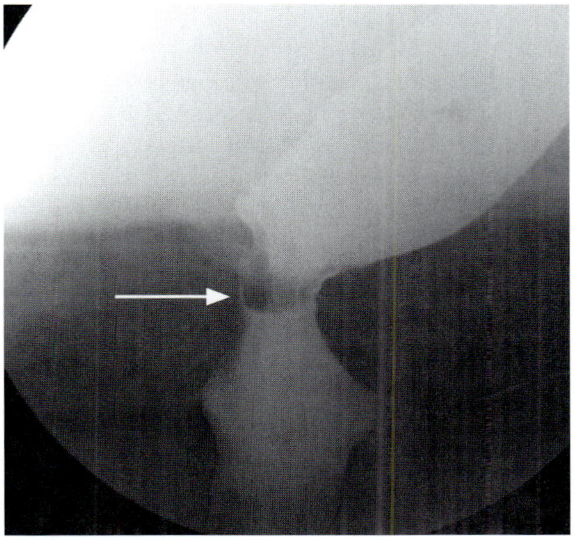

Fig. 7
Mucosal prolapse in a 48-year-old man complaining of faecal incontinence, rectal pain, bleeding and mucous. Anterior protrusion of rectal mucosa into the anal canal (*arrow*), but no widening of the anal canal

nished spontaneously in others [20]. Rectal mucosal prolapse is a proctoscopic diagnosis in which the mucosa of the rectum bulges into the proctoscope during straining, and continues to do so, on withdrawal of the instrument. Mucosal prolapse may be in one rectal mucosal surface or circumferential.

Radiologic findings may be uncertain [21, 22]. Radiologic distinction of circumferential mucosal prolapse from intussusception or normal circumferential rectal folding is difficult based only on morphology of the emptied rectum. Appropriate assessment of the dynamic pattern may help radiologic diagnosis of mucosal prolapse. On straining at evacuation of barium paste, the rectal mucosa glides down into the anal canal without widening of the anorectum, because the mucosal mass consists of soft tissue (Fig. 7). Moreover, the mucosal folding is thicker than normal rectal folds. Differently from proctoscopy, radiology cannot distinguish between mucosal prolapse, internal prolapsed haemorrhoids and mucosal-prolapse-associated haemorrhoids. In our experience, defecography played a major role, changing the physical diagnosis of bulky mucosal prolapse into full-thickness rectal prolapse in 25.6% of cases. Defecography should be performed in patients with overt mucosal prolapse and more severe symptoms to exclude full-thickness rectal prolapse [20, 23] and demonstrate other anorectal disorders coexisting in the same patient who complained of symptoms suggesting obstructed defecation.

Colonic Transit Times

Of 2,837 patients considered, 1,061 underwent radiopaque marker study for the assessment of colonic transit. Although this test is limited by many factors that might contribute to individual differences, colonic transit times are widely used for objective assessment of the progression time of radiopaque markers along the large bowel [24–29]. We based colonic transit study on a technique using ingestion of ten radiopaque markers daily from day 1 to day 10 followed by a single abdominal film on day 11. A few millilitres of a commercial barium paste, given orally on day 9, were employed as the colonic trace for marker count [30]. Classically, the number of total and segmental markers counted was multiplied by 2.4 to calculate transit times in hours [31]. The barium-traced technique reduces the contributory methodological causes of variability in the measurements by monitoring the constipated patients for 10 days and allowing identification of the projective overlap of functionally distant colonic segments (i.e. a low-lying midline cecum confused with rectosigmoid, a low-lying transverse colon confused with sigmoid, or a redundant sigmoid colon confused with right or transverse colon) (Fig. 8). There was no difference in the frequency of normal total colonic transit time and delayed total colonic transit time (43.3% vs. 56.7%) in patients with rectal prolapse. Moreover, rectal prolapse was not associated with typical segmental colonic transit time. Therefore, delayed transit through the colon, especially the proximal colon, indicates that colonic motility is primarily impaired, with patients having both rectal prolapse and colonic inertia. Defecography and transit-time studies should be done on all patients undergoing physiologic testing for rectal prolapse. Preoperative assessment using radiology transit studies is useless from a clinical point of view, because outcome may be improved by correct identification of a coexisting colonic inertia and by offering such patients bowel retraining in intussusception or subtotal colectomy for the treatment of rectal prolapse [32].

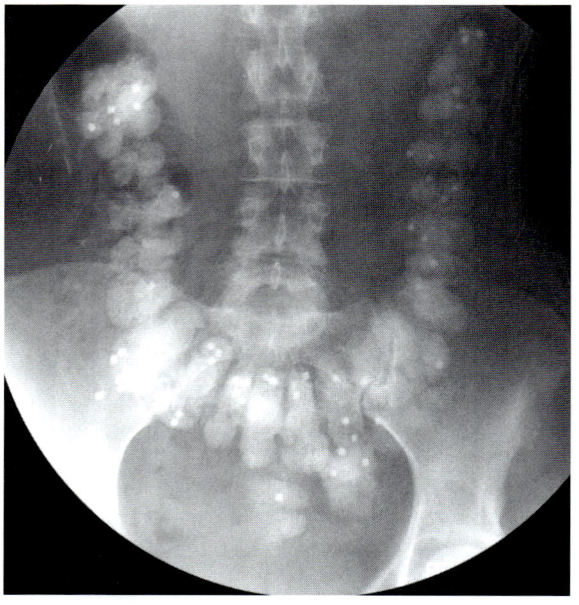

Fig. 8
Colonic transit-time study in a 42-year-old woman with rectal prolapse. Abdominal X-ray obtained 11 days after ingestion of first set of radiopaque markers reveals retention of most of the radiopaque markers in the right and left colon, resulting in a diagnosis of colonic inertia. Note that the low-lying transverse and sigmoid colon overlap each other

Overview of the Literature

Defecography is an integral part of the current diagnostic workup in patients with evacuation disorders. Common indications for performing defecography in patients with constipation or faecal incontinence is to confirm the diagnosis and to quantify the conspicuity and extent of rectal intussusception and prolapse by measuring rectal infolding thickness and depth. Authors found poor correlation regarding intrarectal intussusceptions, because 58.49% of short radiologic intussusceptions were not diagnosed by clinical assessment. However, 72% of patients with long intussusceptions were correctly assessed clinically [33].

Physical diagnosis with the patient in the left-lateral recumbent position and with an empty rectum is compared with defecographic results with the patient in a position similar to the one in which daily evacuation is performed, with the rectum filled with barium paste. The difference in settings is a possible explanation for conflicting clinical and defecographic results [33]. Another possible explanation of the mismatch between clinical examination and radiology is overdiagnosis of intussusception by defecography, because mucosal folds may be misinterpreted as full wall infolding. Considerable confusion arose when defecography studies of asymptomatic subjects unexpectedly showed radiology patterns of rectal intussusception [8, 34, 35]. More specific radiologic criteria for the diagnosis of intussusception and prolapse have been proposed using measurements of rectal infolding thickness, inner and outer intussusception diameter and the ratio between the above two diameters. Rectal infolding thickness in intussusception and prolapse has proved to be broader than rectal folding in asymptomatic subjects [9]. The hypothesis that rectal intussusception in symptomatic patients is more advanced morphologically than that seen in asymptomatic volunteers was later confirmed [13].

To date, defecography has been considered the reference procedure for the diagnosis of rectal intussusception, but there is no gold standard to which defecography can be compared. Some authors chose to quantify the intraobserver variability that exists when diagnosing intussusception and its severity in faecally incontinent patients and found that the level of experience (i.e. over 1,000 defecographies) seems to play a role in diagnosing intussusception [36].

Rectal intussusception has been described as a circular infolding of the rectal wall that is seen to descend in the rectum by varying degrees and may pass into the anal canal. This sequence may be viewed as the first stage of a rectal prolapse if the intussusception protrudes beyond the anus [37]. However, the risk of rectal prolapse developing in patients with a rectal intussusception is very small [15, 38], and operation for intussusception to prevent overt rectal prolapse seems not to be indicated.

Rectal intussusception and rectal prolapse are known causes of feelings of incomplete evacuation, obstructed defecation or faecal incontinence. Despite significant improvement in defecatory symptoms after surgery, many patients had persistent symptoms. It is now well recognised that these patients may have other underlying causes of evacuatory difficulty such as anismus and rectocele, or associated pelvic organ prolapse such as enterocele, sigmoidocele, cystocele, vaginal vault or uterine prolapse or pelvic floor descent that contributed to or caused persistent symptoms and recurrences. These entities will be missed using the classic defecographic technique.

Defecography has evolved from a radiologic technique to evaluate the anorectum for evacuatory dysfunctions to the integrated radiologic approach for evaluating the entire pelvic floor for prolapses [6, 39–41]. The addition of cystography and colpography to defecography has been increasingly adopted to provide a global assessment of pelvic organ prolapse [6, 39–43]. The radiological technique has been called colpocystodefecography [6], dynamic cystoproctography [41] and cystocolpodefecography [9] owing to some methodologic differences. Cystocolpodefecography directly visualises the pelvic organs and has been shown to be more precise in detecting pelvic floor defects and assessing the severity of prolapses than findings obtained during physical examination [1, 33, 44]. The technique contributes additional information in patients with a clinically identified rectal prolapse and as such, allows establishing a preoperative or nonsurgical comprehensive management of the patients.

Clinical Relevance

Despite its popularity, the majority of radiology literature deals with technical defecographic performance. It is relatively easy to obtain evidence about technical and diagnostic performances of a test, which are the first levels of the hierarchical step-by-step models of test efficacy measurement [45–47]. Until recently, little work has been done to investigate the clinical impact of defecography (i.e. does defecography contribute to diagnostic confidence and to delivery of therapy?). Clinical relevance is more difficult to establish, because there is no reference standard to which defecography can be compared. As with all physiologic tests, defecography has limitations, and some interpretations depend more on opinion than objective findings because of the difference in surgical and radiological settings and because histological proof tends to be limited [48]. Many authors have found that symptoms attributed to rectal intussusception or prolapse may persist after surgical repair. It is tempting to extrapolate and say that defecography has not contributed to improve the clinical outcome of patients, but it is very difficult to separate the influence of surgical therapy from radiologic diagnosis.

The best method to assess the percentage of patients improved with defecography versus without defecography is the randomised controlled trial. However, a randomised trial in which 50% of patients were denied a seemingly beneficial defecography would not gain clinical and ethical approval. Acceptable alternative studies on diagnostic and therapeutic impact have been prospective observational studies, relying on questionnaires asking clinicians about "working diagnosis" and "intention to treat" [49]. Some investigators found that defecography (and transit-time studies) was useful to referring clinicians and indicated a definitive diagnosis in 43–53% of cases [50, 51].

Conclusion

Radiology should be systematically performed in the diagnostic work up in patients with rectal intussusception and prolapse. Defecography provides dynamic and morphologic patterns for the explicit diagnosis of rectal intussusception and prolapse and identifies concomitant rectal defects in patients with evacuatory dysfunction. Cystocolpodefecography and colonic transit-time studies identify associated pelvic weakness and colonic dysfunction in patients who strain excessively. Preoperative recognition of all components of pelvic floor disorders helps the surgeon tailor the operative strategy to the patient's particular needs. The aim of pelvic surgical procedures is anatomy restoration and, more importantly, function restoration, which may be more difficult. The major role of the radiologic investigation is to contribute to the diagnostic confidence of referring clinicians in order to offer patients nonsurgical treatment options or a surgical approach.

References

1. Altringer WE, Saclarides TJ, Dominguez JM et al (1995) Four-contrast defecography: pelvic "floor-oscopy". Dis Colon Rectum 38:695–699
2. Siproudhis L, Ropert A, Vilotte J et al (1993) How accurate is clinical examination in diagnosing and quantifying pelvirectal disorders? A prospective study in a group of 50 patients complaining of defecatory difficulties. Dis Colon Rectum 36:430–438
3. Borowitz SM, Sutphen J, Ling W et al (1996) Lack of correlation of anorectal manometry with symptoms of chronic childhood constipation and encopresis. Dis Colon Rectum 39:400–405
4. Grotz RL, Pemberton JH, Talley NJ et al (1994) Discriminant value of physiological distress, symptoms profiles, and segmental colonic dysfunction in outpatients with severe constipation. Gut 35:798–802
5. Merkel IS, Locher J, Burgio K et al (1993) Physiologic and psychologic characteristics of an elderly population with chronic constipation. Am J Gastroenterol 88:1854–1859
6. Hock D, Lombard R, Jehaes C et al (1993) Colpocystodefecography. Dis Colon Rectum 36:1015–1021
7. Liberman H, Hughes C, Dippolito A (2000) Evaluation and outcome of the Delorme procedure in the treatment of rectal outlet obstruction. Dis Colon Rectum 43:188–192
8. Shorvon PJ, McHugh S, Diamant NE et al (1989) Defecography in normal volunteers: results and implications, Gut 30:1737–1749
9. Pomerri F, Zuliani M, Mazza C et al (2001) Defecographic measurements of rectal intussusception and prolapse in patients and in asymptomatic subjects. AJR Am J Roentgenol 176:641–645
10. McGee SG, Bartram CI (1993) Intra-anal intussusception: diagnosis by posteroanterior stress proctography. Abdom Imaging 18:136–140
11. Bartram CI, Turnbull GK, Lennard-Jones JE (1988) Evacuation proctography: an investigation of rectal expulsion in 20 subjects without defecatory disturbance. Gastrointest Radiol 13:72–80
12. Mellgren A, Bremmer S, Johansson C et al (1994) Defecography. Results of investigations in 2,816 patients. Dis Colon rectum 37:1133–1141
13. Dvorkin LS, Gladman MA, Epstein J et al (2005) Rectal intussusception in symptomatic patients is different from that in asymptomatic volunteers. Br J Surg 92:866–872
14. Lowry AC, Simmang CL, Boulos P et al (2001) Consensus statement of definitions for anorectal physiology and rectal cancer: report of the Tripartite Consensus Conference on Definitions for Anorectal Physiology and Rectal Cancer, Washington, DC, May 1, 1999. Dis Colon Rectum 44:915–919
15. Choi JS, Hwang YH, Salum MR el al (2001) Outcome and management of patients with large rectoanal intussusception. Am J Gastroenterol 96:740–744
16. Stoker J, Rociu E, Wiersma TG et al (2000) Imaging of anorectal disease. Br J Surg 87:10–27
17. Bremmer S, Udén R, Mellgren A (1997) Defaeco-peritoneography in the diagnosis of rectal intussusception and rectal prolapse. Acta Radiol 38:578–583
18. Roos JE, Weishaupt D, Wildermuth S et al (2002) Experience of 4 years with open MR defecography: pictorial review of anorectal anatomy and disease. Radiographics 22:817–832
19. Spence-Jones C, Kamm MA, Henry MM et al (1994) Bowel dysfunction: a pathogenic factor in uterovaginal prolapse and urinary stress incontinence. Br J Obstet Gynaecol 101:147–152
20. Altomare DF, Rinaldi M, Chiumarulo C et al (1999) Treatment of external anorectal mucosal prolapse with circular stapler: an easy and effective new surgical technique. Dis Colon Rectum 42:1102–1105
21. Bartram C (2003) Dynamic evaluation of the anorectum. Radiol Clin North Am 41:425–441
22. Stoker J, Bartram CI, Halligan S (2002) Imaging of the posterior pelvic floor. Eur Radiol 12:779–788
23. Pescatori M, Quondamcarlo C (1999) A new grading of rectal internal mucosal prolapse and its correlation with diagnosis and treatment. Int J Colorectal Dis 14:245–249
24. Bouchoucha M, Devroede G, Faye A et al (2006) Colonic response to food in constipation. Int J Colorectal Dis 21:826–833
25. Rao SSC, Ozturk R, Laine L (2005) Clinical utility of diagnostic tests for constipation in adults: a systematic review. Am J Gastroenterol 100:1605–1615
26. Mollen RM, Kuijpers HC, Claassen T (2001) Colectomy for slow-transit constipation: preoperative functional evaluation is important but not a guarantee for a successful outcome. Dis Colon Rectum 44:577–580
27. Nam YS, Pikarsky AJ, Wexner SD et al (2001) Reproducibility of colonic transit study in patients with chronic constipation. Dis Colon Rectum 44:86–92
28. Prokesch RW, Breitenseher MJ, Kattenbach J et al (1999) Assessment of chronic constipation: colon transit time versus defecography. Eur J Radiol 32:197–203
29. Karasick S, Ehrlich SM (1996) Is constipation a disorder of defecation or impaired motility?: distinction based on defecography and colonic transit studies. AJR Am J Roentgenol 166:63–66
30. Pomerri F, Frigo AC, Grigoletto F et al (2007) Error count of radiopaque markers in colonic segmental transit time study. AJR Am J Roentgenol 189:W56–W59
31. Bouchoucha M, Devroede G, Arhan P et al (1992) What is the meaning of colorectal transit time measurement? Dis Colon Rectum 35:773–782
32. Farouk R, Duthie GS (1998) Rectal prolapse and rectal invagination. Eur J Surg 164:323–332
33. Karlbom U, Graf W, Nilsson S et al (2004) The accuracy of clinical examination in the diagnosis of rectal intussusception. Dis Colon Rectum 47:1533–1538
34. Ikenberry S, Lappas JC, Hana MP et al (1996) Defecography in healthy subjects: comparison of three contrast media. Radiology 201:233–238
35. Goei R, van Engelshoven J, Schouten H et al (1989) Anorectal function: defecographic measurement in asymptomatic subjects. Radiology 173:137–141

36. Dobben AC, Wiersma TG, Janssen LW et al (2005) Prospective assessment of interobserver agreement for defecography in fecal incontinence. AJR Am J Roentgenol 185:1166–1172
37. Ihre T, Seligson U (1975) Intussusception of the rectum-internal procidentia: treatment and results in 90 patients. Dis Colon Rectum 18:391–396
38. Mellgren A, Schultz I, Johansson C et al (1997) Internal rectal intussusception seldom develops into total rectal prolapse. Dis Colon Rectum 40:817–820
39. Kelvin FM, Hale DS, Maglinte DD et al (1999) Female pelvic organ prolapse: diagnostic contribution of dynamic cystoproctography and comparison with physical examination. AJR Am J Roentgenol 173:31–37
40. Maglinte DD, Kelvin FM, Fitzgerald K et al (1999) Association of compartment defects in pelvic floor dysfunction. AJR Am J Roentgenol 172:439–444
41. Halligan S, Spence-Jones C, Kamm MA et al (1996) Dynamic cystoproctography and physiological testing in women with urinary stress incontinence and urogenital prolapse. Clin Radiol 1996 51:785–790
42. Kelvin FM, Maglinte DD, Hale DS et al (2000) Female pelvic organ prolapse: a comparison of triphasic dynamic MR imaging and triphasic fluoroscopic cystocolpoproctography. AJR Am J Roentgenol 174:81–88
43. Healy JC, Halligan S, Reznek RH et al (1997) Dynamic MR imaging compared with evacuation proctography when evaluating anorectal configuration and pelvic floor movement. AJR Am J Roentgenol 169:775–779
44. Kenton K, Shott S, Brubaker L (1997) Vaginal topography does not correlate well with visceral position in women with pelvic organ prolapse. Int Urogynecol J Pelvic Floor Dysfunct 8:336–339
45. Thornbury JR (1999) Intermediate outcomes: diagnostic and therapeutic impact. Acad Radiol 6 (Suppl 1):S58–S65
46. Mackenzie R, Dixon AK (1995) Measuring the effects of imaging: an evaluative framework. Clin Radiol 50:513–518
47. Fryback DG, Thornbury JR (1991) The efficacy of diagnostic imaging. Med Decis Making 11:88–94
48. Bartram CI (2005) Functional anorectal imaging. Abdom Imaging 30:195–203
49. Dixon AK (1997) Evidence-based diagnostic radiology. Lancet 350:509–512
50. Harvey CJ, Halligan S, Bartram CI et al (1999) Evacuation proctography: a prospective study of diagnostic and therapeutic effects. Radiology 211:223–227
51. Halverson AL, Orkin BA (1998) Which physiologic tests are useful in patients with constipation? Dis Colon Rectum 41:735–739

SECTION II
Internal Prolapse

6 Rehabilitative Treatment for Internal Rectal Prolapse

Filippo Pucciani

Introduction

Internal rectal prolapse is a full-thickness intussusception of the rectal wall without protrusion beyond the anal canal as demonstrated on defecography [1]. The presence of full-thickness intussusception at defecography may be suspected when intussusception thickness is greater than 3 mm [2]. Internal rectal prolapse is important because it may represent the first stage leading to overt rectal prolapse [3, 4]. Rectal prolapse could be the end point of a full-thickness circumferential intussusception that began as a rectorectal intussusception at ≈8 cm from the anal verge, evolved into a rectoanal intussusception, and finally into an overt rectal prolapse everting outside the perineum. Precise proctography measures indicate that the "take-off" point of the intussusception appears at about 5.5 cm from the anorectal junction anteriorly [5]. In this way, internal rectal prolapse may be related to two different morphological aspects, which are surely a function of the time spectrum, firstly, for example, rectorectal intussusception, and secondly, rectoanal intussusception. Moreover, the clinical condition related to internal rectal prolapse is complex.

Sometimes, rectal intussusception can be found in asymptomatic volunteers. Nevertheless, when symptomatic, it is associated with patients with symptoms and signs of obstructed defecation and/or faecal incontinence [5]. The group of patients affected by internal rectal prolapse is therefore heterogeneous, consisting of patients with multiple pelvic floor symptoms and morphological abnormalities. This is an important point that clarifies why the surgical treatment of internal rectal prolapse has a significant failure rate: both the perineal and abdominal approaches have a failure rate of about 30–40% [6–8]. Surgery to correct internal rectal prolapse in either constipated or incontinent patients is reported to be of doubtful benefit (50% postoperative incidence of constipation or incontinence) [9, 10]. This high postoperative morbidity suggests the need for a therapeutic option other than surgery, offering rehabilitative treatment that may be beneficial in improving the symptoms of obstructed defecation and/or faecal incontinence [11, 12].

Nevertheless, there are some controversial aspects about the rehabilitative treatment of faecal disorders. The evidence-based results of rehabilitative programmes are poor. Several negative factors are present in many studies on rehabilitation of faecal incontinence or constipation, such as confusion between biofeedback and pelvic floor exercises and the wide variety of methods and outcome measures supplied with equipment and training programmes [13, 14]. Furthermore, rehabilitation becomes even more complex in patients affected by rectal intussusception. This is due to the fact that these patients can be further divided into different subgroups, each requiring a different rehabilitation approach: (1) patients with obstructed defecation caused by either rectorectal intussusception or by rectoanal intussusception, (2) patients with faecal incontinence caused by rectoanal intussusception and (3) patients with both incontinence and obstructed defecation caused by rectoanal intussusception. Thus, each patient's rehabilitative programme is based on the rehabilitative techniques employed in the function of his or her own specific pathogenetic profile. Finally the interaction between nurse and patient is the most important variable that may influence the success rate of rehabilitation [12, 15]. Treatment goes on for months, and patients require as point of reference a person who has the ability to combine technical capacities with patience and availability.

As a result of all these factors, it is very difficult to discuss the topic of rehabilitative treatment for internal rectal prolapse due to the risk of being one-sided and incomplete. Thus, the aim of this chapter is to provide only constructive suggestions for the rehabilitative treatment of internal rectal prolapse.

Internal Rectal Prolapse: Rehabilitative Treatment of Obstructed Defecation

Obstructed defecation in patients affected by internal rectal prolapse may have two different pathogenetic pathways depending on intussusception type as described above: symptoms and signs of impaired evacuation may appear both in rectorectal intussusception and in rectoanal intussusception. Rectorectal intussusception is related to pelvic floor dyssynergia caused by paradoxical contraction or inadequate relaxation of the pelvic floor muscles during attempted defecation [16], the latter being associated with an abnormal descending perineum, and a significant relationship ($p<0.003$) has been detected between the length of the rectoanal intussusception and the extent of the perineal descent during straining [17]. Both pelvic floor disorders may be treated through rehabilitation. Pelvic floor dyssynergia is managed by pelvic floor training with an overall success rate of 67–80% [18], whereas descending perineum syndrome may be cured by pelvic floor retraining in the subgroup of patients who have a component of pelvic floor dyssynergia in the early stages of perineal descent (<4 cm) [11, 19]. In this way, pelvic floor dyssynergia is the target of rehabilitative treatment in patients with obstructed defecation caused by internal rectal prolapse.

The up-to-date rehabilitative programme for pelvic floor dyssynergia is based on combined pelviperineal kinesitherapy and biofeedback training ("bimodal rehabilitation") [20]. Pelviperineal kinesitherapy is a specific muscular re-education technique that works on coordinating the levator ani muscles, specifically the puborectalis muscle, by improving muscular performance, extension and elasticity [21]. Biofeedback is an operant conditioning technique because it employs a trial-and-error process by which learning takes place: it seems to work on cortical reconditioning of the defecation reflex [22]. The theory of bimodal rehabilitation is based on the specific assumption that pelviperineal kinesitherapy teaches the patient how to use the single levator ani muscles, whereas biofeedback training strengthens cortical learning.

The cycle of bimodal rehabilitation consists of ten outpatient sessions: each session lasts 1 h and takes place twice a week. The first step is pelviperineal kinesitherapy, in accordance with a standard sequence of exercises, followed by kinesitherapy combined with biofeedback training from the fifth session until the end of the cycle [20]. The results of bimodal rehabilitation are satisfactory: the frequency of bowel movements significantly increases, the need to digitally evacuate the rectum disappears and many patients improve with a decrease in symptoms and signs of obstructed defecation. The overall success rate is about 90%, and the efficacy of treatment is long lasting [23]. Thus, rehabilitation is recommended as a first-line treatment for internal rectal prolapse with pelvic floor dyssynergia caused by paradoxical puborectalis contraction. This approach continues to provide excellent results, and there have been no reports of deterioration following unsuccessful rehabilitation [11]. When rehabilitation fails to offer relief from the obstructed defecation, then other possible coexisting disorders, such as an underestimated enterocele, should be sought.

Internal Rectal Prolapse: Rehabilitative Treatment of Faecal Incontinence

Faecal incontinence related to rectoanal intussusception may be successfully treated with rehabilitation. The usefulness of biofeedback training has been tested in patients with internal rectal prolapse, and a significant reduction in the faecal incontinence score was obtained [11]. Another study demonstrated that improvements in incontinence score were more striking in patients who underwent rehabilitative treatment than in patients who underwent surgery [24]. Nevertheless, some patients show no improvement in incontinence scores after rehabilitative treatment. It is very difficult to state why this is the case, but it is very important to remember that the physiopathology of faecal incontinence is multifactorial. Faecal continence depends on an integrated interaction of many factors: anal sphincters, pelvic floor muscles, sensory and motor activity of the rectum, anal sensation, neural integrity, colonic motility and faecal consistence. All of these factors together interact to maintain continence for gas and stools. Several of them may be simultaneously impaired in incontinent patients with rectoanal intussusception; thus, rehabilitative treatment will not be an efficacious cure if it is not able to correct the defective continence factors. This is also the most important reason why there is no predictive factor of the results of incontinence rehabilitative treatment. Thus, the layout of a rehabilitative plan in these patients should focus on the symptoms of faecal incontinence and not on the morphological degree and size of the rectoanal intussusception.

Multimodal rehabilitation is the latest treatment in rehabilitation of faecal incontinence [25]. This approach involves several techniques: biofeedback, pelviperineal kinesitherapy, volumetric rehabilitation and/or electrostimulation. All of these procedures are guided by manometric data according to a specified algorithm. Biofeedback and pelviperineal kinesitherapy are indicated by low anal resting pressures or weak maximal voluntary contraction. Volumetric rehabilitation (sensory retraining) is indicated for disordered rectal sensation or impaired rectal compliance. Electrostimulation is only a preliminary step when patients need to improve sensation of the anoperineal plane. In this way, each rehabilitative technique used is based on the individual patient's manometric reports, resulting in treatment adapted to the patient given that each rehabilitative technique can modify specific aspects of faecal incontinence. The usual sequence of procedures is: (1) volumetric rehabilitation, (2) electrostimulation, (3) biofeedback and (4) pelviperineal kinesitherapy. Long-term results are satisfactory. The overall mean Jorge–Wexner incontinence score decreases significantly ($p<0.001$); 68% of rehabilitated patients show a significant improvement in incontinence score (≤6), and 31% of all patients become symptom free.

Conclusion

In conclusion, rehabilitation is a useful step for the treatment of internal rectal prolapse. Many patients are cured or, at least, feel better. In any case, nonresponders to rehabilitation may then be selected for other, less conservative, procedures.

References

1. Lowry AC, Simmang CL, Boulos P et al (2001) Consensus statement of definitions for anorectal physiology and rectal cancer, Washington, D.C., May 1, 1999. Dis Colon Rectum 44:915–919
2. Shorvon PJ, McHugh S, Diamant NE et al (1989) Defecography in normal volunteers: results and implications. Gut 30:1737–1749
3. Broden B, Snellman B (1968) Procidentia of the rectum studied with cineradiography. Dis Colon Rectum 11:330–347
4. Ripstein CB (1975) Symposium. Procidentia of the rectum: internal intussusception of the rectum (stage I rectal prolapse). Dis Colon Rectum 18:458–460
5. Dvorkin LS, Gladman MA, Epstein J et al (2005) Rectal intussusception in symptomatic patients is different from that in asymptomatic volunteers. Br J Surg 92:866–872
6. Ihre T, Seligson U (1975) Intussusception of the rectum-internal procidentia: treatment and results in 90 patients. Dis Colon Rectum 18:391–396
7. Barman IR, Harris MS, Rabeler MB (1990) Delorme's transrectal excision for internal rectal prolapse: patient selection, technique, and three year follow-up. Dis Colon Rectum 33:573–580
8. Dodi G, Pietroletti R, Milito G et al (2003) Bleeding, incontinence, pain, and constipation after STARR transanal double stapling rectotomy for obstructed defecation. Tech Coloproctol 7:148–153
9. Christiansen J, Zhu BW, Rasmussen OØ, Sørensen M (1992) Internal rectal intussusception: results of surgical repair. Dis Colon Rectum 35:1026–1029
10. Brown AJ, Anderson JH, McKee RF, Finlay IG (2004) Surgery for occult rectal prolapse. Colorectal Dis 6:176–179
11. Lau CW, Haymen S, Alabaz O et al (2000) Prognostic significance of rectocele, intussusception, and abnormal perineal descent in biofeedback treatment for constipated patients with paradoxical puborectalis contraction. Dis Colon Rectum 43:478–482
12. Hwang YH, Person B, Choi JS et al (2006) Biofeedback therapy for rectal intussusception. Tech Coloproctol 10:11–16
13. Whitehead W, Wald A, Norton J (2001) Treatment options for fecal incontinence. Dis Colon Rectum 44:131–144
14. Heyman S, Jones KR, Scarlett Y, Whitehead WE (2003)

Biofeedback treatment of constipation: a critical review. Dis Colon Rectum 46:1208–1217
15. Tries J (2004) Protocol- and therapist-related variables affecting outcomes of behavioral interventions for urinary and fecal incontinence. Gastroenterology 126 (Suppl 1):S152–S158
16. Pucciani F (2002) Dissinergia del pavimento pelvico e patologie anorettali associate. In: Bove A, Balzano A (eds) La dissinergia del pavimento pelvico. Mediserve, Milano, pp 55–68
17. Tsiaoussis J, Chrysos E, Athanasakis E (2005) Rectoanal intussusception: presentation of the disorder and late results of resection rectopexy. Dis Colon Rectum 48:838–844
18. Rome III Criteria. Bharucha AE, Wald A, Enck P, Rao S (2006) Functional anorectal disorders. Gastroenterology 130:1510–18
19. Harewood GC, Coulie B, Camilleri M et al (1999) Descending perineum syndrome: audit of clinical and laboratory features and outcome of pelvic floor retraining. Am J Gastroenterol 94:126–130
20. Pucciani F, Rottoli ML, Bologna A et al (1998) Pelvic floor dyssynergia and bimodal rehabilitation: results of combined pelviperineal kinesitherapy and biofeedback training. Int J Colorect Dis 13:124–130
21. Di Benedetto P (1995) Chinesiterapia pelvi-perineale: generalità. In: Di Benedetto P (ed) Riabilitazione uroginecologica. Edizioni Minerva Medica, Torino, pp 147–149
22. Papachrhrysostomou M, Smith AN (1994) Effects of biofeedback on obstructive defecation. Reconditioning of the defecation reflex? Gut 35:252–256
23. Bellini M, Pucciani F, Alduini P et al (2000) Bimodal rehabilitation has a long lasting efficacy in pelvic floor dyssynergia. Gastroenterology 118:4374
24. Choi JS, Hwang YH, Salum MR et al (2001) Outcome and management of patients with large rectoanal intussusception. Am J Gastroenterol 96:740–744
25. Pucciani F, Iozzi L, Masi A et al (2003) Multimodal rehabilitation for faecal incontinence: experience of an Italian centre devoted to faecal disorder rehabilitation. Tech Coloproctol l 7:139–147

7 Treatment of Internal Rectal Prolapse by Rectopexy

Hugh M. Paterson, David C.C. Bartolo

Introduction

Internal rectal prolapse (IRP), also known as rectoanal intussusception, occult rectal prolapse or incomplete rectal prolapse, may be described as a full-thickness circumferential infolding arising from the midrectum during straining at defecation and which does not extend beyond the anal canal. However, a consensus clinical definition is lacking, and this makes interpretation of the surgical literature confusing. Most reports are single-unit studies with small numbers accrued over relatively long time periods. A number of procedures have been performed using inconsistent patient selection criteria, and there are no randomised trials. Many authors emphasise conservative therapy as the first line of management in most patients, but we feel that there are good indications for surgery in certain patients: the key is in careful patient selection. What follows is an account of the published results of surgery for IRP, concluding with our own approach to patient selection and operative technique.

Description of and Surgical Approaches to IRP

A number of gradations of IRP severity are described in the literature. Shorvon et al. used defecography to grade IRP by identifying the lowest extent of intussusception in relation to the level of the puborectalis sling (grade I: above puborectalis; grade II: at puborectalis; grade III: into anal canal) [1], whereas Metcalf and Loening-Baucke defined two groups based on length of infolding during straining (greater than or less than 10 mm) [2]. A further morphological refinement relates to the presence or absence of rectosacral separation at defecography, suggesting excessive mesorectal mobility [3, 4]. Although some authors consider IRP to be an early stage in the development of overt rectal prolapse, other evidence suggests that fewer than 5% of patients with defecographic IRP will progress in this way [5, 6]. It is also recognised that IRP is demonstrable by defecography in up to 50% of asymptomatic controls [1, 7]. However, there is evidence that IRP morphology is more advanced in symptomatic patients compared with asymptomatic controls, suggesting there is a subgroup of patients in whom IRP will progress to complete rectal prolapse [8].

Clinical presentation of IRP is variable. It is a component of the spectrum of disorders encompassed by obstructed defecation syndrome and may also be associated with faecal incontinence, perineal heaviness, mucus leakage, a feeling of incomplete evacuation, tenesmus and solitary rectal ulcer syndrome. It is strongly associated with perineal descent [3, 9, 10]. Diagnosis is apparent on physical examination and proctoscopy in only a minority of patients [11, 12], and the most frequently used diagnostic test remains defecography, which is widely available but is often poorly tolerated by patients and requires careful interpretation. Early results of magnetic resonance (MR) defecography are reported to show promising sensitivity in distinguishing true IRP from mucosal prolapse, with the advantage of giving additional information about movement of the entire pelvic floor [13].

Anorectal physiological investigation of patients with IRP demonstrates a number of associated abnormalities of anorectal and pelvic floor dysfunction such that some clinicians consider that the condition is itself an epiphenomenon or consequence of other abnormalities causing obstructed defecation syndrome [14, 15]. IRP may present with incontinence associated with reduced maximum anal resting and squeeze pressures; it is known that sphincter function improves after surgical correction of rectal prolapse [16]. Some patients have reduced rectal compliance [9, 17, 18], although a recent study suggested that in the absence of solitary rectal ulcer syndrome, compliance was normal [19]. Colonic transit time is frequently abnormal [9], and the rectoanal inhibitory reflex may be diminished [2]. Marshall et al. found that IRP was strongly associated with a thickened internal anal sphincter on endoanal ultrasound [20]. Other concurrent findings include rectocele [21–23] and marked perineal descent [24].

Surgical Results

Perineal Approaches

The Delorme procedure has been used by a number of authors in order to avoid the exacerbation of constipation, which is recognised to complicate correction of prolapse by the abdominal approach. Berman et al. [25] found that 15 of 21 patients (71%) with refractory constipation were symptomatically improved following this procedure. These results were replicated by Sielezneff et al. [24], who achieved symptomatic improvement in 68% of a carefully selected group after poor results in his own earlier experience; he found that rectosacral separation at defecography, chronic diarrhoea, faecal incontinence and excessive perineal descent were predictive of adverse outcome. Liberman et al. achieved good results in patients with constipation but found that incontinence fared badly, being improved in only 33% [23]. Dippolito et al. [22] compared circumferential with anterior Delorme and reported patient satisfaction in more than 90%. Their cohort included a high number of patients with rectocele and exclusion of any patient with abnormal anal sphincter function on manometry. Furthermore, only 13/27 (48%) and 18/27 (67%) of patients complained of constipation and incomplete evacuation, respectively, prior to surgery [22] (Table 1).

Abdominal Rectopexy

Results of abdominal surgery for IRP reflect those obtained by surgery for true rectal prolapse. In patients with incontinence, improvement to a variable degree has been noted in most studies [18, 27, 28]. However, constipation-predominant symptoms are minimally improved or even exacerbated in patients undergoing rectopexy alone [12, 29, 30], with the addition of sigmoid colon resection associated with improved results in most reports. Tsiaoussis et al. achieved symptomatic improvement in 80% of patients by resection rectopexy (laparoscopic in most cases). They were careful to select only patients with "large" rectoanal intussusception and noted improvement after surgery in perineal descent, solitary rectal ulcer healing and increased anal resting pressure [9]. Gemsenjager also reported improved symptoms in 65% of patients, though results were better for incontinence than for constipation: 35% with obstructed defecation were not improved by surgery [31]. Brown et al. [28] reviewed results in 74 patients with "occult" rectal prolapse. Their preoperative assessment was unique in the published literature for IRP in including examination under anaesthetic to confirm the degree of rectal wall mobility. However, only 34% underwent resection with rectopexy, which may have contributed to deterioration in constipation from 39% to 50% of patients. Von Papen et al. [32] ex-

Table 1. Results of perineal procedures for internal rectal prolapse

Study	No.	Symptoms	Operation	Symptomatic improvement	Follow-up (months)
Christiansen et al. 1995 [26]	17	ODS	Delorme	5/17 constipation, 3/4 incontinence	24
Berman et al. 1990 [25]	21	ODS	Delorme	15/21 (71%)	36
Dippolito et al. 2005 [22]	27	Mixed	Modified Delorme	92% good to excellent satisfaction	15–32
Sielezneff et al. 1999 [24]	20	Mixed	Delorme	68% improved	8–73
Liberman et al. 2000 [23]	34	ODS	Delorme	88% constipation; 33% incontinence	43

ODS obstructive defecation syndrome

Table 2. Results of abdominal surgery for internal rectal prolapse

Study	No.	Symptoms	Operative technique	Symptomatic improvement	Follow-up (months)
Briel et al. 1997 [33]	13	Incontinence	Sutured rectopexy	5/13 (38%)	67 (10–181)
Ihre and Seligson 1975 [12]	40	Incontinence	Ripstein	Continence restored in 75%	24–120
Schultz et al. 2000 [27]	43	Mixed	Ripstein	Incontinence better; constipation worse	60
Schultz et al. 1996 [18]	42	Incontinence	Ripstein	Continence improved	6
Choi et al. 2001 [6]	10	Mixed	Mixed, mainly sutured rectopexy	6/10 (60%)	45 (12–118)
Brown et al. 2004 [28]	36 29	Incontinence Constipation	Sutured rectopexy Mainly resection rectopexy	Reduced from 49% to 22% Increased from 40% to 50%	48 (12–108)
Tsiaoussis et al. 2005 [9]	27	Constipation	Resection rectopexy	25/27 satisfied/very satisfied at 1 year	45 (12–60)
McCue and Thomson 1990 [29]	12	Mixed	Sponge rectopexy	Good for incontinence, poor for ODS	27
Christiansen et al. 1992 [14]	24	ODS	Wells (9), Orr–Loyge (15) rectopexy	9/24 improved (41%)	12–96
von Papen et al. 2007 [32]	56	Mixed	Laparoscopic resection rectopexy	Improvement in 15/28 with constipation, 16/24 with incontinence	44 (15–92)
van Tets and Kuijpers 1995 [34]	37	Mixed	Abdominal rectopexy	26/37 rendered asymptomatic	12–108

ODS obstructive defecation syndrome

amined results of laparoscopic resection rectopexy for rectal intussusception and found symptomatic improvement in 53% of patients with constipation and 67% of patients with incontinence (Table 2).

Stapled Transanal Rectal Resection (STARR)

Following introduction of the stapled haemorrhoidectomy by Longo, the technique has been adapted for application in IRP, rectocele and internal rectal mucosal prolapse. STARR uses two circular staple guns to perform double-stapled circumferential resection of the lower rectum. Boccasanta et al. [35] were amongst the first to report results of STARR in two studies from the same centre. In 25 patients with perineal descent, IRP and rectocele, symptoms of constipation were improved in all cases at an average follow-up duration of 22 months. A second multicenter trial in 90 patients with obstructive defecation syndrome (ODS) reported similarly impressive results: constipation improved in all cases at 1 year without worsening of incontinence, and the outcome was deemed good or excellent in 90% [36]. Complications included faecal urgency in 17.9% and incontinence to flatus in 8.9%. In 37 patients with ODS, Arroyo et al. [37] recorded improvement in all symptoms at 1 year, with 95% anatomical correction of the structural abnormalities that were noted preoperatively. Ommer et al. published a small prospective study of STARR in 14 patients: defecation scores improved in 13 after mean follow-up of 19 months with one recurrence [38]. Less convincing results were reported by Pechlivanides et al. [39], who found that only nine of 16 patients with ODS were improved after STARR. There have also been reports of significant complications, including suture-line haemorrhage, severe pain, rectal stricture, early symptom recurrence [40] and rectovaginal fistula [41], prompting calls for careful prospective audit [42] and recent publication of a consensus statement on recommendations for the new technique [43] (Table 3).

Other Techniques

External pelvic rectal suspension (EXPRESS procedure) is a novel approach for rectal intussusception and rectocele using Permacol mesh [44]. Briefly, the rectovaginal septum is entered to allow fixation of the T-shaped mesh to the anterior rectal wall. The limbs of the mesh are then fixed to the pubic bone, suspending the rectum. A recto-

Table 3. New operative techniques for internal rectal prolapse

Study	No.	Symptoms	Operative technique	Symptomatic improvement	Follow-up (months)
Williams et al. 2005 [45]	17	Mixed	EXPRESS	ODS improved, incontinence no better	12 (6–20)
Pechlivanides et al. 2007 [39]	16	ODS	STARR	9/16 (56%)	12
Boccasanta et al. 2004 [36]	90	ODS	STARR	ODS reduced from 90% to 19%	12
Ommer et al. 2006 [38]	14	Mixed	STARR	Improved defecation in 13/14	19
Arroyo et al. 2007 [37]	37	ODS	STARR	Clinical improvement 94%	24 (12–60)

ODS obstructive defecation syndrome, *STARR* stapled transanal rectal resection

cele can be repaired by suturing an additional piece of mesh within the rectovaginal septum to the ischium on each side. In the only report published to date, 6-month follow-up in 15 patients found significantly improved evacuation but no improvement in incontinence. Sepsis occurred in three patients, requiring a defunctioning stoma in one [45] (Table 3).

Authors' Experience

Rectocele and IRP demonstrated on defecography have poor correlation with symptoms. Furthermore, IRP varies in severity, and one of the difficulties in interpreting the current literature relates to the variation in degree of IRP between and within studies. From a pragmatic point of view, IRP may be categorised by three diagnostic methods: (1) clinical, (2) proctographic and (3) examination under anaesthetic (EUA).

Cases of clinically apparent IRP, recognised at examination and proctoscopy, are relatively uncommon but tend to be at the more severe end of the spectrum. Care should be taken to distinguish patients incidentally found to have IRP at defecating proctography from genuinely symptomatic patients with incontinence or ODS. For a number of years, we have performed EUA to evaluate the degree of rectal wall prolapse as described by Brown et al. [28] to distinguish defecographic IRP, which has poor correlation with symptoms, from patients who have demonstrable mobility of the midrectum at EUA. This may be analogous to the finding of rectosacral separation on defecography, highlighted by some authors as an important aspect of grading IRP severity [3, 4]. At EUA, the patient is placed in the lithotomy position, and the posterior rectal wall is grasped with Babcock forceps or a similar instrument. Many women will have anterior rectal wall mobility, but the posterior rectal wall is normally fixed and mobility is therefore abnormal. If the posterior rectal wall can be prolapsed at least 2 cm beyond the anorectal margin, then the patient is treated as for complete rectal prolapse by sutured resection rectopexy as the procedure of first choice.

We perform full mobilisation of the rectum to the pelvic floor, including division of the "lateral ligaments" but with careful preservation of hypogastric nerve bundles and *nervi erigentes*. We believe that failure to fully mobilise the rectum is associated with an unacceptable rate of recurrence. We perform full mobilisation of the left colon and splenic flexure, and normally, about 60 cm of the left colon is resected to remove redundancy and avoid constipation secondary to rectal denervation and rectosigmoid angulation. Colonic transit studies may also be useful in guiding the extent of resection if impaired transit is suspected. If, however, at EUA there is rectal wall mobility without complete prolapse, then a judgement must be made as to whether conservative therapy should be pursued or a less invasive surgical option such as the Delorme procedure or STARR undertaken. Symptoms are paramount in this decision, and we favour a more conservative approach in patients with ODS compared with those with incontinence.

Conclusion

In summary, the literature on IRP can be confusing, not least because a satisfactory clinical definition does not exist. It is likely that many published reports refer to complete rectal prolapse that is "occult" because it is not seen but would be

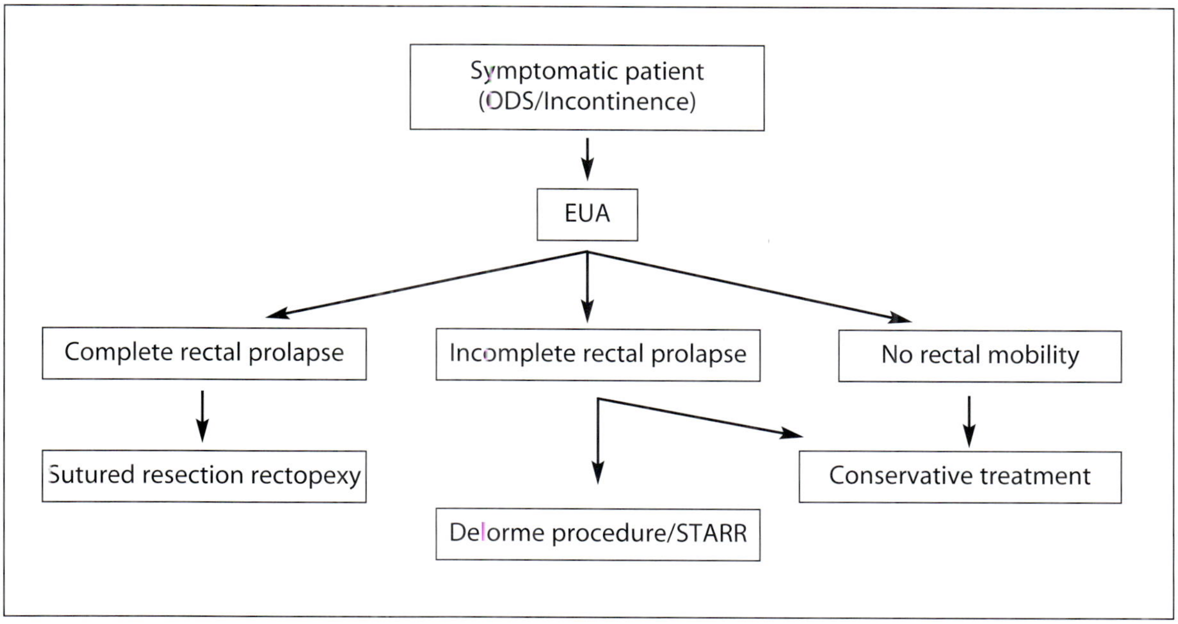

Fig. 1
Algorithm for evaluating internal rectal prolapse. *ODS* obstructive defecation syndrome, *EUA* evaluation under anaesthetic, *STARR* stapled transanal rectal resection

demonstrable at EUA; defecography is not sufficiently reliable in this setting. The algorithm in Figure 1 summarises the approach that we have found to be reliable in evaluating and treating these difficult problems.

References

1. Shorvon PJ, McHugh S, Diamant NE et al (1989) Defecography in normal volunteers: results and implications. Gut 30(12):1737–1749
2. Metcalf AM, Loening-Baucke V (1988) Anorectal function and defecation dynamics in patients with rectal prolapse. Am J Surg 155(2):206–210
3. Berman IR, Manning DH, Dudley-Wright K (1985) Anatomic specificity in the diagnosis and treatment of internal rectal prolapse. Dis Colon Rectum 28(11):816–826
4. Fleshman JW, Kodner IJ, Fry RD (1989) Internal intussusception of the rectum: a changing perspective. Neth J Surg 41(6):145–148
5. Mellgren A, Schultz I, Johansson C, Dolk A (1997) Internal rectal intussusception seldom develops into total rectal prolapse. Dis Colon Rectum 40(7):817–820
6. Choi JS, Hwang YH, Salum MR et al (2001) Outcome and management of patients with large rectoanal intussusception. Am J Gastroenterol 96(3):740–744
7. Bartram CI, Turnbull GK, Lennard-Jones JE (1988) Evacuation proctography: an investigation of rectal expulsion in 20 subjects without defecatory disturbance. Gastrointest Radiol 13(1):72–80
8. Dvorkin LS, Gladman MA, Epstein J et al (2005) Rectal intussusception in symptomatic patients is different from that in asymptomatic volunteers. Br J Surg 92(7):866–672
9. Tsiaoussis J, Chrysos E, Athanasakis E et al (2005) Rectoanal intussusception: presentation of the disorder and late results of resection rectopexy. Dis Colon Rectum 48(4):838–844
10. Sarles JC, Arnaud A, Joly A, Sielezneff I (1991) La procidence interne du rectum. Possibilites therapeutiques, a propos de 47 patients. Gastroenterol Clin Biol 15:124–129
11. Hoffman MJ, Kodner IJ, Fry RD (1984) Internal intussusception of the rectum. Diagnosis and surgical management. Dis Colon Rectum 27(7):435–441
12. Ihre T, Seligson U (1975) Intussusception of the rectum-internal procidentia: treatment and results in 90 patients. Dis Colon Rectum 18(5):391–396
13. Dvorkin LS, Hetzer F, Scott SM et al (2004) Open-magnet MR defaecography compared with evacuation proctography in the diagnosis and management of pa-

tients with rectal intussusception. Colorectal Dis 6(1):45–53
14. Christiansen J, Zhu BW, Rasmussen OO, Sorensen M (1992) Internal rectal intussusception: results of surgical repair. Dis Colon Rectum 35(11):1026–1028; discussion 1028–1029
15. Pescatori M, Spyrou M, Pulvirenti d'Urso A (2006) A prospective evaluation of occult disorders in obstructed defecation using the 'iceberg diagram'. Colorectal Dis 8(9):785–789
16. Farouk R, Duthie GS, Bartolo DC, MacGregor AB (1992) Restoration of continence following rectopexy for rectal prolapse and recovery of the internal anal sphincter electromyogram. Br J Surg 79(5):439–440
17. Duthie GS, Bartolo DC (1992) Abdominal rectopexy for rectal prolapse: a comparison of techniques. Br J Surg 79(2):107–113
18. Schultz I, Mellgren A, Dolk A et al (1996) Continence is improved after the Ripstein rectopexy. Different mechanisms in rectal prolapse and rectal intussusception? Dis Colon Rectum 39(3):300–306
19. Dvorkin LS, Gladman MA, Scott SM et al (2005) Rectal intussusception: a study of rectal biomechanics and visceroperception. Am J Gastroenterol 100(7):1578–1585
20. Marshall M, Halligan S, Fotheringham T et al (2002) Predictive value of internal anal sphincter thickness for diagnosis of rectal intussusception in patients with solitary rectal ulcer syndrome. Br J Surg 89(10):1281–1285
21. Mellgren A, Bremmer S, Johansson C et al (1994) Defecography. Results of investigations in 2,816 patients. Dis Colon Rectum 37(11):1133–1141
22. Dippolito A, Esser S, Reed J 3rd (2005) Anterior modification of Delorme procedure provides equivalent results to Delorme procedure in treatment of rectal outlet obstruction. Curr Surg 62(6):609–612
23. Liberman H, Hughes C, Dippolito A (2000) Evaluation and outcome of the delorme procedure in the treatment of rectal outlet obstruction. Dis Colon Rectum 43(2):188–192
24. Sielezneff I, Malouf A, Cesari J et al (1999) Selection criteria for internal rectal prolapse repair by Delorme's transrectal excision. Dis Colon Rectum 42(3):367–373
25. Berman IR, Harris MS, Rabeler MB (1990) Delorme's transrectal excision for internal rectal prolapse. Patient selection, technique, and three-year follow-up. Dis Colon Rectum 33(7):573–780
26. Christiansen J, Hesselfeldt P, Sorensen M (1995) Treatment of internal rectal intussusception in patients with chronic constipation. Scand J Gastroenterol 30(5):470–472
27. Schultz I, Mellgren A, Dolk A et al (2000) Long-term results and functional outcome after Ripstein rectopexy. Dis Colon Rectum 43(1):35–43
28. Brown AJ, Anderson JH, McKee RF, Finlay IG (2004) Surgery for occult rectal prolapse. Colorectal Dis 6(3):176–179
29. McCue JL, Thomson JP (1990) Rectopexy for internal rectal intussusception. Br J Surg 77(6):632–634
30. Scaglia M, Delaini GG, Ribero F et al (1993) Occult rectal prolapse: functional results after rectopexy. Chir Ital 45(1–6):183–188
31. Gemsenjager E (1996) [Internal rectal prolapse: therapy outcome and current status]. Schweiz Med Wochenschr 126(33):1377–1384
32. von Papen M, Ashari LH, Lumley JW et al (2007) Functional results of laparoscopic resection rectopexy for symptomatic rectal intussusception. Dis Colon Rectum 50(1):50–55
33. Briel JW, Schouten WR, Boerma MO (1997) Long-term results of suture rectopexy in patients with fecal incontinence associated with incomplete rectal prolapse. Dis Colon Rectum 40(10):1228–1232
34. van Tets WF, Kuijpers JH (1995) Internal rectal intussusception—fact or fancy? Dis Colon Rectum 38(10):1080–1083
35. Boccasanta P, Venturi M, Salamina G et al (2004) New trends in the surgical treatment of outlet obstruction: clinical and functional results of two novel transanal stapled techniques from a randomised controlled trial. Int J Colorectal Dis 19(4):359–369
36. Boccasanta P, Venturi M, Stuto A et al (2004) Stapled transanal rectal resection for outlet obstruction: a prospective, multicenter trial. Dis Colon Rectum 47(8):1285–1296; discussion 1296–1297
37. Arroyo A, Perez-Vicente F, Serrano P et al (2007) Evaluation of the stapled transanal rectal resection technique with two staplers in the treatment of obstructive defecation syndrome. J Am Coll Surg 204(1):56–63
38. Ommer A, Albrecht K, Wenger F, Walz MK (2006) Stapled transanal rectal resection (STARR): a new option in the treatment of obstructive defecation syndrome. Langenbecks Arch Surg 391:32–37
39. Pechlivanides G, Tsiaoussis J, Athanasakis E et al (2007) Stapled transanal rectal resection (Starr) to reverse the anatomic disorders of pelvic floor dyssynergia. World J Surg 31(6):1329–1335
40. Dodi G, Pietroletti R, Milito G et al (2003) Bleeding, incontinence, pain and constipation after STARR transanal double stapling rectotomy for obstructed defecation. Tech Coloproctol 7(3):148–153
41. Bassi R, Rademacher J, Savoia A (2006) Rectovaginal fistula after STARR procedure complicated by haematoma of the posterior vaginal wall: report of a case. Tech Coloproctol 10(4):361–363
42. Jayne DG, Finan PJ (2005) Stapled transanal rectal resection for obstructed defaecation and evidence-based practice. Br J Surg 92(7):793–794
43. Corman ML, Carriero A, Hager T et al (2006) Consensus conference on the stapled transanal rectal resection (STARR) for disordered defaecation. Colorectal Dis 8(2):98–101
44. Dench JE, Scott SM, Lunniss PJ et al (2006) Multimedia article: external pelvic rectal suspension (the express procedure) for internal rectal prolapse, with or without concomitant rectocele repair: a video demonstration. Dis Colon Rectum 49(12):1922–1926
45. Williams NS, Dvorkin LS, Giordano P et al (2005) External Pelvic Rectal Suspension (Express procedure) for rectal intussusception, with and without rectocele repair. Br J Surg 92(5):598–604

8 Treatment of Rectal Intussusception by Internal Delorme Procedure

Ezio Ganio, Iacopo Giani

Introduction

Tuttle first described a rectoanal intussusception in 1903 [1]. Since that time, several authors have described this anatomical condition in different ways – internal intussusception, internal procidentia, intrarectal prolapse, internal prolapse of the rectum, occult rectal prolapse – with the purpose of delineating a "circumferential descent (funnel-shaped infolding) of the rectal wall that does not pass beyond the anal canal".

Symptoms of obstructed defecation are frequently related to the presence of rectal intussusception, but whether internal intussusception of the rectum is the cause or a secondary phenomenon of the problem is unknown, and conservative management towards surgery should be adopted. Moreover, some authors consider rectoanal intussusception as a normal variety of the anatomical structure [2–7]. However, patients refractory to conservative treatment may be candidates for surgical options. Surgical treatment of functional outlet obstruction in patients with rectal intussusception may include abdominal, perineal or transrectal approaches.

Indications for the Delorme procedure, which was first described in 1900 as a surgical option for the treatment of rectal prolapse [8], has been expanded to include rectal outlet obstruction secondary to internal rectal prolapse. Of the 21 patients treated by Berman et al. [9] in 1990 with the Delorme transrectal excision for internal rectal prolapse, 71% achieved sustained and maintained symptomatic relief at a 3-year follow-up. Also, Liberman et al. [10], in 2000, reported a favourable experience with the Delorme procedure in the treatment of internal rectal prolapse or a combination of internal rectal prolapse and rectocele, with an overall 75% patient satisfaction sustained at a mean follow-up of 43 months. In 2005, Dippolito et al. published their results with the Delorme procedure in comparison with a less invasive anterior modification of the technique for the treatment of internal intussusception with or without rectocele. In the medium term, the anterior Delorme procedure showed a success rate of 92.3%, and positive results with the Delorme procedure reached 100% [11].

Regardless of these good results, some complications must be noted. With the decreased of rectal compliance and capacitance, some degree of incontinence – from soiling to urgency – has been reported in the first months, usually with complete recovery within 1 year. There is also the possibility of anal stenosis secondary to suture fibrosis, rectal bleeding and urinary retention after surgery; the incidence of these morbidities was between 29.6% and 38.2% [9–11].

Defecography

Although rectoanal intussusception may be observed during physical examination, it is much more likely to be detected during defecography, which remains the most useful and diffuse diagnostic tool if applied to symptomatic subjects (Fig 1). Defecography is crucial to document the presence of anatomical changes stemming from the symptoms of obstructed defecation. In particular, it is fundamental in order to distinguish between rectoanal intussusception and rectal internal mucosal prolapse [12] and to describe and quantify rectoanal intussusception. It also reveals the presence of other abnormalities, such as the presence of a rectocele or weakened pelvic floor with perineal descent, or failure of the puborectalis to relax during straining and evacuation, which is often associated with pelvic perineal dyssynergia.

Rectoanal intussusception, as reported in the literature examining 2,816 patients, appears to be the main reason for obstructed defecation in 31% of cases [3, 4, 6, 13]. Colpodefecography seems to be the examination of choice because it allows assessment not only of the rectum but also of the rectovaginal space and the vagina in order to investigate the presence of an associated enterocele or medium and anterior compartment failure. However it should be noted that a transient infolding of the rectal wall can occur during evacuation, even in asymptomatic subjects: 44% of men and 45% of women in the Shorvon et al. experience of 1989 [5]. Also, the possibility of grading rectoanal intussusception permitted by the introduction of defecography has introduced new classifications based on the depth of infolding. According to Choi et al., a large rectoanal intussusception may be defined as an intussusception ≥10 mm extending into the anal canal, which is useful data in the management of such patients [6]. In 1989, Fleshman et al. categorised intussusception and prolapse from grade I to V, adopting parameters such as rectal mobility, intussusception and anal sphincter relaxation [7]. In more complex cases in which all pelvic compartments are involved, the introduction of dynamic magnetic resonance imaging has opened up the possibility of better understanding the relationships between the pelvic floor organs and the structures involved [14].

As seen in the literature and in our experience, patients with rectoanal intussusception may have a great variety of symptoms and morphological or functional anomalies. In cases where, in addition to symptoms of obstructed defecation, patients complain of various degrees of faecal incontinence, endoanal ultrasound is useful to help detect sphincter defects and to highlight redundancy of rectal mucosae; pelviperineal neurophysiological tests (electromyographic recordings of the anal sphincters) and anorectal manometry are also useful, particularly to evaluate sphincter tone. Anorectal manometry is a very important in all cases with signs – both during physical examination than during defecography – that indicate pelviperineal dyssynergia, in which it is the basic parameter for diagnostic definition and selection for possible pelviperineal rehabilitation.

However, asymptomatic subjects can also show features of dyssynergic defecation during anal manometry.

Treatment

Anatomofunctional abnormalities can be independent from clinical symptoms, and their surgical treatment must be carefully considered. The risk following careful morphological and physiological investigation is overestimation of the disturbances and overindication for treatment. Stool softeners, laxatives and behavioural measures help some patients but often do not offer satisfactory long-term results. Pelviperineal rehabilitation programmes may correct pelvic dyssynergia, correcting paradoxical contraction of pelvic muscles. However, the most severely symptomatic patients with a high degree anatomofunctional abnormalities may be candidates for surgical options via either a perineal or an abdominal ap-

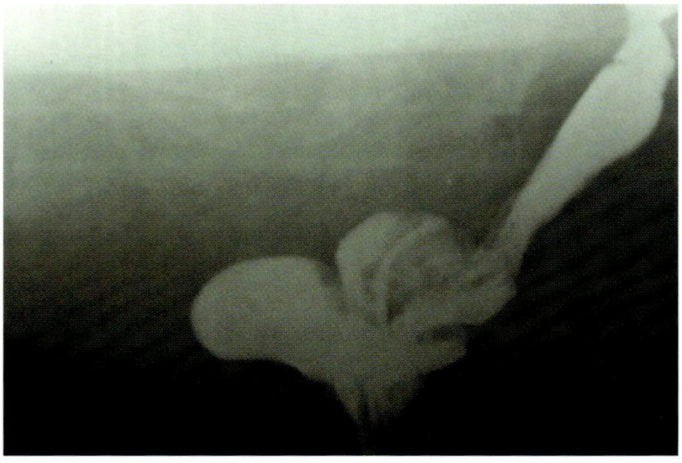

Fig. 1
Preoperative defecography showing rectocele and intussusception

proach, but the utility of surgical correction of internal intussusception for functional disorders remains unproven [15]. Because abdominal procedures often result in unrelieved symptoms, we decided to investigate the possibility of the Delorme procedure to evaluate whether therapy improved functional outcome. We choose to remove the circular infolding of the rectal wall, a feature that may create a "ball-valve" type of obstruction [16] during defecation. Thus, the reason for using the Delorme procedure is that it allows the possibility of removing the cause of the prolapse. However, even with the Delorme procedure, it may be difficult to completely remove the upper portion of intussusception, and there is also the risk of dangerous stretching of the anal sphincter. For these reasons, we modified the external Delorme procedure to an endorectal procedure.

Endorectal Proctopexy

It has been a decade since we introduced the endorectal proctopexy (ERPP) procedure, a technique basically derived from the Delorme procedure. This technique allows correction of rectoanal intussusception under visual control. It may be associated with levatorplasty in cases of a weakened pelvic floor to achieve correction not only of the rectal intussusception but also of the other associated pelvic floor disorders responsible of obstructed defecation symptoms.

With the patient in the lithotomy position under epidural anaesthesia and using a specially designed disposable anoscope fixed to the perineum by stitches, the rectal intussusception or prolapse is easily visualised. The anoscope is equipped with a rotating valve, and through the anoscope, the rectal submucosa is infiltrated with 1:200,000 adrenaline saline solution. A circular mucosal incision 2 cm above the dentate line is made, and the mucosa is dissected for 8–15 cm according to the entity of rectal intussusception or prolapse. The circular rectal musculature is then plicated to "bellows" using eight reabsorbable 2/0 stitches. A mucomucosal suture completes the endorectal anastomosis.

Procedure

A gentle anal exploration is performed to assess anal canal elasticity before the introduction of an Eisenhammer anal retractor. The rectal ampulla is cleaned using saline and then Betadine solution. A specially designed disposable anoscope (Changzhou Kangdi Medical Stapler Co., Ltda, Changzohou, China) is inserted and fixed using four stitches to ensure good access to the lower rectum. Adrenaline saline infiltration is performed on the submucosa of the infolding rectum, beginning at the anorectal junction. Using diathermy, a circumferential mucosal incision is started 1.5–2 cm above the dentate line (Fig. 2).

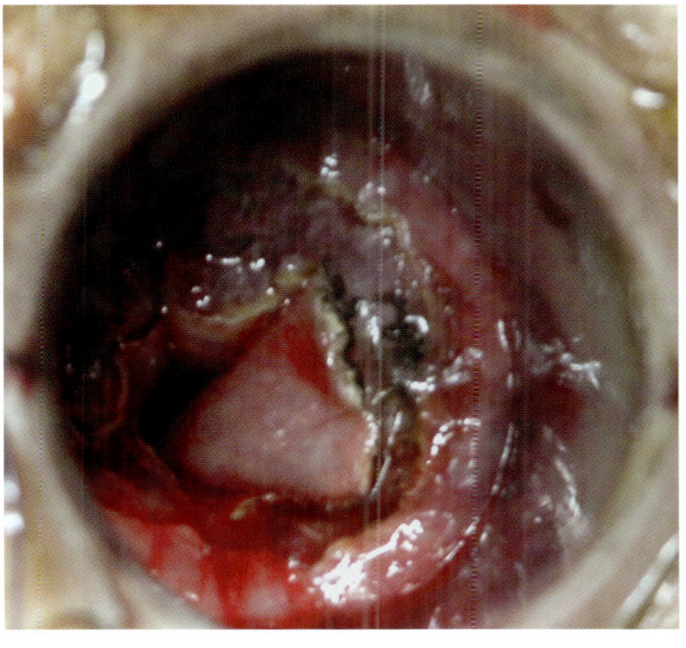

Fig. 2
Circumferential mucosal incision started 1.5–2 cm above the dentate line

The white rectal inner muscle layer is identified. The dissection should be progressive and pursued in a uniform manner throughout the circumference using diathermy (Fig. 3). The mucosal cylinder is gently pulled down with Klemmer clamps (Fig. 4). It is not usually necessary to use a retractor. Attention to ensure haemostasis of the muscular vessels is important. Injection of adrenaline solution may be useful. Dissection is continued throughout the entire internal rectal wall prolapse, preserving the mucosal cylinder.

Muscle plication is achieved by subdividing the anal circumference into four quadrants (anterior, posterior and right and left sides) by placing four stitches (3, 6, 9 and 12 o'clock) (Figs. 5 and 6), with the first stitch at 12 o'clock. The stitch must include the distal mucosal margin, therefore achieving a progressive rectal circular muscle plication, with four to six steps in the proximal direction until reaching the proximal mucosal margin. The described suture is repeated on the other three quadrants, allowing a shortening in the "bellows" of the rectal muscle wall, with correction of rectoanal intussusception and approximation of mucosal margins. At this point, the mucosal cylinder is interrupted, and the last mucosal suture point is positioned from the outside in.

The anastomosis is completed with two to three mucosal stitches in between the previous stitches (Figs. 7 and 8). The procedure can be associated with a levatorplasty if a type II–III rectocele or an enterocele is associated, particularly in cases of a weakened pelvic floor [17]. The procedure provides good anatomical correction.

ERPP Safety

Safety has been evaluated in a group of 53 patients with a median age of 52.4 years. No patients died as a result of the procedure. We observed no septic complications, but anastomotic dehiscence was observed in five patients (9.4%). Four of these patients later presented with an anastomotic substenosis, and surgical revision was required in two of them (3.8%). Furthermore, a septum haematoma occurred in one patient. Faecal urgency and soiling occurred in 39% of patients in the first 2 weeks after surgery; at 1 month, only 7.5% complained of urgency, and the problems disappeared within 6 months. No patient complained of major faecal incontinence.

ERPP Results

In the last 10 years, more than 120 patients have undergone ERPP. A retrospective analysis assessed 53 cases (average age 52.5 years) operated between February 2003 and August 2006 and with a mean follow-up of 23.4 (12–42) months. Of these patients, 51 have shown anatomical and, in particular, functional improvement, with a success rate of 96.2%. The straining score decreased from

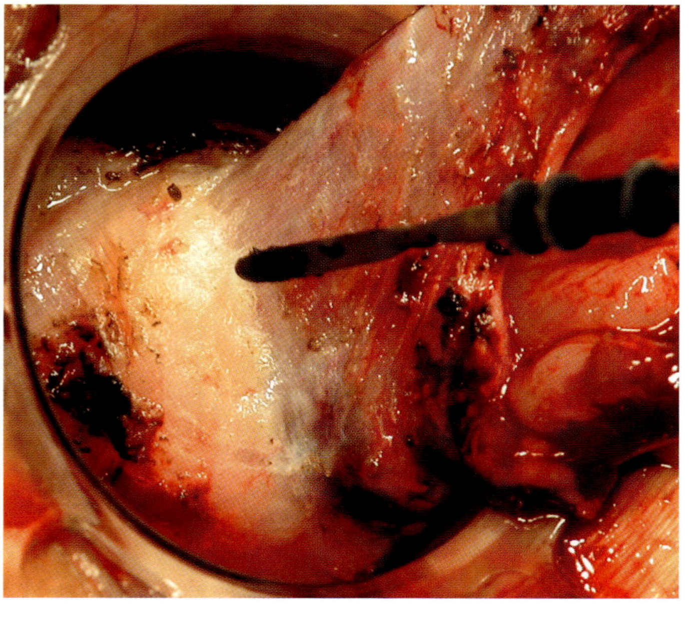

Fig. 3
Mucosectomy performed with diathermy

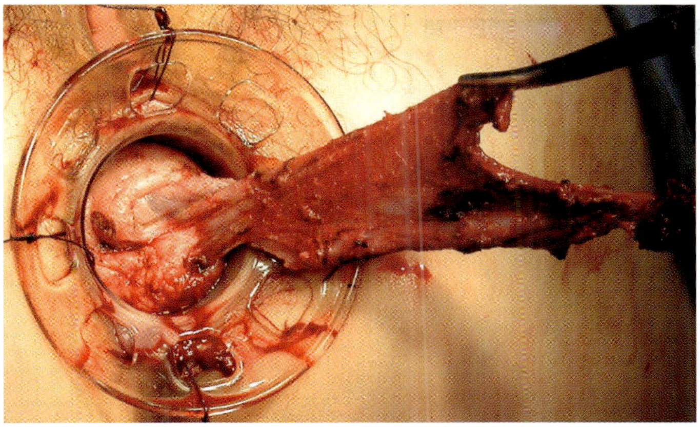

Fig. 4
Entity of mucosectomy depends on intussusception width

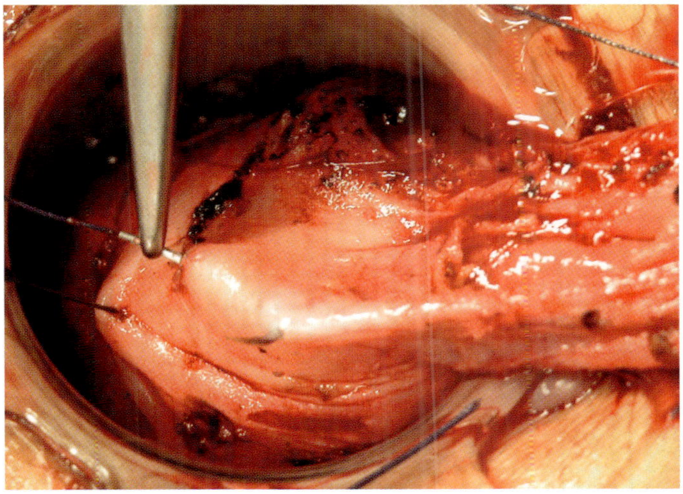

Fig. 5
Rectal muscular layer is plicated using a 2/0 reabsorbable suture

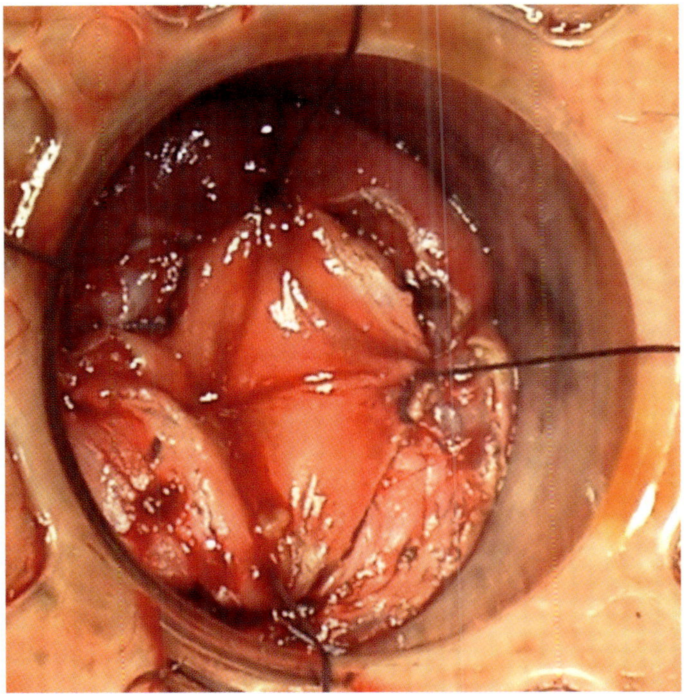

Fig. 6
The first four stitches (3, 6, 9, 12 o'clock). After removing the mucosal cylinder, anastomosis was carried out with 12 2/0 reabsorbable stitches

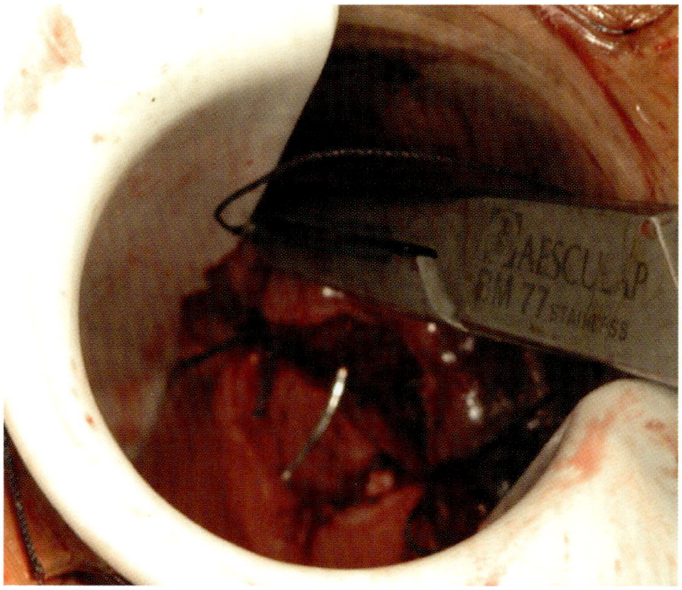

Fig. 7
Anastomosis is completed with two to three only mucosal stitches in between the previous stitches

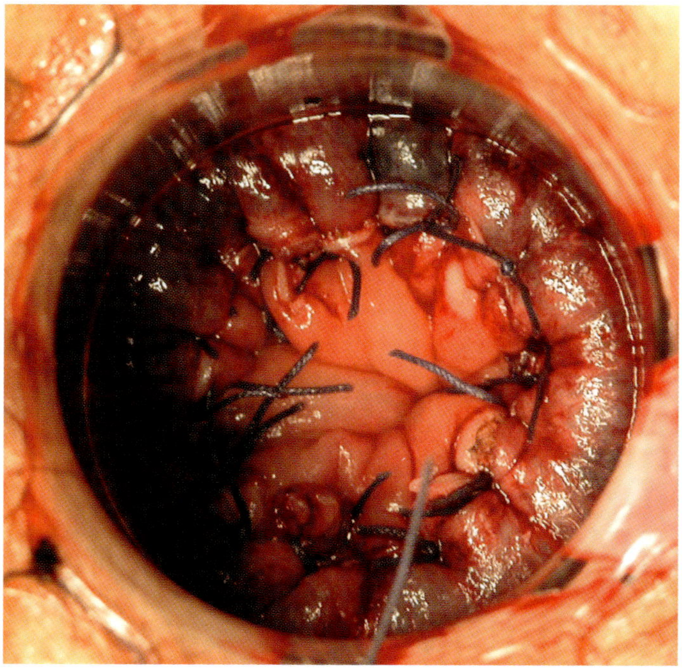

Fig. 8
A complete circular mucomucosal suture completes the endorectal anastomosis

7.1 to 0.6, the Cleveland Clinic constipation score [18] from 5.7 to 1.9, and the mean number of evacuations per week increased from 9.2 to 12.6 (Table 1).

In another group of patients, we compared ERPP with stapled transanal rectal resection (STARR) with or without associated levatorplasty. All groups were compared according to the straining score, the Cleveland Clinic constipation score [18], bowel-habits diary (number of defecations per day) and incontinence score. Patients were evaluated after 3 months and 1 year using

Table 1. Functional evaluation at baseline and last follow-up: straining score

	Baseline	Postoperative	*P* value
Straining score	7.1 ± 4.6	0.6 ± 1.4	<0.001
Cleveland Clinic constipation score	5.7 ± 3.4	1.9 ± 2.1	<0.001
Evacuation/week	9.2 ± 7.2	12.6 ± 8.1	NS

Straining score is the sum of a punctuate from 1 to 3 of an evacuation questionnaire that includes difficulties in evacuation, feeling of dissatisfaction, number of episodes of daily unsuccessful evacuation, time spent in the bathroom and the need for digitisation

Table 2. Comparison of functional results following endorectal proctopexy (ERPP) and stapled transanal rectal resection (STARR)

	Straining score			Cleveland Clinic constipation score		
	Baseline	Last FU	*P* value	Baseline	Last FU	*P* value
STARR	9.00 ± 5	1.70 ± 0.58	<0.001	6.80 ± 3.67	2.35 ± 2.81	<0.001
ERPP	8.65 ± 3.71	0.68 ± 1.39	<0.001	5.74 ± 2.71	1.59 ± 1.96	<0.001
LP–STARR	7.82 ± 3.09	0.45 ± 1.18	<0.001	6.09 ± 3.22	1.77 ± 2.15	<0.001
LP–ERPP	8.95 ± 5.09	0.89 ± 2.31	<0.001	6.39 ± 3.33	1.84 ± 2.53	<0.001

FU follow-up, *LP* levatorplasty

Table 3. Complications following endorectal proctopexy (ERPP) and stapled transanal rectal resection (STARR)

	LP + ERPP	LP + STARR	ERPP	STARR
Persisted obstructed defecation	7.9%	9.1%	4.3%	20%
Haematoma	2.6%	9.1%	0%	5%
Anastomotic leakage	5.3%	9.1%	8.7%	5%
Second intervention	2.6%	4.5%	0%	10%
Anastomotic stenosis	2.6%	4.5%	4.3%	5%

Postoperative complications did not differ statistically between the four treatment groups.
LP levatorplasty

the straining score and Cleveland Clinic constipation score, with attention to postsurgical complications. A total of 103 procedures was performed. Median patient age was 56.1 years. We performed 60 levatorplasties, of which 38 were associated with ERPP and 22 with STARR; 23 patients underwent ERPP and 20 underwent the STARR procedure. Constipation symptoms and scores significantly decreased in all groups (Table 2). Functional results between the procedures were similar.

In our experience, symptoms of persistent obstructed defecation were more frequent after the STARR procedure (Table 3). The other most common complications observed did not differ significantly between the groups. Urgency was more frequent after the STARR procedure: 15% at 3 months vs. 4.3% in the ERPP group ($P < 0.01$), whereas at 1 year, urgency continued only in one patient after STARR (5%).

Conclusion

Discussions in recent years regarding surgery for rectoanal intussusception prompted us to reconsider the role of the Delorme procedure. The modified technique presented here allows correction of rectoanal intussusception under visual control. When the technique was compared with the STARR technique, we observed no significant difference in functional outcome. ERPP completes the possibilities of treatment for rectal intussusception; correction is adjustable to the entity of the pathology. ERPP reduces costs and effectively improves symptoms of obstructed defecation. If the technique is properly performed, expected functional results are good, and constipation and symptoms of obstructed defecation related to rectoanal intussusception can be corrected in more than 90% of cases.

References

1. Tuttle JP (1903) A treatise on the diseases of the anus, rectum and pelvic colon. Appleton, NY, p 961
2. Christiansen J, Zhu BW, Rasmussen OO, Sorensen M (1992) Internal intussusception: results of surgical repair. Dis Colon Rectum 35:1026–1029
3. Ihre T, Seligson U (1975) Intussusception of the rectum-internal procidentia: treatment and results in 90 patients. Dis Colon Rectum 18:391–396
4. Mellgren A, Schultz I, Johansson C, Dolk A (1997) Internal rectal intussusception seldom develops into total rectal prolapse. Dis Colon Rectum 40:817–820
5. Shorvon PJ, McHugh S, Diamant NE et al (1989) Defecography in normal volunteers: results and implications. Gut 30:1737–1749
6. Choi JS, Hwang YH, Salum MR et al (2001) Outcome and management of patients with large rectoanal intussusception. Am J Gastroenterol 96:740–744
7. Fleshman JW, Kodner IJ, Fry RD (1989) Internal intussusception of the rectum: a changing perspective. Neth J Surg 41:145–148
8. (1985) Classic articles in colonic and rectal surgery. Edmonde Delorme 1847–1929: on the treatment of total prolapse of the rectum by excision of the rectal mucous membranes or recto-colic. Dis Colon Rectum 28(7):544–553
9. Berman IR, Harris MS, Rabeler MB (1990) Delorme's transrectal excision for internal rectal prolapse: patient selection, technique, and three-year follow-up. Dis Colon Rectum 33:573–580
10. Liberman H, Hughes C, Dippolito A (2000) Evaluation and outcome of the Delorme procedure in the treatment of rectal outlet obstruction. Dis Colon Rectum 43:188–192
11. Dippolito A, Esser S, Reed J 3rd (2005) Anterior modification of Delorme procedure provides equivalent results to Delorme procedure in treatment of rectal outlet obstruction. Curr Surg 62:609–612
12. Pomerri F, Zuliani M, Mazza C et al (2001) Defecographic measurements of rectal intussusception and prolapse in patients and in asymptomatic subjects. AJR Am J Roentgenol 176:641–645
13. Hoffman MJ, Kodner IJ, Fry RD (1984) Internal intussusception of the rectum: diagnosis and surgical management. Dis Colon Rectum 27:435–441
14. Lienemann A, Anthuberc, Baron A, Reiser M (1997) Dynamic MR colpocystorectography assessing pelvic floor descent. Eur Radiol 7:1309–1317
15. Christiansen J, Hesselfeldt P, Sorensen M (1995) Treatment of internal rectal intussusception in patients with chronic constipation. Scand J Gastroenterol 30:470–472
16. Van Tets WF, Kuijpers JHC (1995) Internal rectal intussusception—fact or fancy? Dis Colon Rectum 38:1080–1083
17. Marti MC (1989) Rectocele. Ann Gastroenterol Hepatol 25:309–311
18. Agachan F, Chen T, Pfeifer J et al (1996) A constipation scoring system to simplify evaluation and management of constipated patients. Dis Colon Rectum 39:681–685

9 The STARR Procedure for Internal Rectal Prolapse

Paul-Antoine Lehur, Guillaume Meurette, Marco La Torre

Introduction

Internal rectal prolapse associated with rectocele is frequently observed in patients complaining from outlet obstruction, also called obstructive defecation syndrome (ODS) after Antonio Longo [1]. There are three potential surgical approaches in the management of disordered defecation in relation with internal rectal prolapse and rectocele: abdominal, transvaginal and transanal. Each of these has its indications, advantages, risks and potential failures and drawbacks. The STARR procedure (stapled transanal rectal resection) belongs to the group of procedures performed through the anal canal (transanal approach). It is a relatively new option developed by Longo on the basis of a better understanding of ODS and specifically the part played by internal rectal prolapse (or intussusception) in the syndrome [2].

Surgical Technique

Here we describe the STARR procedure as we routinely perform it. A new option using a newly designed device is also described.

Procedure Goals

The objective of the procedure is to resect the internal rectal prolapse by means of staplers inserted into the anal canal. This is part of the growing surgical trend known as natural orifice surgery (NOS). The procedure was initially described using two circular PPH 01 staplers (Ethicon Endo-Surgery). The major part of our experience relies on this procedure. The STARR procedure, along with resection of the internally prolapsed rectum, can anatomically correct a rectocele. More "normal" rectal anatomy, capacity and compliance are therefore reestablished, allowing for better function. A significant modification of the technique is discussed, with the use of a reloadable, curved cutting stapler, the contour trans-STARR (Ethicon Endo-Surgery). Preoperative measures are summarised in Table 1.

The STARR Procedure Step by Step

Step 1: Exposure

This step consists of (a) placement of the circular anal dilator (CAD33), (b) assessment of the prolapse and (c) insertion of the spatula and the anoscope. The procedure begins with gentle dila-

Table 1. Preoperative measures – STARR procedure

Bowel preparation	No full bowel prep; a cleansing enema is given to empty the rectum
Anaesthesia	General, locoregional or caudal
Antibiotic prophylaxis	Cefotaxime 2 g + metronidazole 500 mg i.v. at induction of anaesthesia
Position	Lithotomy position to check completely, at the same time, the vagina and anal sphincters
Operative material	PPH 01 (Ethicon Endo-Surgery): two sets each containing a circular stapler, a disposable circular anal dilator with obturator, a windowed anoscope, a metallic spatula and a suture threader
Suture material	1-0 Ethibond for fixation of anal dilator (2) 2-0 Prolene 75 cm with rounded-tip 3/6 needle for purse-string sutures (5–7) 3-0 Vicryl for hemostasis (2–3)

tion of the anal canal and relaxation of the anal sphincter muscle. Repeated insertion of the lubricated obturator is recommended before insertion of the anal dilator, which is then fixed by four stitches to the anal skin. The mucosa of the lower rectum has to be clearly exposed, with the anal dilator protecting the anal mucosa. The prolapsed rectum is pulled back with a gauze swab through the anal dilator. If the pulled-out rectal wall protrudes more than half-way out of the anal dilator, this indicates a pronounced prolapse, leading to the placement of three to four purse-string sutures along the anterior rectal wall; if the prolapse is less pronounced, two purse-string sutures will be sufficient. The anal dilator provides a specific posterior window to allow placement of a metallic spatula (malleable retractor) of 8–10 cm, which is inserted into the rectum and will protect the posterior rectal wall when the PPH 001 circular stapler is closed and fired. The spatula must be inserted with care, inserting a finger into the rectum to move the prolapsing rectal wall, thus avoiding injury or perforation of the rectal wall. Then the anoscope is introduced into the anal dilator, showing the anterior aspect of the rectal wall from the right to the left side (Fig. 1).

Step 2: Anterior Stapled Rectal Resection

This step consists of (a) placement of the anterior half-purse-string sutures, (b) performance of the anterior stapling and (c) control of the staple line. There are several methods of placing the purse-strings sutures, the goal being to attract the rectal prolapse and the everted rectocele into the fully open PPH 001 stapler to transect the full rectal wall. Whichever method is used, the sutures are placed deep in the rectal wall to include enough tissue to exert a significant traction. In case of a thin rectovaginal wall, it is of utmost importance to avoid inclusion of the vagina in the purse-string sutures.

- Transverse purse-string suturing: A mean of three half-purse-string sutures using Prolene 2-0 are inserted above the dentate line 1- to 2-cm apart, from right to left (Fig. 2). They should include the top of the rectocele and the rectal procidentia. The first semicircular suture is placed 2- to 3-cm above the base of the haemorrhoidal tissue, and the anoscope is turned accordingly. The second transverse suture should be carried out approximately 2- to 2.5-cm above the first suture. The last suture is placed 2- to 2.5-cm above. The free ends of the three sutures are knotted at the right and left, allowing for even traction of the prolapse when stapling it.
- Vertical purse-string suturing: It has been recently shown that the same results can be achieved with greater ease by placing vertically three to five purse-string sutures on the everted anterior rectal wall including the prolapse. The free ends of the sutures are similarly knotted on each side to allow traction on the prolapse during stapling.

The PPH 01 circular stapler is then inserted fully open. The ends of the two threads are pulled anteriorly to make space to the stapler. The head of the device is positioned right above the purse-string sutures, posteriorly in contact with the spatula. The ends of the semicircular suture threads are pulled out through the lateral holes of the casing using the suture threader. The stapler is

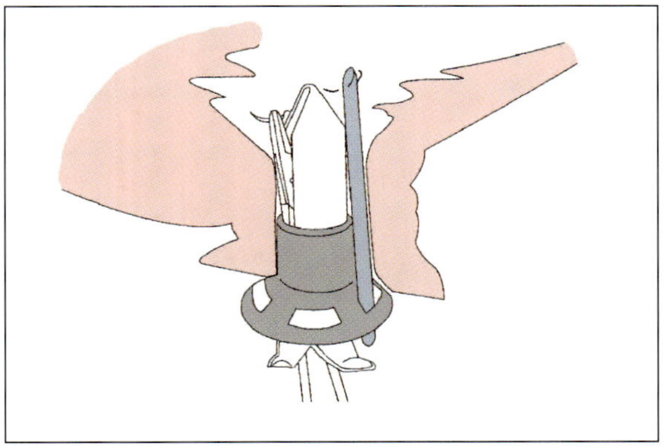

Fig. 1
Exposure (*in blue*: metallic spatula)

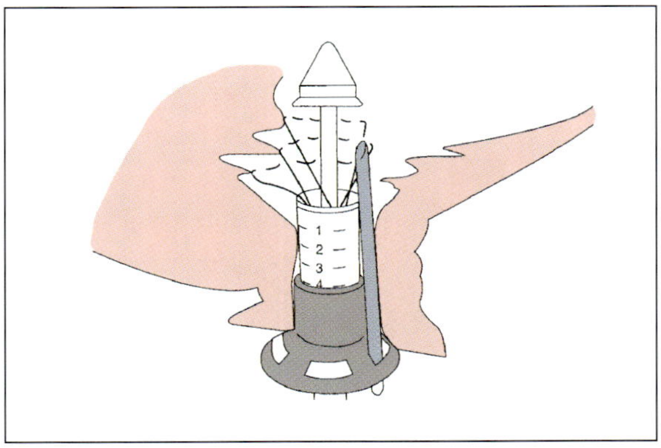

Fig. 2
Transverse placement of the anterior purse-string sutures

then closed slowly to 2 cm, with its head well positioned above the semicircular sutures and in front of the spatula. Moderate traction is applied on the suture ends, which are clamped together at the back side of the axis of the stapler, and the stapler is gently pushed further into the rectum until the black-painted casing is inserted 4 cm into anal dilator. Further traction is exerted on the sutures, and the stapler is tightened until full (vascular) closure. In female patients, we insert two fingers into the vagina. By pushing against the posterior vaginal wall, we make sure that the maximum amount of prolapse is drawn into the casing. When the stapler is closed, it is always observed that the vagina is expelled out of the jaws of the stapler. If not, the sutures have to be checked and the stapling performed differently. The stapler is then fired well in the axis of the rectum (Fig. 3).

The stapler is opened by giving it a one-quarter or a half turn and withdrawn. The anterior semicircular staple line is then controlled (Fig. 4).

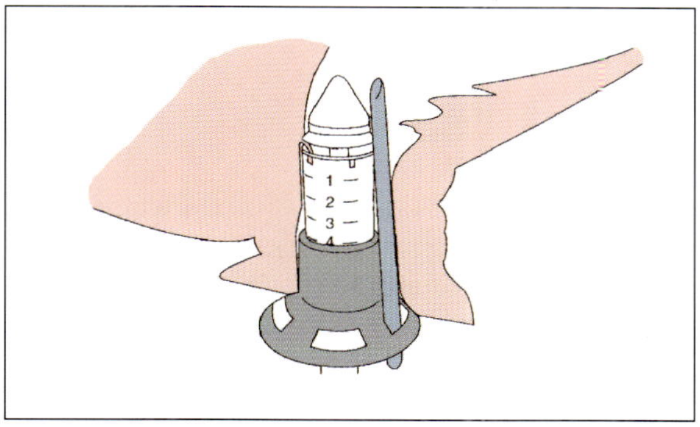

Fig. 3
Stapling of the anterior rectal wall

Frequently, the stapler at the posterior side, right in front of the metallic spatula, creates a "mucosal bridge". Significant traction on the purse-string sutures allows the mucosa to be included circumferentially inside the casing of the stapler and the two edges of the anterior anastomosis to be connected. During this procedure, the spatula is important to avoid total occlusion of the rectal lumen. The bridge made of staples must be cut with scissors.

Step 3: Posterior Stapled Rectal Resection

The same procedure is performed on the posterior aspect of the rectal procidentia using a second circular PPH 01 stapler. As the procidentia usually predominates anteriorly, some have considered this second resection unnecessary. We personally include systematically the second stapling when STARR is selected for a patient. The posterior rectal resection allows bringing the shape of the rectal ampulla into equilibrium after the first anterior resection.

The same metallic spatula is carefully placed through the anterior window of the anal dilator for approximately 8–10 cm into the rectum to protect the anterior rectal wall and the anterior staple line (Fig. 5). The anoscope is then introduced into the anal dilator to expose the posterior rectal wall.

Two or three half-purse-string sutures with Prolene 2-0 are prepared above the dentate line, starting on the left side (3 o'clock position). The first semicircular suture is placed 2- to 3-cm above the haemorrhoidal tissue, from right to left side. The two "dog ears" created by the anterior staple line in the right and left rectum are landmarks for placement of these posterior half-

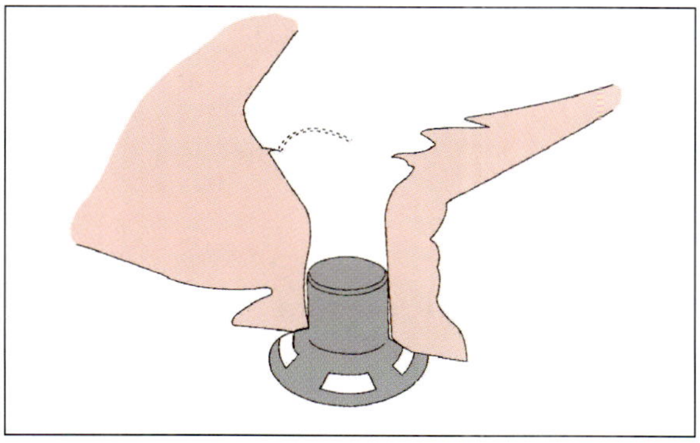

Fig. 4
Aspect of the anterior staple line

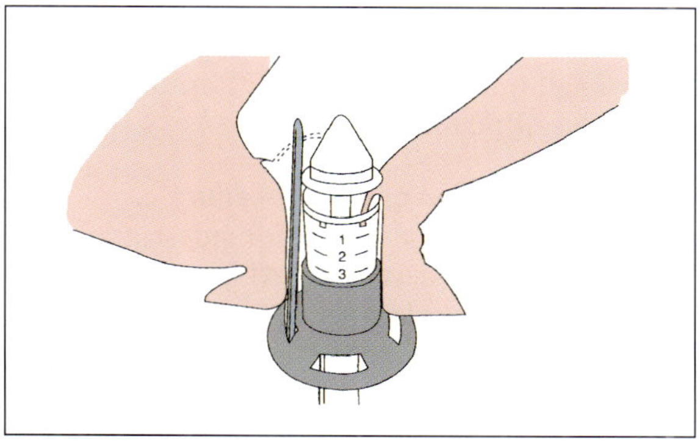

Fig. 5
Stapling of the posterior rectal wall

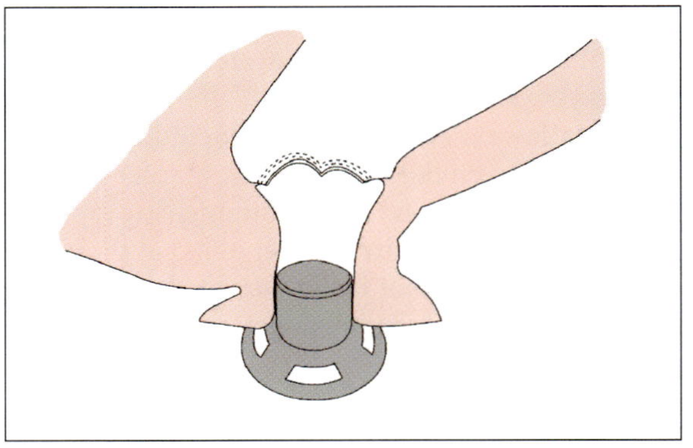

Fig. 6
Final aspect after STARR procedure

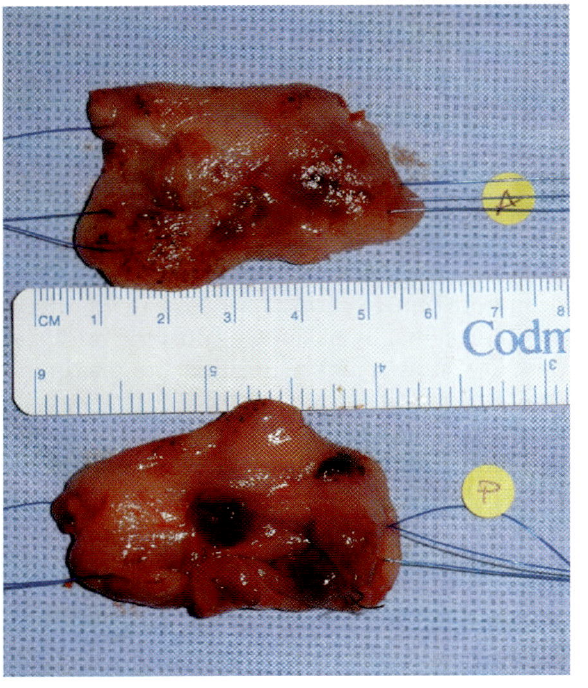

Fig. 7
Aspect of anterior (*A*) and posterior (*P*) hemidoughnuts following the STARR procedure

purse-string sutures. The first is positioned under the base of the 3 o'clock fold to the 9 o'clock fold. The second transverse suture should be placed above the folds and more laterally to insert the redundant prolapse into the casing. If necessary, another suture is placed 2- to 2.5-cm above.

The unified ends of the purse-string sutures are pulled anterior to mobilise the rectal redundancy. The stapler is inserted completely open, and the head of the device is positioned right above the semicircular sutures. The ends of the threads are pulled out with the suture threader through the lateral holes of the casing and placed anterior to the axis of the stapler. The stapler is then closed to 2 cm, making sure that its head remains positioned above the semicircular purse-string sutures and in contact with the spatula placed anteriorly. Constant traction is applied to the sutures, and the stapler casing is inserted into the anoscope to close the stapler without excessive tension. The PPH 01 is fully closed and fired in the axis of the rectum (Fig. 5). After a few seconds, the stapler is opened by giving it a one quarter or a half turn and removed. If it is too far open, removal is difficult.

Step 4: Completion of the Procedure

A mucous bridge at the anterior side, right below the metallic spatula, is searched for and transected, if present. The dog-ears on each edge of the staple line are sutured onto the rectal wall laterally with 3-0 absorbable sutures, using the anoscope for exposure. The anastomosis is examined carefully over its entire circumference, checking for bleeding (Fig. 6). For bleeders, we recommend the use of a deep X absorbable suture, including the staple line (no electrocautery).

The initial "prolapse test" (inserting and then pulling the gauze swab) can show correction of the procidentia compared with the preoperative aspect when the procedure is successful. Then the anal dilator can be removed.

The procedure usually lasts 30–45 min. We avoid performing it with other anorectal or perineal procedures to keep it quick and simple. However, some tension-free vaginal tape (TVT) techniques for urinary stress incontinence have been associated when indicated.

The semicircular doughnuts are extracted from the two staplers, measured and sent for pathology examination (Fig. 7). Postoperative care is summarised in Table 2.

The Trans-STARR Procedure

It is understandable that the circular stapler is not the perfect design for performing optimal resection of an internal rectal prolapse on demand and on its full circumference. The dog-ears indicate

Table 2. Postoperative care – STARR procedure

Bleeding prevention	Foley catheter inserted in the rectum for 12 h, with 50 ml saline irrigation (allows identification of bleeding), or lubricated gauze mesh taken out after 4–6 h
Bladder catheter	No
Fasting/diet	No
Medications	Pain killers and anti-inflammatory drugs according to local practice; oral laxatives
Hospital stay	1–3 days; vaginal and rectal examination when leaving the hospital
First postoperative visit	6 weeks; at 3 months, clinical examination, anal manometry and defecography

the asymmetric resection resulting from the application of the two PPH 01 staplers used as described earlier.

A new device is progressively being launched by the Ethicon Endo-Surgery Company throughout Europe – the contour trans-STARR – the purpose of which is to perform transanal rectal resection in a different and probably more efficient manner. This device of the new "contour" generation of stapling machines is a disposable/reloadable curved cutting stapler (Fig. 8). It allows insertion on a curved line two staple rows on the patient's side and one on the specimen, with a cutting line in between. Successive application of about five to seven cartridges permits resection of a circular doughnut corresponding to the internal prolapse (Fig. 9).

The technique involved in using the trans-STARR is still evolving, and it is premature to go into details. Even though the concept of transanal rectal resection is similar, this new tool demands new skills and therefore readapted training and experience. However, the first procedures have

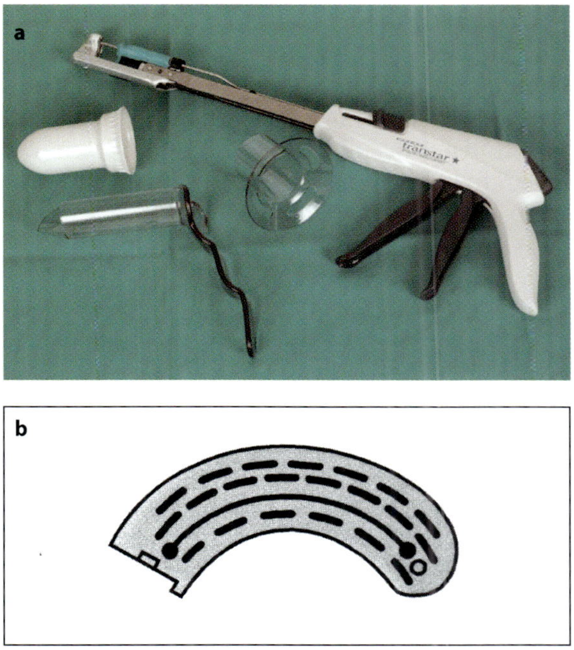

Fig. 8a, b
Contour trans-STARR device (Ethicon Endo-Surgery) (**a**) and its staple-line shape (**b**)

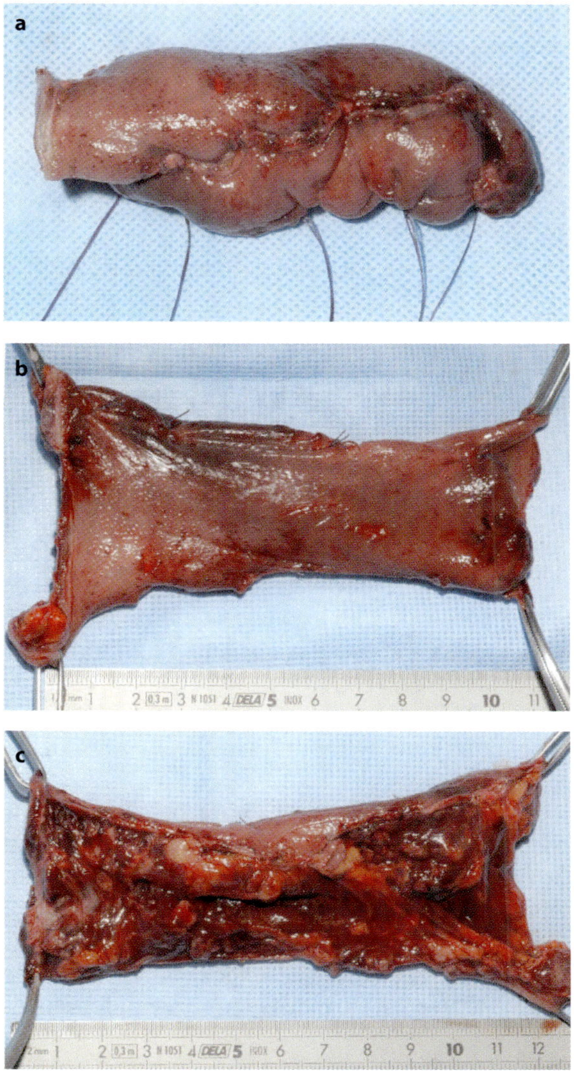

Fig. 9a-c
Single "doughnut" obtained following contour trans-STARR application for rectal internal prolapse – initial experience. Doughnut closed (**a**) Doughnut open: mucosa face (**b**) Doughnut open: external face (**c**)

proven safe and promising in term of feasibility. More cases and longer-term follow-up are needed to confirm that STARR done with the PPH 01 should be replaced by the contour trans-STARR technique in the near future.

Personal Experience

Our experience with the STARR procedure consists of more than 70 procedures over a period of 5 years. This procedure has been performed over this period with two PPH 01 staplers, as described earlier. We are starting the new procedure using the contour trans-STARR stapler, following training and under procedural guidance. Therefore, the majority of the following comments refer to our PPH 01 experience. Our general feeling is that:

- The procedure is safe if done by a surgeon having experience with staplers and properly trained for the STARR procedure.
- It is an easily reproducible technique, and we consider the learning curve to be three two four procedures for a trained colorectal surgeon.
- The key point for success is certainly based on appropriate patient selection.
- Intra- or postoperative complications, although possible, have been limited and, in our experience, never severe.
- Functional results in the long term are not yet available in controlled series.

All surgeons with experience in this field know how assessment of ODS patients is difficult and suffers from subjectivity. However, if correctly selected, patients can be ensured improvement in their symptoms, without too great a risk of problems.

From July 2002 to September 2005, we operated on 65 female patients [mean age ± standard deviation (SD) 59±9] complaining of ODS in whom rectocele and internal procidentia were identified. This series included our initial experience with the procedure. Concomitant procedures were TVT (four), anoplasty (two), hemorrhoidectomy (one pile) (one) and excision of exposed intravaginal mesh (one). Mean procedure duration, done under general anaesthesia in 90% of cases, was 30±15 min. No intraoperative complications were observed. Postoperative complications (except urinary tract infection) occurred in three patients: bleeding (two – one reoperated on; no blood transfusion) and rectal stenosis (one – treated by digital dilation). Pain and discomfort were evaluated as limited and easy to control. Mean hospital stay was 3.5±1 days.

During a mean follow-up of 19 months, six patients had to be reoperated: two under local anaesthesia on for pile excision (one) and staple-line granuloma (one), and three under general anaesthesia for enterocele (two laparoscopic mesh suspension and one vaginal suspension through perineal approach). Another patient was diagnosed with an enterocele, but surgical treatment was deferred.

Thirty patients from this group were prospectively assessed for anorectal function after STARR, with a median follow-up of 12.3 months. Assessment was based on preoperative and postoperative self-administrated questionnaires collected on a standard form, including ODS score (none: 0; maximum: 24), faecal incontinence [Cleveland Clinic Florida (CCF)] score (none: 0; maximum: 20), and Symptoms Severity Index (none: 0; maximum: 90). Quality of life was assessed through Patient Assessment of Constipation Quality of Life (PAC QoL) questionnaire. Anal physiology and defecography were routinely performed preoperatively and at a mean 4 month postoperatively. STARR resulted in significant improvement of the ODS (p<0.0001) and PAC QoL (p=0.027) scores. Continence was not significantly modified, even if in the immediate postoperative weeks a tendency for urge and minor faecal incontinence occurred (Fig. 10). Modification of the individual symptoms in favour of improvement is shown in Figure 11.

Anatomical correction of the rectocele and internal procidentia was specifically assessed for this series. A significant decrease was demonstrated in the three parameters measured on defecography: depth (p=0.007), perimeter (p<0.0001) and neck (p=0.001). Correction of the internal procidentia was obtained in six out of eight cases where high procidentia was identified. Improvement in the completeness of rectal emptying was also clearly demonstrated as a significant anatomical alteration of rectal shape.

Modification of perineal descent following STARR was more difficult to objectively assess. The staple line location (anterior and/or posterior) was not easy to locate. In some cases, a rectal anterior plication could indicate the staple line.

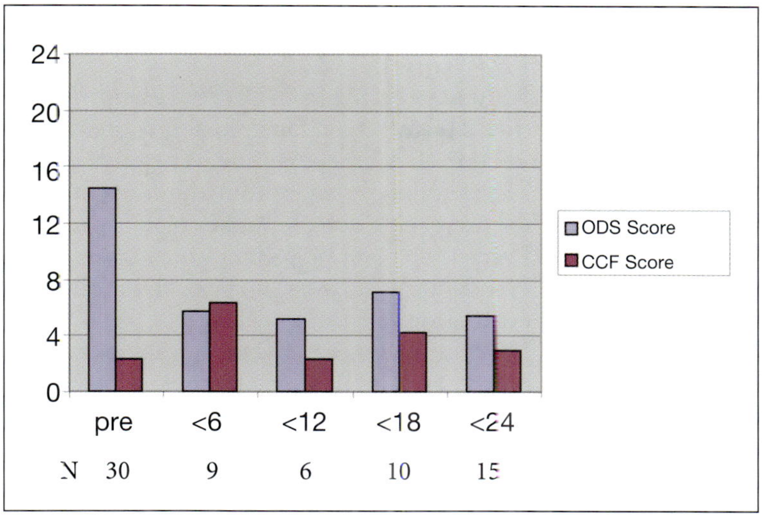

Fig. 10
Function following STARR in a prospective series of 30 patients (*N* number of patients at each time period – in months). *ODS* obstructive defecation syndrome, *CCF* Cleveland Clinic Florida

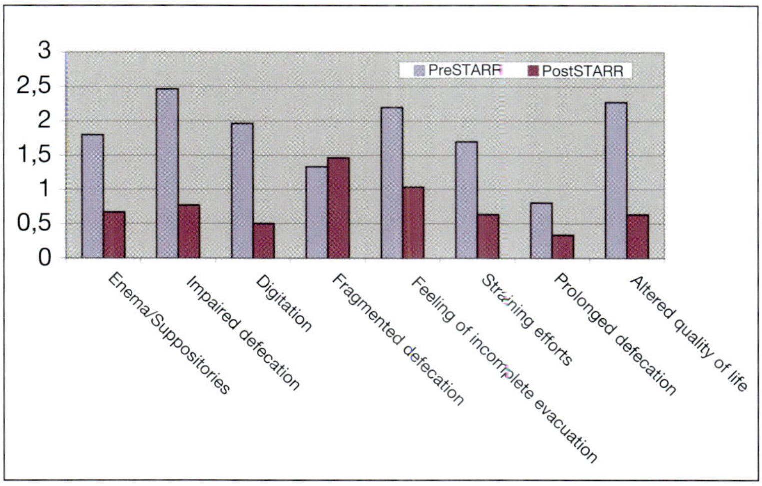

Fig. 11
Symptom severity index following STARR in a prospective series of 30 patients

Minor residual rectocele was often seen below. Correlation between function and anatomy was investigated but was not significant, probably due to the limited number of cases. Physiology tests showed that anal pressures were not significantly modified, whereas rectal maximal tolerated volume significantly decreased (Table 3).

We concluded from this study that at 1-year follow-up, the efficacy of STARR on rectal emptying is (partly) explained by anatomical correction of the rectocele and procidentia and a reduction of rectal volume.

Table 3. Results of physiology tests in a series of 30 obstructive defecation syndrome patients treated with STARR procedure[a]

Parameters	Pre-STARR[b]	Post-STARR[b]	P value
Resting pressure (mmHg)	63 (18)	65 (19)	NS
Voluntary contraction (mmHg)	81 (92)	83 (43)	NS
Contraction duration (s)	31 (27)	26 (16)	NS
Rectal max tolerable volume (ml)	229 (82)	121 (45)	<0.0001

NS not significant
[a]Personal unpublished results, [b]mean [standard deviation (SD)]

Overview of the Literature

Over the last 5–7 years, many European centres have included the STARR procedure as a treatment option for ODS. As members of the international working party (June 2005), we participated in developing a consensus on the application of STARR to the treatment of certain rectal conditions, including internal rectal prolapse. Recommendations concerning the potential applicability of this new approach have been made, and some trends are presently accepted by the surgical community [1]. However, the procedure has been submitted to only limited objective analysis. Evaluation of the current status of the procedure in terms of functional results in the long term remains weak, and as Jayne and Finan stated, the indications for STARR have yet to be clearly defined [2].

If some concerns about safety of the procedure were expressed at the beginning of the experience [3], it is now apparent that if done accordingly to the described standards, STARR is a safe procedure. In a multicentre study published in 2004 on 90 patients, there was no mortality, no sepsis, 4.4% bleeding and 3.3 % rectal stenosis treated by digital dilation. Hospital stay was 2.1±1 days and a 10±4-day sick leave [4]. In a smaller unicentre series from Spain, a similar morbidity rate was observed, with one postoperative bleeding and one stenosis over 37 operated patients [5]. That paper mentioned better results in terms of intraoperative bleeding and staple-line granulomas following the use of a PPH 03 device normally devoted to stapled anopexy, as the size of the staples is shorter than in the PPH 01 stapler. However, we consider it risky to use a STARR in full-thickness rectal resection.

Function after STARR has been assessed in two series. Good to excellent results were observed in 89% of cases for Boccasanta et al [4], with a significant improvement in all ODS symptoms and with no incontinence or dyspareunia. A bitter and critical analysis of the results was done in the invited commentary to this paper, written by R.K.S Phillips. However, the second paper [5], in which a functional success rate of 94.6% was found, and our own experience confirmed the results produced in the Italian multicentre study [4]. Results from randomised controlled trials coming soon will allow greater certitude regarding the outcome of the STARR procedure [6].

Indications for STARR – Patient Selection

Individuals suffering from ODS have a normal desire to defecate but an impaired ability to evacuate the rectum in a timely manner. They usually express the following symptoms and are best assessed by specific questionnaires (1):

- Evacuation by prolonged or repeated straining
- Frequent calls to defecate prior to or following evacuation
- Use of digital means to effect evacuation
- Sense of incomplete evacuation
- Excessive time spent in the toilet
- Pelvic pressure, rectal discomfort and perineal pain

Findings associated with ODS symptoms include rectal internal prolapse with mucosal prolapse and rectocele.

The combination of the characteristic history and the examination findings leads to offering the patient the STARR procedure when medical management – which includes explanation of the nature of the disease, fibre-rich diet, laxatives and suppositories or small enemas and pelvic floor retraining and biofeedback done by a specialist – has failed. Assessment prior deciding upon surgery includes:

- Clinical examination
- Proctosigmoidoscopy
- Colonoscopy
- Defecography with concomitant small-bowel filling; alternatively, dynamic magnetic resonance imaging (MRI) can be used
- Colonic transit time using radiopaque pellets to assess slow-transit constipation
- Anal manometry, including rectal compliance
- Genitourinary workup, with a voiding cystourethrogram

In our group, the typical patient for STARR is a woman between the ages of 45 and 65 years having had vaginal delivery, suffering from ODS, with normal faecal continence and no prolapse of the anterior compartment. Significant rectocele and internal rectal prolapse are demonstrated on defecography (Fig. 12). Associated anismus is not considered as a contraindication. Exclusion criteria include external full-thickness rectal prolapse, enterocele (Fig. 13) and anal stenosis that precludes insertion of the stapling device. Rectocele expressing as a vaginal bulge without ODS is not an indication for STARR but for a vaginal ap-

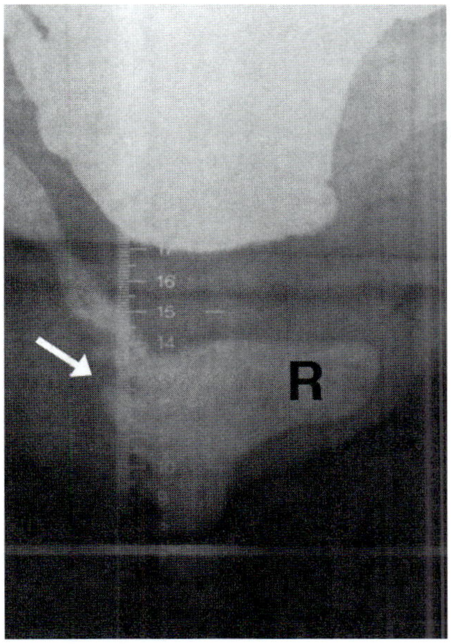

Fig. 12
Defecography: rectocele (R) and internal rectal prolapse (*arrow*). Indication for a STARR procedure

proach with sacrospinous fixation according to Richter [7]. As well, significant associated gynaecologic/urinary prolapse requires a *combined* treatment. Other contraindications are self evident: perineal infection (abscess, fistula), rectovaginal fistula, inflammatory bowel disease, radiation proctitis and prior colorectal anastomosis due to modification of the rectal blood supply. The presence of foreign material adjacent to the rectum (e.g. mesh) following rectopexy indicated the need for caution; however, in our experience, it has been possible to safely perform STARR on the lower rectum in patients with persisting ODS after cure of enterocele.

Conclusion

After more than 5 years of experience with STARR, we consider it to be an innovative, technically safe and minimally invasive procedure useful in carefully selected and well-informed patients. Collection of data, best done in a registry, is critical to the process of evaluating the safety and efficacy of the STARR procedure, as there is still a need to define selection criteria and indications, to compare surgical options objectively, to better understand the way STARR cures patient suffering due to ODS and to determine long-term results.

We will enter a new era with the contour trans-STARR device, but if the tool changes, the concept is still similar, and the knowledge accumulated with the PPH 01 procedure is not wasted and remains useful, especially when long-term outcome is concerned.

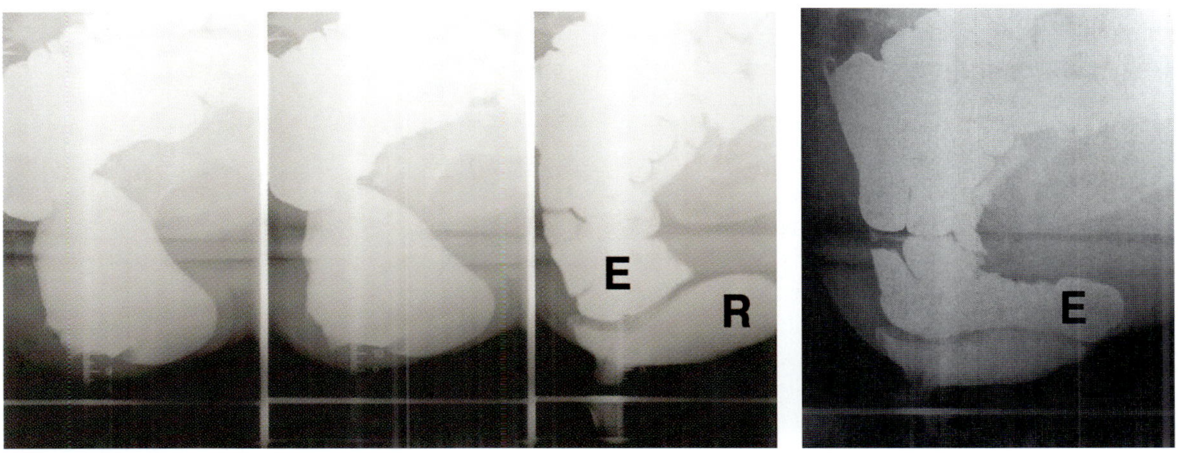

Fig. 13
Defecography: enterocele (*E*) with rectocele (*R*). A contraindication for a STARR procedure

References

1. Corman ML, Carriero A, Hager T et al (2006) Consensus conference on the stapled transanal rectal resection (STARR) for disordered defaecation. Colorectal Dis 8:98–101
2. Jayne DG, Finan PJ (2005) Stapled transanal rectal resection for obstructed defaecation and evidence-based practice. Br J Surg 92:793–794
3. Dodi G, Pietroletti R, Milito G et al (2003) Bleeding, incontinence, pain and constipation after STARR transanal double stapling rectotomy for obstructed defecation. Tech Coloproctol 7:148–153
4. Boccasanta P, Venturi M, Stuto A et al (2004) Stapled transanal rectal resection for outlet obstruction: A prospective, multicenter trial. Dis Colon Rectum 47:1285–1296
5. Arroyo A, Perez-Vicente F, Serrano P et al (2007) Evaluation of the stapled transanal rectal resection technique with two staplers in the treatment of obstructive defecation syndrome. J Am Coll Surg 204:56–63
6. European STARR trial group (2006) How is the profile of the patients submitted to STARR for obstructed defaecation syndrome? Preliminary report of a multicentre controlled trial comparing STARR vs. biofeedback. Oral poster presentation. Colorectal Dis 8(Suppl 4):19
7. Lehur PA, Hamy A (2000) Cure chirurgicale des rectocèles par voie périnéo-vaginale: plicature rectale, sacro-spinofixation vaginale et périnéorraphie postérieure. J Chir 137:165–169

10 The EXPRESS Procedure for Internal Rectal Prolapse

Pasquale Giordano, Norman S. Williams

Introduction

External pelvic rectal suspension (EXPRESS procedure) is a newly developed operation aimed at restoring the anatomical position of the internal rectal prolapse whilst hopefully improving the underlying physiological abnormality. The procedure is carried out transperineally with limited rectal mobilisation, and where appropriate, it can be combined with surgical correction of a rectocele. The operation consists of "hitching up" the rectum and reinforcing the rectovaginal wall utilising a commercially available, long-lasting collagen biomaterial (Permacol, Tissue Science Laboratories plc, Aldershot, UK).

Patient Selection

The procedure is offered to patients with severe rectal evacuatory dysfunction who have been shown on proctography to have a circumferential, full-thickness intussusception that impedes rectal evacuation. All patients must have tried a course of optimal conservative management and a supervised bowel-retraining programme prior to consideration for surgery. An associated rectocele is repaired only if greater than 2 cm in diameter and contains residual barium after evacuation on proctography.

Surgical Technique

The patient is prepared with a phosphate enema on the day of the operation to ensure that the rectum is empty before the procedure. The operation is carried out under either general or regional anaesthesia with the patient placed in the Lloyd-Davies position on the operating table. A dose of cefuroxime 750 mg and metronidazole 500 mg is administered at induction, and a urinary catheter is inserted in the bladder. After infiltration in the rectovaginal plane with 1 in 300,000 adrenaline saline solution, a crescent skin incision is made in the perineum midway between the vagina and the anus. The dissection starts in a plane just anterior to the external anal sphincter and extends cranially to enter the rectovaginal plane, taking care not to injure the sphincter complex, the rectum or the vagina. A Lone Star anal retractor applied to the edges of the wound facilitates the dissection. Meticulous haemostasis is performed, as bleeding from the vaginal venous plexus is common. Once the rectovaginal plane is entered, the dissection is extended up to the posterior vaginal fornix to the level of Denonvilliers fascia. The posterior wall of the vagina is retracted anteriorly and the medial borders of the levator ani muscle exposed. The anterior rectal wall is gently dissected from the puborectalis muscle on both sides to achieve rectal mobilisation as lateral as possible. Lateral retraction of the puborectalis muscle may help the lateral rectal dissection. This dissection allows access to approximately 12–15 cm of the anterolateral aspect of the distal rectum. In the male patient, a similar dissection is performed extending behind the prostate. Close dissection to the rectal wall is of paramount importance, especially at the inferolateral aspect of the prostate, to minimise hazard to the pelvic nerves.

Once the perineal dissection is completed, two 2-cm skin incisions are made just medial and above the level of the pubic tubercle on both sides. Two 0 PDS sutures on a J needle are inserted into the periosteum and tendinous insertions overlying the pubis on both sides. These sutures are left long with their needles in tact and clipped. The

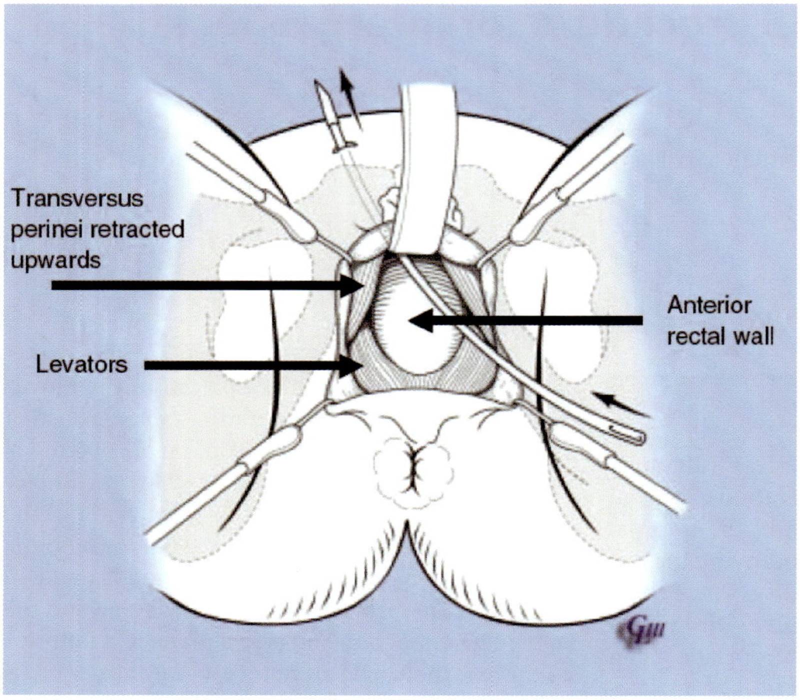

Fig. 1
External pelvic rectal suspension (EXPRESS) procedure for intussusception. A purpose-designed tunneller is inserted via the perineal wound (lateral to the vagina) upwards behind the pubic bone to emerge through the suprapubic wound, taking great care to prevent injury to the bladder. Reproduced with permission from [1]. Permission is granted by John Wiley & Sons Ltd on behalf of the BJSS Ltd

incisions are deepened to gain access to the retropubic space. A purpose-designed tunneller is inserted via the perineal wound lateral to the vagina, upwards and anterior to the bladder through the retropubic space of Retzius and behind the pubic bone to emerge through the suprapubic wound (Fig. 1). The plane is delineated by blunt dissection as far as possible from above and below to guide the tip of the tunneller as it is advanced upwards, thus preventing injury to the bladder and vagina.

The sharp point of the tunneller is replaced by a plastic olive, which has attached to it a T-shaped strip of Permacol (Fig. 2). This strip is then drawn down to the perineal wound and its transverse part, measuring 2 cm in width, is sutured to the anterolateral rectal wall with a 2.0 polydioxanone suture (PDS, Ethicon, Edinburgh, UK), with its lower edge at approximately 6–8 cm above the superior border of the sphincter complex (Fig. 3). The vertical part of the strip is left emerging from the suprapubic wound, with an artery forceps attached. This manoeuvre is repeated on the opposite side. Once the strips are in place, vertical traction is exerted on them via the suprapubic wounds. When firm but not excessive traction of the rectal wall is achieved, the proximal part of the T-shaped Permacol strips are sutured to the periosteum of the pubic bone with the two interrupted 0 PDS sutures previously placed (Fig. 4). If a rectocele is also present, it can be repaired at the same time using a patch of Permacol. The patch is 5 × 5 cm with two extensions on the lateral sides. It is sutured over the anterior rectal wall with interrupted 2.0 PDS sutures (Fig. 5). The lateral wings are routed behind the puborectalis and sutured with two 0 PDS sutures on a J needle to the periosteum overlying the medial aspect of the ischium in line with the rectocele on either side. This is performed from within the perineal wound, the rationale being to reinforce the rectovaginal septum and at the same time limit the anterior protrusion and ballooning effect of the anterior rectal wall causing the rectocele.

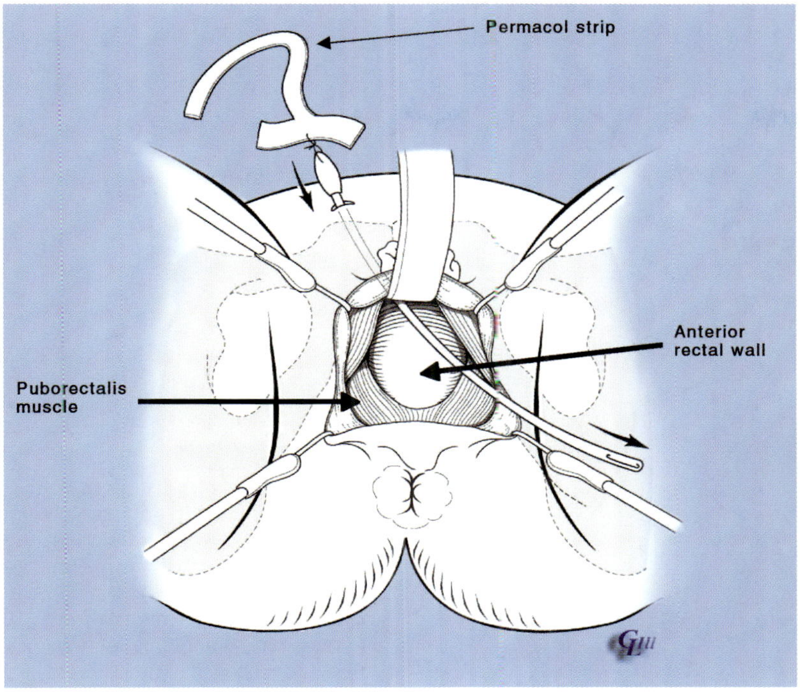

Fig. 2
External pelvic rectal suspension (EXPRESS) procedure for intussusception. The sharp point of the tunneller is replaced by a plastic olive, which has attached to it a T-shaped strip of Permacol. Reproduced with permission from [1]. Permission is granted by John Wiley & Sons Ltd on behalf of the BJSS Ltd

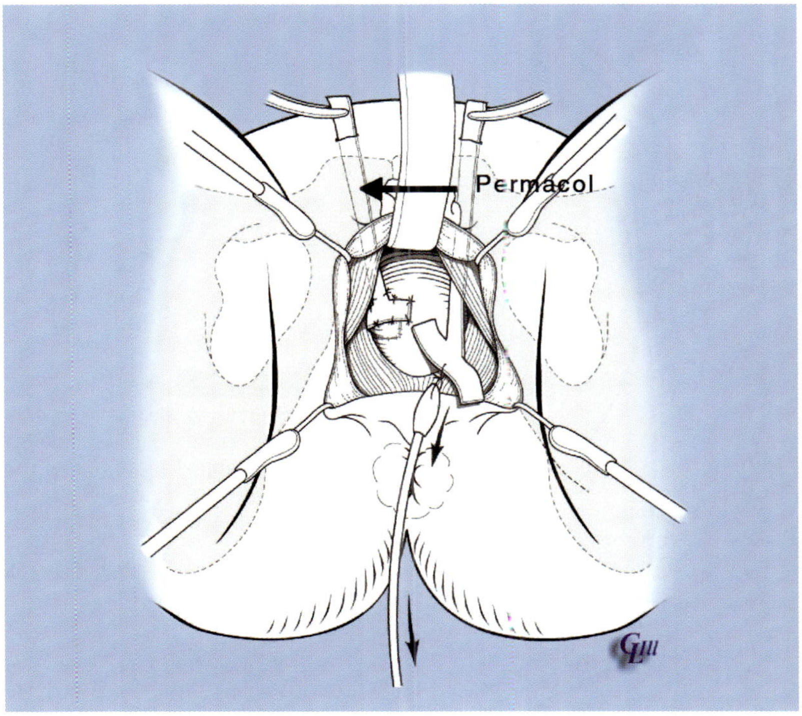

Fig. 3
External pelvic rectal suspension (EXPRESS) procedure for intussusception. The Permacol strip is drawn down to the perineal wound and positioned so the transverse part of the strip lies on the anterolateral wall of the rectum approximately 8 cm above the superior border of the sphincter complex. The second strip is similarly placed on the opposite side. Reproduced with permission from [1]. Permission is granted by John Wiley & Sons Ltd on behalf of the BJSS Ltd

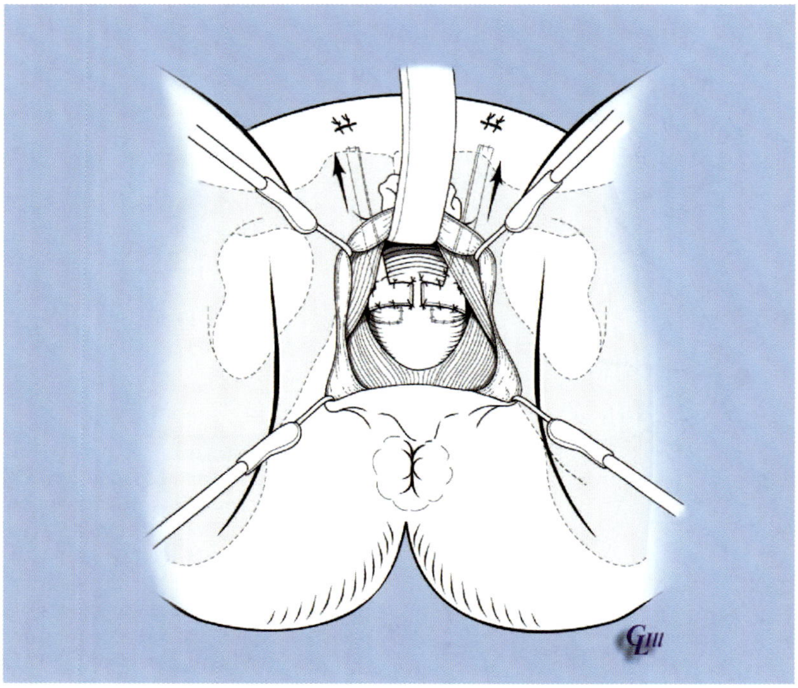

Fig. 4

External pelvic rectal suspension (EXPRESS) procedure for intussusception. After gentle upward traction on the Permacol strips, they are sutured to the periosteum of the pubic bon. Reproduced with permission from [1]. Permission is granted by John Wiley & Sons Ltd on behalf of the BJSS Ltd

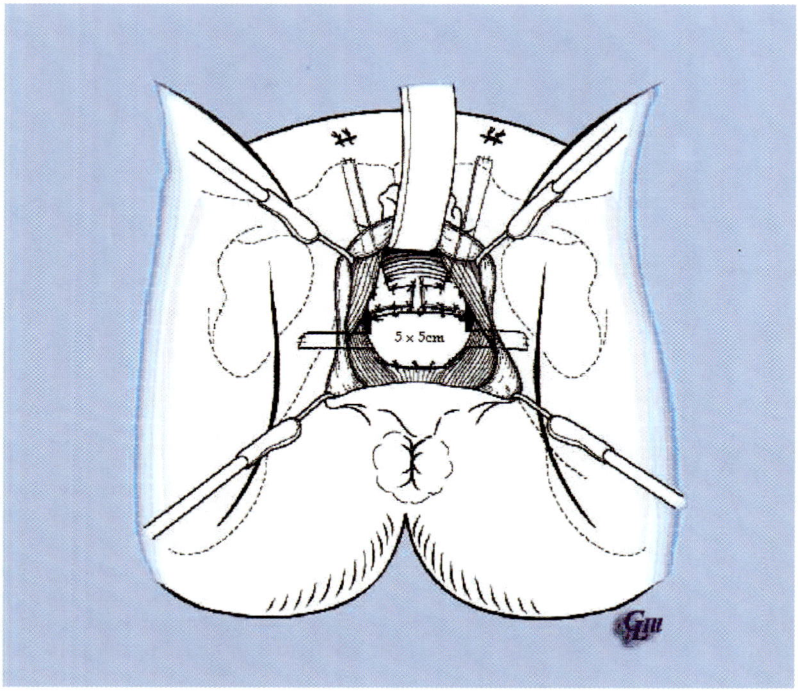

Fig. 5

Concomitant rectocele repair. A patch of Permacol is sutured over the defect in the rectovaginal septum, and the wings are sutured to the ischial tuberosities. Reproduced with permission from [1]. Permission is granted by John Wiley & Sons Ltd on behalf of the BJSS Ltd

Results

Our initial experience included 17 patients [1]. Thirteen patients (all women) had a concomitant rectocele repair. Clinical details are summarised in Table 1. Median follow-up was 12 (6–20) months.

There were no major intraoperative complications. One patient in whom the anterior rectal wall was injured and repaired at the time of the operation, subsequently developed sepsis in the rectovaginal plane, which required drainage and a

Table 1. Patient demographics and symptoms. For age, parity and symptom duration, values represent median (range). The frequency of each symptom is represented by the number of patients (out of 17) reporting that symptom.

Rectal intussusception (n = 17)	
Patient characteristics	**Demographics**
Age	47 (20–67)
Gender M:F	4:13
Symptom duration (months)	36 (5–400)
Previous pelvic surgery	6
Gracilis neosphincter	2
Colposuspension	4
Hysterectomy	3
Parity	3 (0–5)
Symptom	
Obstructed defecation	16
Straining	13
Anorectal pain	8
Prolapse	7
Bleeding per rectum	7
Toilet revisiting	7
Mucus per rectum	6
Faecal incontinence	5
Urinary incontinence	5

defunctioning stoma. Two other patients developed local sepsis, one requiring surgical drainage. Despite the sepsis, none of the patients required Permacol removal. Postoperative complications included neuralgic pain ($n = 3$), which resolved in all cases during follow-up. No patient reported any changes in sexual function and in particular none of the women reported dyspareunia.

When reviewed at 6 months, all patients reported a significant improvement in symptoms related to prolapse and evacuatory function. Incontinence did not deteriorate in any of the patients. Quality of life also significantly improved. Anorectal physiology demonstrated a significant reduction in maximum tolerable volume and pelvic floor descent. All other measurements remained unchanged. Fourteen patients underwent postoperative proctographic evaluation. In ten, the intussusception appeared improved by surgery. Eleven of the 14 patients who underwent postoperative proctography had undergone a rectocele repair: eight had no evidence of rectocele on postoperative proctography. In the remaining three, who all presented with very large rectoceles (8 cm, 8 cm, 6.5 cm), rectocele size was markedly reduced postoperatively (3 cm, 2.5 cm, and 2.5 cm, respectively). Postoperative functional outcome did not differ significantly in patients with and without postoperative radiological improvement.

Discussion

Patients with rectal evacuatory dysfunction may present with a variety of symptoms, often nonspecific and with very variable impact on quality of life. In these patients, defecography is used to demonstrate possible morphological abnormality. However, similar morphological abnormalities can be identified also in normal subjects [2] and therefore cannot be used on their own as an indication for surgery. Furthermore, as confirmed in our experience, improved symptoms following surgical intervention does not necessarily correlate with improved anatomical appearance on postoperative evacuatory proctography. Nevertheless, it is our belief that in patients without pelvic floor dyssynergia in whom severe symptoms have failed to respond to optimal conservative treatments, gross anatomical abnormalities revealed on evacuatory proctography may contribute to their symptoms. Notwithstanding these limitations, the basis of this new technique is to correct the anatomical abnormalities in a way that is less invasive and more effective than traditional approaches.

Rectal intussusception is normally initiated by an anterior takeoff point at approximately 6–8 cm from the anorectal junction [3, 4]. Our aim was to fix this area to prevent the process of intussusception. To reach this area via an abdominal approach, rectal mobilisation to the pelvic floor is necessary. Such mobilisation carries potential hazard to the pelvic autonomic nerves and may contribute to postoperative constipation [5]. Furthermore, incomplete rectal mobilisation during abdominal rectopexy may result in inadequate fixation and lead to unsatisfactory results. The EXPRESS procedure through the perineal approach allows relatively easy access to the crucial area of the takeoff point without violating the peritoneal cavity and hopefully with less risk to pelvic nerves. In our experience, it is not associated with worsening incontinence. The insertion of Permacol strips to the anterior rectal wall to prevent the initial takeoff of the rectal wall also provides structural support to the entire pelvic floor, as confirmed by a significant reduction in pelvic floor descent. Further, the Permacol patch in the rectovaginal plane, with its lateral attachments to the ischium, buttresses the anterior rectal wall and successfully corrects the associated rectocele, as demonstrated on postoperative proctography.

Dissection of the rectovaginal plane required with the EXPRESS procedure can be challenging, and perforation of the vagina or rectum may occur. Despite repair of such defects, it was feared that the presence of foreign material would impair healing and result in extrusion, as has been the case with synthetic mesh in rectocele repair (unpublished observations). In the authors' experience, even when local sepsis developed, implant extrusion or erosion never occurred, and the Permacol never had to be removed [1, 6].

References

1. Williams NS, Dvorkin LS, Giordano P et al (2005) EXternal Pelvic REctal SuSpension (Express procedure) for rectal intussusception, with and without rectocele repair. Br J Surg 92:598–604
2. Pomerri F, Zuliani M, Mazza C et al (2001) Defecographic measurements of rectal intussusception and prolapse in patients and in asymptomatic subjects. AJR Am J Roentgenol 176:641–645
3. Brodén B, Snellman B (1968) Procidentia of the rectum studied with cineradiography. A contribution to the discussion of causative mechanism. Dis Colon Rectum 11:330–347
4. Ihre T (1990) Intussusception of the rectum and the solitary ulcer syndrome. Ann Med 22:419–423
5. Huber FT, Stein H, Siewert JR (1995) Functional results after treatment of rectal prolapse with rectopexy and sigmoid resection. World J Surg 19:138–143
6. Williams NS, Giordano P, Dvorkin LS et al (2005) External pelvic rectal suspension (the Express procedure) for full-thickness rectal prolapse: evolution of a new technique. Dis Colon Rectum 48:307–316

SECTION III
External Prolapse

11 Perineal Approach to External Rectal Prolapse: The Delorme Procedure

Gian Andrea Binda, Alberto Serventi

Introduction

The Delorme procedure is a perineal technique for repair of full-thickness rectal prolapse first described by the French military surgeon Edmond Delorme in 1900 [1]. This procedure includes stripping the mucosa of the prolapsed rectum and sutured plication of the bare muscle remnant, which collapses the wall like an accordion. The mucosa is then reapproximated to seal the anastomosis. The technique Delorme described is simple, may be performed under regional anaesthesia, is performed through a perineal approach and does not require a bowel resection and anastomosis. However, the Delorme procedure was not commonly used until a report by Uhlig and Sullivan [2] in 1979, after which it gained increased popularity. The simplicity of the approach and lack of major complications have made it popular with both surgeons and patients over the past 20 years and has led to its use as a primary operation for rectal prolapse.

Surgical Technique

The operation [3–6] is performed with the patient in the lithotomy position after mechanical preparation of the rectum, urinary catheterisation, short-term antibiotic and deep venous thrombosis prophylaxis. It can be performed under general or spinal anaesthesia or light sedation with local anaesthetic infiltration. Where possible, the rectal prolapse and anal canal are everted; a Lone-Star retractor is placed to expose the anal verge. A solution of saline/adrenaline 1/200,000 is injected into the submucous layer above the dentate line to reduce bleeding and define the plane of dissection. A circumferential incision is made in the rectal mucosa usually 1–1.5 cm proximal (orad) to the dentate line (Fig. 1a) to preserve a sensitive area of rectal mucosa and to simplify anastomosis.

A plane of dissection between the mucosa and the internal sphincter and circular muscle of the rectum is developed, and a sleeve of mucosa is

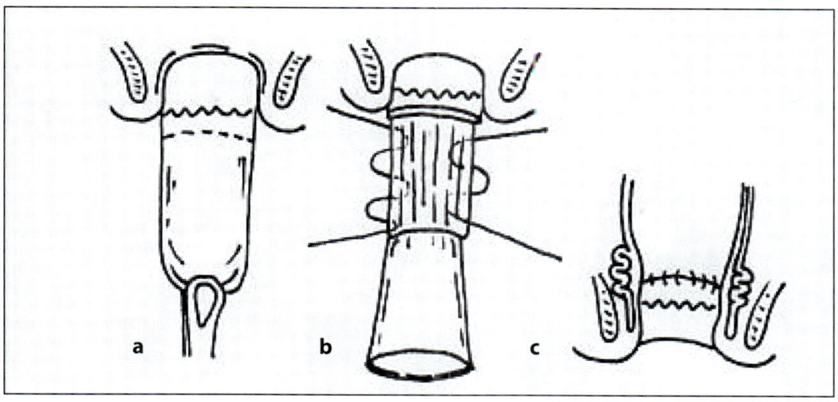

Fig. 1a-c
Delorme procedure: mucosal incision (**a**), muscular plication (**b**) and anastomosis (**c**). Modified from [6], with permission from Elsevier

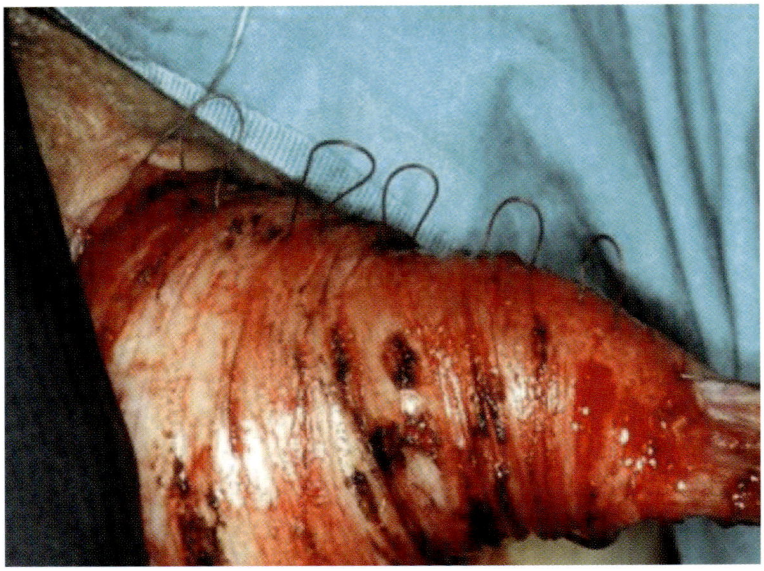

Fig. 2
Delorme procedure: rectal muscle plication

mobilised. The dissection is occasionally difficult to get started, especially if the patient has had scarring from long-standing prolapse or haemorrhoidectomy. The bright circular muscle is an important landmark, and the plane of dissection becomes more apparent as one proceeds upwards. The upwards dissection is completed when the rectal mucosa cannot be pulled down any further; typically, a sleeve of mucosa of 10–15 cm is mobilised but in some cases may reach more than 30 cm in length. Careful haemostasis is necessary to keep the field clear, and a number of transmural vessels have to undergo regularly diathermy; very seldom is it necessary to tie a vessel.

The rectal muscle is then longitudinally plicated in four quadrants with 2/0 absorbable sutures (Fig. 1b), starting at the apex of the dissection and continuing down to the distal cut edge of mucosa in the anal canal (Fig. 2); we suggest including the mucosal layer at the end of the suture, with four cardinal stitches, to reinforce plication. These sutures are placed and tagged, and additional sutures are placed in between for a total of eight sutures. As they are tied, the muscle is plicated. The excess mucosa is then excised, and an interrupted mucosa-to-mucosa anastomosis with 3/0 absorbable sutures is performed (Fig. 1c).

To improve anatomical and functional results, Lechaux et al. [7] proposed a modified extended technique that aims at performing a total pelvic floor repair. After stripping the mucosa to the apex of the prolapse, the prolapsed pouch of Douglas is exposed through a transverse incision of the anterior rectal musculature, excised and sutured as high as possible by two pursestring absorbable sutures. To perform a rectopexy, the presacral space is entered through the intersphincteric plane displayed by blunt dissection between the initial mucosal incision and the circular rectal muscle, and an absorbable mesh is inserted to enhance rectal adhesion to the sacral fascia. Diastasis of the levator ani is corrected by preanal and postanal repair (Fig. 3). Postanal repair is performed by approximating the puborectalis muscles through a posterior intersphincteric approach. Repair of the perineal body is accomplished by preanal levatorplasty effected through anterior muscular exposure, with two or three transversal nonabsorbable sutures. Rectocele that is a constant feature is repaired according to Uhlig and Sullivan [2] by vertical suture of the anterior transverse muscular incision and anterior plication in one or two layers of the circular muscle in the vertical axis. The urinary catheter is removed on the first postoperative day, and the patient can be discharged according to his or her general condition.

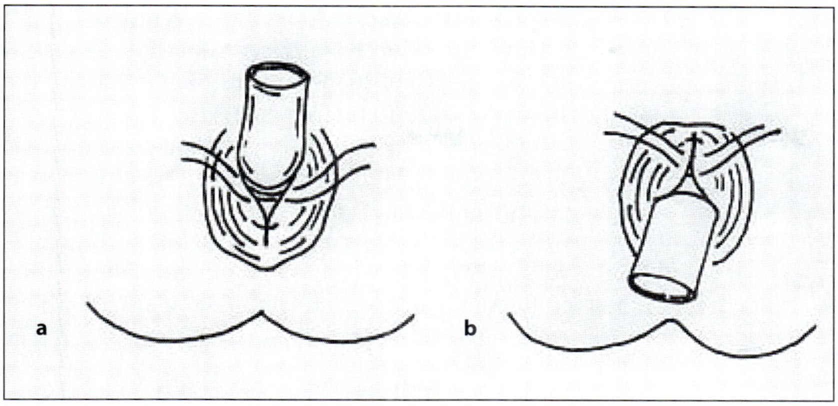

Fig. 3a, b
Delorme procedure: postanal and preanal repair according to Lechaux et al. [7]

Patients and Methods

In the last 10 years, we treated 44 patients (one man; 43 women) with a perineal procedure. Mean patient age was 76 (range 35–97) years. Faecal incontinence and constipation were present in 75% and 59% of patients, respectively. The surgical procedure was performed in 21 cases with the Delorme technique (in 11 with associated levatorplasty as described by Lechaux et al. [7]), whereas in 23, we used the Altemeier technique (in 18 with levatorplasty, as suggested by Prasad et al. [8]). In 41 cases (93%), the procedure was performed under spinal anaesthesia and in three cases (7%) under general anaesthesia. Mean hospital stay was 7 days [8.5 (min. 2, max. 10) days in the Altemeier group, and 5.4 (min. 3, max 21) days in the Delorme group].

Overall complication rate was 18% (8/44): 9% (2/21) in the Delorme group and 26% (6/23) in the Altemeier group. Specifically, there was one anastomotic stenosis treated with ambulatory dilatation and one rectal bleeding necessitating reintervention in the Delorme group, and two anastomotic stenosis – one hydroureteronephrosis in a patient treated for an associated ureteral prolapse, one urinary retention, one pneumonia and one pelvic haematoma medically managed – in the Altemeier group. Levatorplasty did not significantly influence morbidity: 24% (7/29) in the levatorplasty group and 6% (1/15) in the no levatorplasty group (Fishers test = n.s.).

A 35-year-old woman with Down syndrome who was treated with a Delorme procedure without levatorplasty died from pulmonary embolism in the first postoperative day (mortality: 2%). At a mean follow-up of 38 (range 3–113, median 32) months, 12 patients were dead for nonrelated causes and without recurrence.

We observed recurrence in 9/44 patients, with an overall recurrence rate of 20% (19% Delorme, 22% Altemeier). Recurrence rate was 10.3% and 40% in patients with or without levatorplasty, respectively (p = 0.02, Fisher's test) (Table 1). Six (four Delorme and two Altemeier) of these nine patients were treated with the Altemeier procedure, one with a laparoscopic resection–rectopexy, whereas the others refused further treatment.

Patients in the Delorme group experienced improvement in faecal incontinence and constipation at a rate of 64% and 58%, respectively, whereas patients in the Altemeier group experienced improvement at a rate of 68% and 71%, respectively. Faecal incontinence improved in 68% and 64% of patients in the levatorplasty and no levatorplasty groups, respectively, whereas consti-

Table 1. Role of levatorplasty in reducing recurrence

	With levatorplasty		
Procedure	***n***	**Recurrence**	**%**
Altemeier	18	2	11
Delorme	11	1	9
Total	29	3	10.3
	Without levatorplasty		
Procedure	***n***	**Recurrence**	**%**
Altemeier	5	3	60
Delorme	10	3	30
Total	15	6	40

Table 2. Functional results

Faecal incontinence improvement		
Procedure	**n**	**%**
Altemeier	13/19	68
Delorme	9/14	64
Total	22/33	67
Constipation improvement		
Procedure	**n**	**%**
Altemeier	10/14	71
Delorme	7/12	58
Total	17/26	65

pation improved in 62% and 69% of patients, respectively (Table 2).

Only one patient with normal bowel habit who underwent the Altemeier procedure experienced postoperative constipation; this man showed no sexual dysfunction.

Discussion and Review of Literature

There are approximately 100 surgical procedures described for the treatment of complete rectal prolapse performed by either a perineal or an abdominal approach. The choice between an elective abdominal or perineal procedure was traditionally determined by the patient's general condition. In the past, perineal repair was considered only in elderly and debilitated patients unfit for an abdominal approach because it was reported to result in poorer anatomic and functional outcome and a high recurrence rate of up to 50% [9]. During the last decade, however, results of improved technique in relation to recurrence, mortality and residual function have raised renewed interest in the perineal approach and in particular for the Delorme and Altemeier procedures [10].

Recent series using the Delorme procedure [7, 11–22] (Table 3) confirmed its safety, with reported mortality rates of 0–4.8% and morbility rates of 12–14%. In our experience, Delorme's morbidity was 9%. Most of the complications described in the literature were treatable with an ambulatory or medical approach, and reintervention was seldom necessary.

Recurrence rates vary from 0% to 38%. This wide range may be related to the length of follow-up, to variations in case mix and patient selection, to the effects of coexisting medical conditions, and to the difficulty of assessing outcomes in an elderly population; combining these factors, the "true" recurrence rate is about 15–20%. Watts and Thompson [14] showed that patient age and gender, grade of incontinence, presence of diverticular disease and length of mucosal resection did not affect recurrence. However, recurrence was significantly more common following secondary operation, suggesting that prolapses recur in a subgroup of patients who have a more pernicious condition, but this is not confirmed by other authors.

In the experience of Lechaux et al. [7], best results (5% recurrence rate) were obtained in younger patients with good pelvic floor musculature, whereas in elderly patients with a weak pelvic floor, the recurrence rate was 21%.

In a study by Sielezneff et al. [23], factors associated with failure of the Delorme procedure included proximal procidentia with retrosacral

Table 3. Results of the Delorme procedure for rectal prolapse

Source	Number	Mortality n (%)	Continence %	Constipation %	Recurrence n (%)	Follow-up months
Pascual et al. [11]	21	0	87 (+)	+	2 (9.5)	34
Marchal et al. [12]	60	4 (7)	42 (+)	54 (+)	14 (23)	88
Serventi et al. [13]	21	1 (4.8)	64 (+)	58 (+)	4 (19)	38
Watts and Thompson [14]	101	4 (4)	25 (+)	13 (+)	30 (27)	36
Liberman et al. [15]	34	0	32 (+)	88 (+)	0	43
Pescatori et al. [16]	33	0	+	44 (+)	6 (18)	39
Yakut et al. [17]	27	0	NS	NS	4 (4.2)	38
Agachan et al. [18]	8	0	+	NS	3 (38)	24
Kling et al. [19]	6	0	67 (+)	100 (+)	1 (17)	11
Lechaux et al [7]	85	1 (1.2)	45 (+)	100 (+)	11 (14)	33
Oliver et al. [20]	41	1 (2.4)	58 (+)	NS	8 (22)	47
Senapati et al. [21]	32	0	46 (+)	50 (+)	4 (12.5)	21
Tobin and Scott [22]	43	0	50 (+)	NS	11 (26)	20

+ improvement, *NS* not stated

separation on defecography, faecal incontinence, chronic diarrhoea and major perineal descent (>9 cm on straining). The authors concluded that in the absence of these factors, the Delorme procedure provided a satisfactory and durable outcome.

Different authors stress the importance of associated levatorplasty in reducing recurrence: Lechaux et al. [7] and Uhlig and Sullivan [2] reported recurrence rates of 13.5% and 6.8%, respectively, in patients treated with the Delorme modified technique. In our experience, levator repair significantly reduced risk of recurrence from 30% to 9% without significantly increasing mortality, morbidity or hospital stay.

Regarding functional outcome, overall postoperative incontinence is improved by the Delorme procedure in up to 87% of cases. This result is somewhat surprising, as it has been shown that there is no change in anal sphincter pressure, and there is a reduction of rectal compliance after the operation [24], but the outcome is confirmed in all studies examined. To improve these good functional results, Pescatori et al. [16] combined the Delorme procedure with sphincteroplasty in 33 patients: continence improved in 70%, and in 44%, constipation was cured. The authors concluded that the Delorme procedure combined with sphincteroplasty seemed indicated when both clinical and physiological findings showed a concomitant severe pelvic floor dysfunction.

The Delorme procedure also improves constipation. This may result from the decreased compliance of the rectum and from the improved continence and consequently reduction of use of loperamide or similar agents; furthermore, rectal mucosectomy may have an important effect on proximal colonic motility, with more frequent rectal filling [24]. This effect seems to be one of the advantages of the Delorme procedure compared with an abdominal procedure, for which postoperative constipation has been reported in up to 50% of cases [25, 26]. Division of the lateral ligaments [27] and posterior dissection that lead to partial denervation of the rectum might be responsible [28]. Resection of the redundant sigmoid, associated with abdominal rectopexy [29], reduces the risk of severe constipation but increases the magnitude of the procedure [30].

Regarding the choice of operation and the indications to perform a Delorme procedure, Agachan et al. [18] compared the Delorme procedure, the perineal rectosigmoidectomy (Altemeier procedure) and perineal rectosigmoidectomy with levatorplasty (Altemeier–Prasad procedure [8]), obtaining results comparable with our experience. The recurrence rate was highest with the Delorme procedure; however, postoperative continence was improved in all three procedures. The postoperative incontinence score was lowest in patients with the Altemeier–Prasad procedure. Recurrence rates were 38% for the Delorme procedure, 13% for the Altemeier procedure and 5% for the Altemeier–Prasad technique. Postoperative anorectal function and anorectal physiological characteristics were similar for all groups. The authors concluded that perineal rectosigmoidectomy with levatorplasty was a safe procedure, resulting in significantly better short-term outcome than either the Altemeier procedure alone or the Delorme procedure. Concomitant levatorplasty achieves not only a more significant improvement in continence but also a lower short-term recurrence rate.

Yakut et al. [17], evaluating their results of the Delorme procedure and of abdominal resection with or without rectopexy, noted that the most important complications were sexual problems in men who underwent posterior rectopexy procedures. Also, the Altemeier procedure, which requires complete isolation of the rectum and division of its lateral ligaments, could cause sexual dysfunction in young men [31]. As shown for others procedures, pelvic surgery causes adhesions and can reduce fertility in young women [32].

Extensive diverticular disease may prohibit perineal rectosigmoidectomy and a complete and effective proximal mucosectomy in the Delorme procedure. Inadequate resection may predispose to early prolapse recurrence [20]. As perineal rectosigmoidectomy is difficult to perform in patients with a small prolapse and those whose prolapse is not full thickness in its entire circumference, Takesue et al. [33] suggested that if the prolapsing rectal segment is shorter than 4–5 cm, a modification of the Delorme procedure is a better approach than perineal rectosigmoidectomy. An Italian consensus on rectal prolapse published in 2000 [34] agrees with this assessment

Another indication we suggest for Delorme procedure is ascites; Delorme intervention, unlike the Altemeier or abdominal procedures, doe not requires peritoneum opening, thus avoiding the risk of ascites leakage or infection.

Conclusion

In conclusion, the Delorme procedure has a major recurrence risk but has different advantages versus the Altemeier technique: it avoids the hazards of a coloanal anastomosis; respects internal sphincter innervation and rectal sensitivity can be performed under local anaesthesia; and has a similar functional outcome to that of the Altemeier technique. The Delorme procedure should be considered as a primary procedure for patients with ascites or for frail and elderly persons with prolapse associated with constipation and/or not longer than 5 cm [35]. The Delorme procedure can also be proposed to young women of child-bearing age or to young men to avoid the risk of sexual dysfunction.

References

1. Delorme E (1900) Sur le traitement des prolapsus du rectum totaux par l'excision de la muquese rectale au rectal-colique. Bull Mem Soc Chir Paris 26:499–518
2. Uhlig BE, Sullivan ES (1979) The modified Delorme operation: its place in surgical treatment for massive rectal prolapse. Dis Colon Rectum 22:513–521
3. Lechaux JP (2002) Trattamento chirurgico del prolasso rettale completo dell'adulto. Encycl Med Chir. Tecniche Chirurgiche-Addominale. Elsevier, Paris, Pub med 40–710
4. Karulf RE, Madoff RD, Goldberg SM (2001) Rectal prolapse. Curr Probl Surg 38:771–832
5. Houry S (2000) Opération de Delorme pour prolapsus rectal. J Chir 137:338–341
6. Jacobs LK, Lin YJ, Orkin BA (1997) The best operation for rectal prolapse. Surg Clin North Am 77:49–70
7. Lechaux JP, Lechaux D, Perez M (1995) Results of Delorme's procedure for rectal prolapse: advantages of a modified technique. Dis Colon Rectum 38:301–307
8. Prasad ML, Pearl RK, Abcarian H et al (1986) Perineal proctectomy, posterior rectopexy, and postanal levator repair for the treatment of rectal prolapse. Dis Colon Rectum 29:547–552
9. Friedman R, Muggia-Sulam M, Freund HR (1983) Experience with one-stage perineal repair of rectal prolapse. Dis Colon Rectum 26:789–791
10. Madiba TE, Baig MK, Wexner SD (2005) Surgical management of rectal prolapse. Arch Surg 140:63–73
11. Pascual Montero JA, Martinez Puente MC, Pascual I et al (2006) Complete rectal prolapse clinical and functional outcome with Delorme's procedure. Rev Esp Enferm Dig 98:837–843
12. Marchal F, Bresler L, Ayav A et al (2005) Long-term results of Delorme's procedure and Orr-Loygue rectopexy to treat complete rectal prolapse. Dis Colon Rectum 48:1785–1790
13. Serventi A, Sallustio P, Lobascio P, Binda GA (2005) Role of levatorplasty in total rectal prolapse treatment using perineal approach. II Joint Meeting ECCP/EACP. I Congress SICCR. Medimond, Bologna, pp 155–157
14. Watts AMI, Thompson MR (2000) Evaluation of Delorme's procedure as a treatment for full thickness rectal prolapse. Br J Surg 87:218–222
15. Liberman H, Hughes C, Dippolito A (2000) Evaluation and outcome of the Delorme procedure in the treatment of rectal outlet obstruction. Dis Colon Rectum 43:188–192
16. Pescatori M, Interisano A, Stolfi VM et al (1998) Delorme's operation and sphincteroplasty for rectal prolapse and faecal incontinence. Int J Colorectal Dis 13:223–227
17. Yakut M, Kaymakciioglu N, Simsek A et al (1998) Surgical treatment of rectal prolapse: a retrospective analysis of 94 cases. Int Surg 83:53–55
18. Agachan F, Reissman P, Pfeifer J et al (1997) Comparison of three perineal procedure for the treatment of rectal prolapse. South Med 90:925–932
19. Kling KM, Rongione AJ, Evans B et al (1996) The Delorme procedure: a useful operation for complicated rectal prolapse in the elderly. Am Surg 62:857–860
20. Oliver GC, Vachon D, Eisenstat TE et al (1994) Delorme's procedure for complete rectal prolapse in severely debilitated patient: an analysis of 41 patients. Dis Colon Rectum 37:461–467
21. Senapati A, Nicholls RJ, Thomson JPS et al (1994) Results of Delorme's procedure for rectal prolapse. Dis Colon Rectum 37:456–460
22. Tobin SA, Scott IHK (1994) Delorme operation for rectal prolapse. Br J Surg 81:1681–1684
23. Sielezneff I, Malouf A, Cesari J et al (1999) Selection criteria for internal rectal prolapse repair by Delorme's transrectal excision. Dis Colon Rectum 42:367–373
24. Plusa SM, Charig JA, Balaji V et al (1995) Physiological changes after Delorme's procedure for full-thickness rectal prolapse. Br J Surg 82:1475–1478
25. Mann CV, Hoffman C (1988) Complete rectal prolapse: the anatomical and functional results of treatment by an extended abdominal rectopexy. Br J Surg 75:34–37
26. McCue JL, Thompson JPS (1991) Clinical and functional results of abdominal rectopexy for rectal prolapse. Br J Surg 78:921–923
27. Speakman CT, Madden MV, Nichols RJ et al (1991) Lateral ligament division during rectopexy causes constipation but prevents recurrence: results of a prospective randomised study. Br J Surg 78:1431–1433

28. Delemarre JB, Gooszen HG, Kruyt RH (1991) The effect of posterior rectopexy on fecal continence. Dis Colon Rectum 34:311–316
29. Frykman HM, Goldberg SM (1969) The surgical treatment of rectal procidentia. Surg Gynecol Obstet 129:1225–1230
30. McKee RF, Lauder JC, Poon FW et al (1992) A prospective randomized study of abdominal rectopexy with and without sigmoidectomy in rectal prolapse. Surg Gynecol Obstet 174:145–148
31. Meyers JO, Wong WD, Rothenberg DA et al (1990) Rectal prolapse in male. Implications for management. Dis Colon Rectum 33:28
32. Gorgun E, Remzi FH, Goldberg JM et al (2004) Fertility is reduced after restorative proctocolectomy with ileal pouch anal anastomosis: a study of 300 patients. Surgery 136:795–803
33. Takesue Y, Yokoyama T, Murakami Y et al (1999) The effectiveness of perineal rectosigmoidectomy for the treatment of rectal prolapse. Surg Today 29:290–293
34. Altomare DF, Boccasanta P (2000) Algoritmo decisionale per il trattamento del prolasso rettale completo. UCP News 4:43–44
35. Gourgiotis S, Baratsis S (2007) Rectal prolapse. Int J Colorectal Dis 22:231–243

12 Perineal Approach to External Rectal Prolapse: The Altemeier Procedure

Donato F. Altomare, Marcella Rinaldi

Introduction

The perineal approach to treating full-thickness external rectal prolapse was adopted in the first attempt to cure this condition due to the risk posed by the intraperitoneal approach in the pre-antibiotic era and before adequate anaesthesiological support became available. The first rectosigmoidectomy reported in the literature was an emergency amputation of the rectum for an irreducible rectal prolapse with gangrene, performed by Auffret in 1882 [1]. Then in 1888, Mikulicz [2] described a series of six cases of rectal amputation for incarcerated complete rectal prolapse, with no mortality or recurrence, so that the operation was long associated to his name (as reported in Gabriel's textbook on rectal surgery, dated 1949 [3]). Following other occasional reports, Miles [4] made a detailed description of the technique in 1933, but the name of Altemeier [5] was finally linked to this operation after his paper describing his procedure on elderly and debilitated patients was published in the *Archives of Surgery* in 1952.

Surgical Procedure

Patient Preparation and Position

As for any operation on the colon, the patient will undergo mechanical cleansing of the bowel using polyethylene glycol solution by mouth the day before surgery, antibiotic prophylaxis and antithrombotic prophylaxis 1 h before surgery. A Foley catheter is inserted in the bladder.

The patient's position during this operation is still controversial, as many surgeons in Europe still prefer the original position described by Mikulicz and Altemeier, the lithotomy position, with a slight degree of Trendelenburg. In the USA, and in my personal experience, the jacknife position is preferred because it offers the operators more advantages and makes the operation itself easier for at least two reasons: firstly, the mesorectal small vessels entering the posterior part of the rectum can be controlled and cauterised more easily because they are in direct view of the surgeon; secondly the venous blood pressure at the perineum is decreased because of the position of the right atrium of the heart below the perineum. This makes the prolapse and haemorrhoids less oedematous and congested and can reduce intraoperative bleeding. In addition, the small bowel is moved into the peritoneal cavity.

Anaesthesia

Epidural (low spinal) anaesthesia is optimal for this perineal approach, particularly for patients with pulmonary problems. The duration of the effect of the anaesthesia also can fit the operating time, which lasts between 1 and 2.5 h in almost all the series. In selected cases, locoregional perianal anaesthesia has been performed [6] in an outpatient setting, whereas general anaesthesia is preferred by many anaesthetists. The operation is virtually painless, and epidural or i.v. analgesia is not necessary postoperatively.

Procedure

With the patient in the jacknife position, the glutei are kept apart with tape, and the prolapse is exposed by gentle traction on the apex of the prolapse with Babcock forceps. This manoeuvre can be facilitated by inviting the patient (if under spinal anaesthesia) to make a Valsalva manoeuvre. Adoption of a Lone Star self-retractor greatly

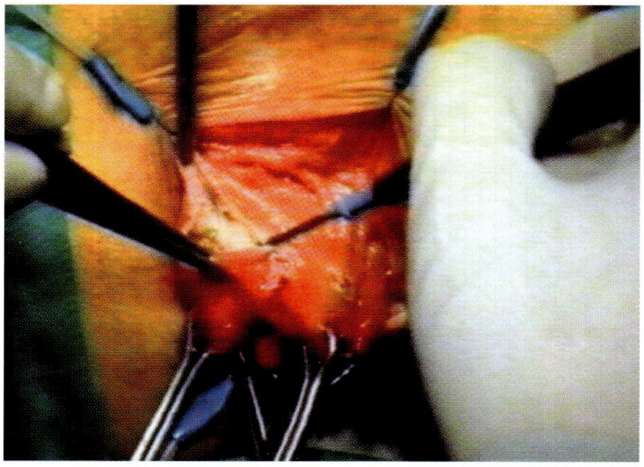

Fig. 1
Diathermy incision of full-thickness rectal prolapse exposed with the help of a Lone Star self-retractor

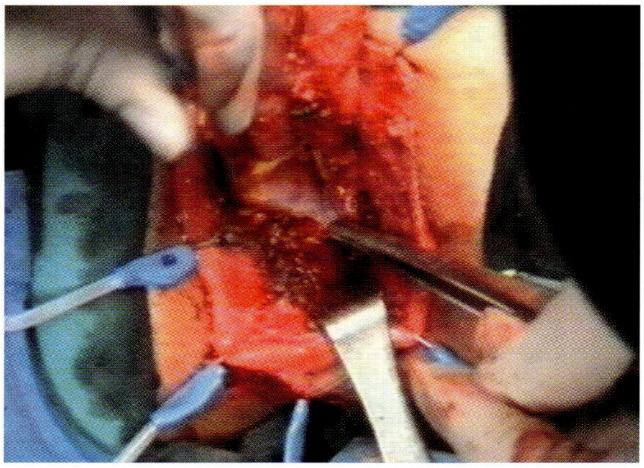

Fig. 2
Opening the pelvic pouch of the peritoneum (patient in jacknife position)

facilitates the procedure. The hooks of the retractors are placed initially between the everted rectum and the anus and, after full incision of the rectum, inside the inner ring of the mucosa.

The dissection site is identified about 2–4 cm proximal to the dentate line and marked with a diathermy. The level of the incision should not include the internal anal sphincter and should be more distal (about 4 cm from the dentate line) (Fig. 1) if a stapled anastomosis is planned, because about 1 cm of tissue is resected by the stapler. If these length ranges are not respected, repositioning of the anastomosis inside the pelvis at the end of the operation is not possible and, vice versa, postoperative protrusion is more probable. Infiltration of the submucosa with 1:200,000 adrenaline solution is suggested by some authors to reduce bleeding, but it is not strictly necessary and can alter the dissection plane. A circumferential diathermy incision is then made including all the layers of the rectal wall in order to reach the submuscular adipose tissue. Haemostasis can be easily achieved with diathermy. At this time, only the extraperitoneal rectum is exteriorised and can be fully mobilised by cauterisation of the small vessels entering the rectal wall from the mesorectum. This step can also be performed using radiofrequency ligation (Ligasure, Tyco) or ultrasound dissectors (Ultracision, Ethicon). The dissection of the rectum from the vagina must be performed with great care, as it can sometimes be difficult if the appropriate plane of dissection is not identified. Once the extraperitoneal rectum is fully mobilised, the pouch Douglas is opened (Fig. 2), allowing entrance into the peritoneal cavity. The presence of adhesions or an enterocele can be evaluated at this time and treated if necessary.

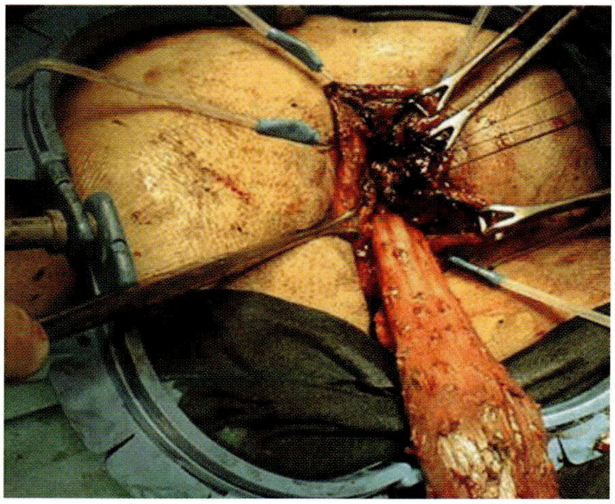

Fig. 3
Full mobilisation of the rectum and sigmoid colon

The exteriorisation of the rectum and sigmoid colon is continued by progressive ligation (or cauterisation) of the small mesenterial vessels just before their entrance into the sigmoid wall. The amount of colon to be resected depends on how easy it is to exteriorise it (Fig. 3). Sometimes, this can be preoperatively determined by a barium enema. However, isolation of the colon must be interrupted when it cannot be drawn out of the pelvis without tension.

The hook retractors are then placed within the anal ring to expose the peritoneum and allow evaluation of the hiatus of the levators ani, which

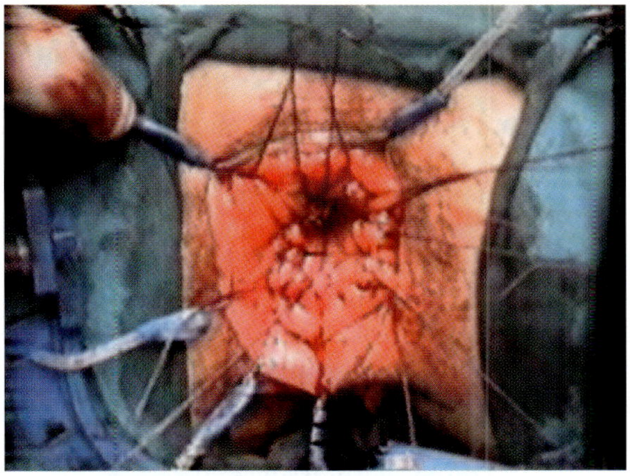

Fig. 4
Coloanal anastomosis by interrupted stitches

must be narrowed by posterior muscle plication using two to three nonabsorbable interrupted stitches (2/0 Prolene). Sometimes, one or two more stitches can be applied anteriorly. The sutures should allow a finger to be passed easily between the colon and the plicated muscles. The peritoneum of the pouch of Douglas does not necessarily need to be reclosed and could be left open or trimmed and sutured if it is redundant.

The colonic wall is then incised anteriorly in order to place the first 3/0 Vicryl stitch between the anorectum and the colonic mucosa. After further interruption of the rectal wall, the stitches are placed at the right and left quadrant and, after complete resection of the elongated colon, the last anterior quadrant is sutured. Such a procedure should prevent any twisting of the anastomosis. Care should be taken to include in these sutures not only the mucosa but also the muscular wall. This step of the operation could be easily contaminated by faecal material coming out from the incised colon, and attention must be paid to prevent this, and particularly to prevent contamination of the pouch of Douglas. The anastomosis is completed by applying at least two interrupted sutures between each cardinal point (Fig. 4). An excessive number of sutures or an uninterrupted suture could favour the occurrence of anastomotic stricture. Once the exteriorised anastomosis is completed and the haemostasis controlled, the colon can be replaced inside the peritoneal cavity, concluding the procedure.

The anastomosis can be performed with a circular stapler (31, 33 or 34 mm), although no advantages have been demonstrated [7, 8], whilst this certainly increases the cost of the procedure. In this case, a continuous 2/0 Prolene purse-string suture should be placed on the edge of the proximal colon and on the anorectum. After introduction of the stapler into the anus, the proximal suture is tied first and the anorectal suture after. The stapler is then closed completely, fired and withdrawn. A haemostatic absorbable sponge could be left within the anus. There is no need for postoperative medication; antibiotics are continued for 2–3 days, and oral feeding can be started within 1–2 days.

The Italian Experience

A review of the experience from seven major colorectal centres of the Italian Society of Colorectal Surgery was recently carried out [9]. Seventy-eight American Society of Anaesthesiologists (ASA) III and IV patients (female:male ratio 9:4, mean age 71 years, range 26–93) underwent perineal rectosigmoidectomy according to Altemeier associated with levatorplasty in 86% of the cases under general (21 cases), spinal (50 cases) or locoregional (seven cases) anaesthesia, with the patient in the prone (29 cases) or lithotomy (49 cases) position. In 11 patients (14%), the prolapse had previously been treated by the Delorme procedure (eight cases), Ripstein rectopexy (one case) or the stapled transanal rectal resection (STARR) procedure (two cases). The mean duration of the operation was 90 min, and the mean length of the rectocolonic resected specimen was 20 cm (range 7–40 cm).

The coloanal anastomosis was fashioned manually in all but three cases in which a 31-mm circular stapler was used; 80% of them suffered from major faecal incontinence, 6% from soiling and 14% were not incontinent. In the postoperative period, incontinence improved in 16 cases (30%) (soiling or no incontinence), whereas in three patients, it deteriorated. Four patients with normal preoperative continence had postoperative soiling.

Although there was no postoperative mortality, six (7.7%) major complications (pelvic haematomas in three patients, one requiring surgical revision; anal strictures in two; anastomotic dehiscence requiring surgery in one), and eight minor complications (four transient anal pain and burning sensation; two high temperature; two urinary retention) were recorded.

After a mean follow-up of 45 (range 2–93) months, the overall recurrence rate was 23% but varied significantly – from 0% to 47%. Recurrences were treated with a new Altemeier procedure in eight cases, a Delorme procedure in one, a Wells' rectopexy in one, post anal repair in one, anal bulking agents in two and sacral nerve electrostimulation in one.

In this experience, perineal rectosigmoidectomy for full-thickness rectal prolapse proved to be a relatively safe and effective treatment with acceptable postoperative morbidity, particularly for frail and elderly patients, although the recurrence rate is not negligible and continence restoration remains unpredictable. In cases of failure, a repeat Altemeier operation is still possible.

Perineal Rectosigmoidectomy (Altemeier Procedure): A Review of the Literature

After the first publication of clinical results with perineal rectosigmoidectomy by Altemeier [9] in the 1970s, the procedure was widely adopted in the USA and in some European countries but less commonly in Italy and Eastern countries. The majority of data published, in fact, derive from US institutions. Nevertheless, they are very inhomogeneous because of some differences in the operative procedure (with or without levatorplasty, length of resected bowel, hand-sewn or stapled anastomosis and addition or not of a colonic pouch) and in preoperative and postoperative functional evaluation (almost all patients are defined as "incontinent", without manometric data or other details about the morphology of the anal sphincters being specified). Even evaluation of results is complicated by the different interpretation of "mucosal prolapse", recorded as recurrence of rectal prolapse in some studies. An overview of the data available in the literature shows that the Altemeier procedure is usually performed in patients of advanced age (mean 73.6 years), often with associated respiratory or cardiovascular problems; approximately four out of five are women, with associated faecal incontinence and with an overt rectal prolapse exceeding 10 cm.

The clinical outcomes of reported series of perineal rectosigmoidectomy are summarised in Table 1 [6, 8, 10–25], which lists the relatively few papers (only 18) published so far on this topic. Some papers from the same institutions (53% from the USA) reviewing different periods were omitted, as only the most recent are reported.

Complications

The procedure is accomplished with relatively low morbidity (from 5% to 24%) and mortality (from

Table 1. Results of perineal rectosigmoidectomy

Authors	Year	Patients (n)	Mean age	Follow-up (months)	Recurrence (%)	Incontinent patients (%)	Improvement (%)
Altemeier et al. [10]	1971	106	64	-	3	-	-
Porter [11]	1971	110	-	12-60	58	66	10
Friedman et al. [12]	1983	27	61	-	50	-	-
Gopal et al. [13]	1984	18	76	12	6	-	-
Prasad et al. [14]	1986	25	71	36	0	-	88
Vasilevsky and Goldberg [15]	1987	66	-	31	0	41	78
Ramanujam et al. [16]	1987	41	-	20	5	100	78
Finlay and Atchison [17]	1991	17	82	24	6		
Williams et al. [18]	1992	114	78	12	10	58.8	
Johansen et al. [19]	1993	20	82	26	0	70	25
Deen et al. [20]	1994	10	72	17	30	100	80
Kim et al. [21]	1999	183	-	-	16	-	-
Takesue et al. [22]	1999	10	79	42	10	70	71
Kimmins et al. [6]	2001	63	79	21	6.3	71	70
Zbar et al. [23]	2002	80	69	22	3.8	5	100
Chun et al. [24]	2004	109	76	29	16.5	-	100
Habr-Gama et al. [25]	2006	44	76	49	7.1	-	85.7
Boccasanta et al. [8]	2006	40	71	28	12.5	100	100

0% to 6%, the latter for unrelated events) rates despite the very elderly and frail patient population. Most of the early complications are medical, such as pneumonitis, cystitis, cardiac failure and so on. Complications directly related to the procedure include local or pelvic abscesses due to rupture of the suture line, hematomas for anastomotic bleeding, anastomotic stricture, rectovaginal fistulas anal pain. All these complications are anecdotal, unlike coloanal anastomosis performed for other reasons.

Recurrence

The recurrence rate in the literature ranges widely from 0% to 58% (without levatorplasty), and this remains the main drawback of this operation. This widely variable success is not easy to explain, even if some technical changes in the procedure, such as the association of a levatorplasty (which was firstly proposed by Gopal et al. [13] and subsequently modified by Ramanujam et al [16] and Prasad et al. [14]), could improve the results, as confirmed in many studies. Particularly, the role of levatorplasty was considered by Chun et al. [24] in a retrospective evaluation of 109 patients, showing that the recurrence rate was reduced and the time to recurrence was significantly longer in the levatorplasty group; continence improved in both groups, but particularly in the levatorplasty group. Certainly, the surgeon's experience could play a role, and the length of follow-up should be considered [26], although a pooled analysis of the studies available so far does not show any relationship between recurrence and length of follow-up. This is in agreement with other authors who have reported almost all recurrences within 2 years of the operation [6, 27]. Another critical point could be the length of the resected specimen. In fact, the presence of a weak pelvic floor with a residual mobile sigmoid colon could favour a recurrence. However, the definition of recurrence is a major cause of confusion, as in some series, even a minor rectal mucosal prolapse or a wet anus is considered as such.

Functional Results

As far as the functional postoperative results are concerned, the data presented in almost all studies are of poor quality. Scoring systems to quantify the severity of faecal incontinence or constipation are used only in two papers [8, 24], whereas a dedicated quality-of-life questionnaire is never mentioned.

One of the major functional problems associated with rectal prolapse is faecal incontinence, which is estimated to occur in about 80% of cases in most studies. In some cases, the impending prolapse itself can cause or contribute to incontinence due to the relaxing effect on the anal sphincter, but in most cases, there is a weak pelvic floor with a patent patulous anus and evident hiatus of the pelvic diaphragm (puborectalis muscles), which cannot be normalised with any operation. Pudendal neuropathy has been claimed to play a role by some authors who consider both the prolapse and the pelvic weakness as an expression of the same neuromuscular deficiency [28]. However, the role of pudendal neuropathy is controversial, as in other experiences, no relationship was found between clinical outcome and the presence of pudendal neuropathy [19]. Furthermore, with this operation, the rectal ampulla is resected, and therefore rectal compliance is diminished, thus contributing to faecal incontinence. This point is controversial, as rectal resection for cancer of the proximal rectum is rarely associated with faecal incontinence unless the pelvic nerves are injured during pelvic dissection, but the issue is considered relevant and some authors prefer a colonic-pouch anal anastomosis instead of direct coloanal anastomosis [29].

The addition of levatorplasty to perineal rectosigmoidectomy, previously discussed for its role in the prevention of recurrence, is associated with a significant improvement in continence in the two studies comparing the addition or not of a levatorplasty [24, 26].

Conclusion

Perineal rectosigmoidectomy is the operation of choice for elderly, high-risk patients affected by full-thickness rectal prolapse exceeding 5 cm, because the procedure is relatively safe and painless, with no need for general anaesthesia, an early resumption of normal activities and short in-hospital stay. However, in sexually active men with a full-thickness rectal prolapse, the perineal approach should be considered despite the higher risk of recurrence because it carries less risk of pelvic nerve injury and sexual dysfunction [18]. Finally, in cases of recurrence, there are no contraindications to a repeat procedure.

References

1. Auffret M (1882) Un cas de procidence du gros intestine d'une lenguer de 90 centimetres: operation per excision: double range de suture; mort. Progr Med 10:650
2. Mikulicz J (1889) Zur operative Behandlung des prolapsus recti et coli invaginali (1889) Arch Klin Chir 38:74–79
3. Gabriel WB, Lond MS eds (1949) The principle and practice of rectal surgery. H.K. Lewis, London, p 120
4. Miles WE (1933) Rectosigmoidectomy as a method for procidentia recti. Proc R Soc Med 26:1445–1452
5. Altemeier WA, Giuseffi J, Hoxworth P (1952) Treatment of extensive prolapse of the rectum in aged and debilitated patients. Arch Surg 65:72–80
6. Kimmins MH, Evetts BK, Isler J, Billingham R (2001) The Altemeier repair: outpatient treatment of rectal prolapse. Dis Colon Rectum 44:565–570
7. Vermeulen FD, Nivatvongs S, Fang DT et al (1983) A technique for perineal rectosigmoidectomy using autosuture devices. Surg Gynecol Obstet 156:85–86
8. Boccasanta P, Venturi M, Barbieri S, Roviaro G (2006) Impact of new technologies on the clinical and functional outcome of Altemeier's procedure. A randomized controlled trial. Dis Colon Rectum 49:652–660
9. Marino F, Binda GA, Ganio E (2007) Long-term outcome of Altemeier's procedure for full thickness rectal prolapse. A survey of 6 colorectal units. Tech Coloproctol 11:172–173 Abstr
10. Altemeier WA, Culbertson WR, Schowengerdt C, Hunt J (1971). Nineteen years' experience with the one-stage perineal repair of rectal prolapse, Ann Surg 173:993–1006
11. Porter N (1971) Surgery for rectal prolapse. BMJ 3:113
12. Friedman R, Muggia-Sulam M, Freund HR (1983) Experience with the one stage perineal repair of rectal prolapse. Dis Colon Rectum 26:789–791
13. Gopal KA, Amshel AL, Shonberg IL, Eftaiha M (1984) Rectal procidentia in elderly and debilitated patients. Experience with the Altemeier procedure. Dis Colon Rectum 27:376–381
14. Prasad ML, Pearl RK, Abcarian H et al (1986) Perineal proctectomy, posterior rectopexy and postanal levator repair for the treatment of rectal prolapse. Dis Colon Rectum 29:547–552
15. Vasilevsky CA, Goldberg SM (1987) The use of the intraluminal stapling device in perineal rectosigmoidectomy for rectal prolapse. In: Ravitch MM, Stephen MM (eds) Principles and practice of surgical stapling. Year Book Medical Publishers, Chicago, pp 480–486
16. Ramanujam PS, Venkatesh KS (1988) Perineal excision of rectal prolapse with posterior levator ani repair in elderly high-risk patients. Dis Colon Rectum 31:704–706
17. Finlay IG, Atchison M (1991) Perineal excision of the rectum for prolapse in the elderly. Br J Surg 78:687–689
18. Williams JG, Rothenberger DA, Madoff RD, Goldberg SM (1992). Treatment of rectal prolapse in the elderly by perineal rectosigmoidectomy. Dis Colon Rectum 35:830–834
19. Johansen OB, Wexner SD, Daniel N et al (1993) Perineal rectosigmoidectomy in the elderly. Dis Colon Rectum 36:767–772
20. Deen KE, Grant E, Billingham C, Keighley MRB (1994) Abdominal resection rectopexy with pelvic floor repair versus perineal rectosigmoidectomy and pelvic floor repair for full thickness rectal prolapse. Br J Surg 81:302–303
21. Kim D-S, Tsang CBS, Wong WD et al (1999) Complete rectal prolapse: evolution of management and results. Dis Colon Rectum 42:460–469
22. Takesue Y, Yokoyama T, Murakami Y et al (1999) The effectiveness of perineal rectosigmoidectomy for the treatment of rectal prolapse in elderly and high-risk patients. Surg Today 29:290–293
23. Zbar AP, Takashima S, Hasegawa T, Kitabayashi K (2002) Perineal rectosigmoidectomy (Altemeier's procedure): a review of physiology, technique and outcome (2002) Tech Coloproctol 6:109–116
24. Chun SW, Pikarsky AJ, You SY et al (2004) Perineal rectosigmoidectomy for rectal prolapse: role of the levatorplasty. Tech Coloproctol 8:3–9
25. Habr-Gama A, Jacob CE, Jorge JM et al (2006) Rectal procidentia treatment by perineal rectosigmoidectomy combined with levator ani repair. Hepatogastroenterology 53:213–217
26. Agachan F, Pfeiffer J, Joo JS et al (1997) Results of perineal procedures for the treatment of rectal prolapse. Am Surgeon 63:9–12
27. Rothenberger DA (1989) Anal incontinence. In: Cameron JL (ed) Current surgical therapy, 3rd edn. BC Decker. Philadelphia, pp 186
28. Steele SR, Goetz LH, Minami S et al (2006) Management of recurrent rectal prolapse: surgical approach influences outcome. Dis Colon Rectum 49:440–445
29. Yoshioka K, Ogunbiyi OA, Keighley MRB (1998) Pouch perineal rectosigmoidectomy gives better functional results than conventional rectosigmoidectomy in elderly patients with rectal prolapse. Br J Surg 85:1525–226

13 Surgery for Rectal Prolapse: Functional Outcome from the Perineal Approach – An Overview

Steven D. Wexner, Amit Khanna

Introduction

Numerous approaches to the treatment of rectal prolapse have been described throughout the history of medicine. Rectal prolapse is often associated with functional disorders such as constipation and/or incontinence [1]. Recognition of this association and careful evaluation of baseline function is critical to providing appropriate therapy. Both abdominal and perineal variants of rectal prolapse repair have been examined in a growing body of literature. These reports have intended to determine both short- and long-term functional outcomes associated with a multitude of approaches to rectal prolapse surgery. This overview provides evidence to aid the clinician in surgical decision making when faced with the patient in need of operative repair. Surgical therapy of rectal prolapse is often not standard, but rather, tailored after careful consideration of the patient's operative risk, life expectancy, associated functional disorders, and previous operative history.

Much debate has centered on the specific pathophysiology of rectal prolapse. The specific causation has yet to be fully elucidated. However, there are some specific observations that may aid in therapy. Landmark cinedefecography performed by Broden and Snellman revealed rectal prolapse as a circumferential intussusception of the rectum [2]. Parks et al. [3], in 1966, demonstrated abnormal perineal descent leading to possible traction injury of the pudendal nerves and denervation of the pelvic floor muscles and sphincter. Reports by Kiff et al. [4] added more evidence, to suggest a possible role of pudendal nerve injury in patients with perineal descent. Functional disturbances associated with rectal prolapse seem to represent a multifactorial and complex process that may include chronic sphincter stretch, denervation of pelvic muscles, impairment of sensation, and rectoanal inhibitory reflex (RAIR) inhibition. Although several studies have measured and characterized these abnormalities, the exact initiating event in rectal prolapse remains uncertain. Some authors have proposed that intussusception in the midrectum associated with chronic straining in combination with slow-transit constipation may lead to rectal prolapse [5]. This complexity poses challenges in designing specific therapy targeted at improving functional outcomes. Nonetheless, there have been some significant advances in the surgical management of rectal prolapse with regard to optimization of postoperative function. In the following pages, we review the available functional outcomes following rectal prolapse repair using the perineal approach.

Functional Evaluation of the Patient with Rectal Prolapse

Prior to embarking on the functional assessment of a patient with rectal prolapse, the general health status of the patient is of paramount importance. Preoperative risk stratification is critical for the surgeon to select patients who will not only have the most durable repair but one with limited morbidity. Perhaps no disease in colorectal pathology requires more individual adjustment or "customization" of procedures than that of rectal prolapse.

At Cleveland Clinic Florida, the patient with rectal prolapse will generally undergo a series of baseline functional tests, with the most critical tool being a detailed history and physical examination. A comorbid history of genitourinary dysfunction should be obtained, along with validated assessments of functional status. For measuring fecal incontinence, the internationally used Wexner scoring system is employed using a 20-point system [1]. A detailed history of bowel habits is also obtained with regard to evidence of constipation, as this is often coincident with the presence of rectal prolapse. Among patients with rectal prolapse, incontinence is noted in 40–80% [1]. Other important historical factors may include previous anorectal surgery, prolapse repairs, and presence of neurological disease.

Physical examination often begins with the recreation of the environment in which the prolapse commonly occurs, namely, on a commode. Therefore, we routinely ask our patients to strain while seated on a commode to evaluate the extent of prolapse in the physiologic evacuatory setting. A careful digital examination should be performed to evaluate for evidence of sphincter integrity and approximate resting and squeeze pressures. In addition, anoscopy and full colonoscopy should be performed to exclude other sources of rectal bleeding or masses that may initiate an intussusception. Finally, achieving high patient satisfaction is dependent upon both understanding the patient's predominant complaints and setting appropriate expectations of suggested therapy (Table 1).

Although there is considerable variation by institution, the functional evaluation of the patient who presents with rectal prolapse should aid in selection of patients for specific therapy, define severity of constipation, and define the need for other nonsurgical adjunct therapies (Table 2). Cinedefecography is performed, although not specifically to demonstrate the prolapse–which can most often be seen with a physical examination–but rather to evaluate for the concomitant presence of enterocele, paradoxical puborectalis contraction, and internal intussusception that may be responsive to biofeedback therapy. Pudendal nerve terminal motor latency (PNTML) assessment is often performed and can help elucidate inappropriate puborectalis contraction, and has been used by some authors to predict postoperative anal incontinence [6]. Colonic transit studies in patients with severe constipation can also alter the planned operation in favor of combined resection and rectopexy.

Anorectal manometry is usually abnormal in the incontinent rectal prolapse patient; most often, patients will present with decreased resting and squeeze pressures that are normal to low [7]. The predictive value of these tests has been evaluated in a review by Glasgow et al. [8] at Washington University. All patients treated at that institution by perineal repair for rectal prolapse from 1995–2004 ($n = 45$) were examined with respect to anal manometry and PNTML for a median follow-up of 33.8 months. All patients underwent perineal rectosigmoidectomy (PRS) mostly with levatorplasty. Using a predictive model, the authors found that patients with preoperative squeeze pressure >60 mmHg had improved fecal continence relative to lower pressures [positive predictive value (PPV) of 89.5%]. In addition, they did not find that pudendal nerve function accurately predicted postoperative incontinence. They also reported an 8.9% recurrence rate, whereas the overall incontinence rate improved from 77.8% to 35.6%. Mean preoperative resting pressure and pudendal neuropathy did not correlate with functional outcome. Only 6.9% of the rectal prolapse population had normal manometric findings. In addition, other reviews have confirmed that at significantly low levels of function, such as preoperative resting anal pressures <10 mmHg and maximum voluntary contraction pressure <50 mmHg, incontinence tends to persist postoperatively [9]. However, it remains unclear what role PNTML plays in the preoperative evaluation of rectal prolapse patients.

Several functional abnormalities have been suggested in patients with rectal prolapse, including altered function in both internal and external sphincter muscles, lower anal resting pressures suggesting a damaged internal sphincter muscle, inhibited RAIR, and reduced maximal contraction indicating damage to the puborectalis

Table 1. Historical aspects

Medical risk stratification
Functional historical approach to rectal prolapse
Wexner Incontinence Scoring System
History of constipation
Comorbid conditions
Genitourinary dysfunction or prolapse
Patient expectations and prioritization

Table 2. Potential tests performed in patients with rectal prolapse

Rectal examination
Anoscopy
Colonoscopy
Cinedefecography
Anorectal manometry
Pudendal nerve terminal motor latency assessment
Anal electromyography
Colonic transit time in the setting of constipation

and external anal sphincter muscles. Possible etiologies for impaired function associated with rectal prolapse include chronic sphincter stretch, denervation of pelvic muscles, sensation impairment, and RAIR inhibition.

Perineal Approaches to Rectal Prolapse: A Functional Perspective

The two most commonly performed perineal approaches to rectal prolapse are the Delorme procedure and the PRS [10, 11]. These approaches have been classically advocated for the medically high-risk or elderly patient whose operative risk may be significant from an abdominal approach. Tsunoda et al. performed a review targeted to evaluate the anorectal physiology of the Delorme procedure for rectal prolapse [12]. The authors reviewed 31 consecutive patents at Showa University Hospital between 1994 and 2002 for a median duration of 39 months. They performed anorectal physiology testing prior to operation and at 6 months. They measured resting pressure, squeeze pressure, volume at first sensation, and maximum tolerated volume. They also graded fecal incontinence using the Wexner incontinence score. The median preoperative incontinence score improved after the Delorme procedure from 11.5 to 6.0 after operation, with improvement in maximum resting pressure (from 21 to 23.5 cm H_2O). The squeeze pressure also improved from 64 to 108 cm H_20, and a decrease in volume at rectal sensation fell from a median of 100 to 70 ml (p <0.002). Maximum tolerable volume also decreased from 260 to 160 ml (p <0.05). However, the authors conceded that in patients older than 80 years, a 33% recurrence rate was noted. Overall, continence improved in 63% of the cohort after operation.

Another series by Senapati et al. [13] from St. Mark's Hospital from 1978 to 1990 reviewed their outcomes after Delorme procedure on 32 patients with complete rectal prolapse. Mean follow-up was 24 months, whereas a recurrence rate of 12.5% was noted. No newly developed constipation was reported postoperatively, and 50% of the constipated patients reported improvement, and incontinence improved in 46%. The authors cited the importance of long-term follow-up in determining the true recurrence rate of Delorme repairs. They estimated the recurrence rate to be somewhere between 5% and 20% which is generally higher than following abdominal approaches [14].

A more recent review by Marchal et al. [15] in 2005 retrospectively reviewed patients undergoing Delorme rectal prolapse procedures at the University of Nancy. They recorded an overall complication rate with the Delorme procedure of 15% and a recurrence rate of 23% with a median follow-up of almost 6 years. They reported that of the 24 patients undergoing a Delorme procedure with a preoperative history of constipation, approximately 54% improved after repair. An additional 12.5% worsened, and 33.5% were unchanged. Of the patients with incontinence, 42% reported improved symptoms.

A large series reported by Kim et al. [16] reviewed the University of Minnesota experience in the management of complete rectal prolapse. They retrospectively reviewed 372 patients from 1976 to 1994 with a mean follow-up of 98 months who underwent resection rectopexy (RR) or PRS. They were able to locate only 49% in follow-up for evaluation of functional results and found that there was no significant difference in morbidity between the two approaches (14% vs. 20%). Thirty percent of the RR group had medical problems as opposed to 61% of the perineal group, indicating a lower health status in the PRS group. The most common complication reported was small-bowel obstruction. Perineal procedures had, as expected, a higher recurrence rate of 16% vs. 5%. Recurrences were noted to be the highest in the age groups of patients younger than 40 and older than 65 years, and most recurrences were noted within 3 years. Functional improvement was not significantly different between the two groups. Improvement in continence was 55% and 53%, respectively, for RR and PRS, and improvement in constipation was 43% overall. The authors further made the assertion that perineal repair may be preferable in specific populations, even though high recurrence rates occur. They also suggested that young men might be good candidates for PRS secondary to nerve-injury risk and older age groups due to coexisting morbidities.

The first 7 years of the Cleveland Clinic Florida experience was reviewed in 1997 with an analysis of three perineal procedures for the treatment of rectal prolapse [17]. Sixty-one patients who underwent Delorme, PRS, or PRS with levatorplasty between 1988 and 1995 were assessed, and their outcomes evaluated at a median of

24–29 months' follow-up. No difference was found in mean squeeze and resting pressures, capacity, or sensitivity. Concomitant levatorplasty was associated with significant improvement in postoperative continence. The study concluded that PRS with levatorplasty has an acceptably low morbidity rate and results in lower recurrence and better short-term functional outcome when compared with Delorme or PRS alone. Several other investigators confirmed improved continence when levatorplasty was added to PRS [18, 19].

Conclusion

The surgical management of rectal prolapse is complex and best tailored to the individual patient. This assertion seems to be realized in a recent meta-analysis by Bachoo et al. [20] in that there was insufficient evidence to determine which approach had the best outcomes. Certainly, there is no procedural panacea, as the heterogeneity of patients who present with rectal prolapse must be emphasized in determining which of the surgical approaches will lead to improved functional outcome with the minimal associated morbidity. Future developments in the area of minimal-access surgery have challenged some of the established paradigms in limiting higher-risk patients to perineal procedures over abdominal rectopexy, but further study must be undertaken to determine the long-term durability of these minimally invasive approaches.

References

1. Jorge JM, Wexner SD (1993) Etiology and management of fecal incontinence. Dis Colon Rectum 36:76–97
2. Broden B, Snellman B (1968) Procidentia of the rectum studied with cineradiography: a contribution to the discussion of causative mechanism. Dis Colon Rectum 11:330–347
3. Parks AG, Porter NH, Hardcastle J (1966) The syndrome of the descending perineum. Proc R Soc Med 59:477–482
4. Kiff ES, Barnes PRH, Swash M (1984) Evidence of pudendal neuropathy in patients with perineal descent and chronic straining at stool. Gut 25:1279–1282
5. Fazio VW (2005) Current therapy in colon and rectal surgery. Mosby, Philadelphia, pp 131–134
6. Birnbaum EH, Stamm L, Rafferty JF (1996) Pudendal nerve terminal motor latency influences surgical outcome in treatment of rectal prolapse. Dis Colon Rectum 39(11):1215–1221
7. Matheson DM, Keighley MR (1981) Manometric evaluation of rectal prolapse and faecal incontinence. Gut 22:126–129
8. Glasgow SC, Birnbaum EH et al (2006) Preoperative anal manometry predicts continence after perineal proctectomy for rectal prolapse. Dis Colon Rectum 49:1052–1058
9. Williams JG, Wong WD, Jensen L et al (1999) Incontinence and rectal prolapse: a prospective manometric study. Dis Colon Rectum 34:209–216
10. Delorme E (1985) On the treatment of total prolapse of the rectum by excision of the rectal mucous membranes or rectocolic. Dis Colon Rectum 28:544–553
11. Altemeier WA, Culbertson WR, Schowengerdt C, Hunt J (1971) Nineteen years' experience with the one-stage perineal repair of rectal prolapse. Ann Sur 173:993–1006
12. Tsunoda A, Yasuda N, Yokoyama N et al (2003) Delorme's procedure for rectal prolapse: clinical and physiological analysis. Dis Colon Rectum 46:1260–1265
13. Senapati A, Nicholls RJ, Thompson JP, Phillips RK (1994) Results of Delorme's procedure for rectal prolapse. Dis Colon Rectum 37:456–460
14. Raftopoulos Y, Senagore AJ, Di Giuro G et al (2005) Recurrence rates after abdominal surgery for complete rectal prolapse: a multicenter pooled analysis of 643 individual patient data. Dis Colon Rectum 48: 1200–1206
15. Marchal F, Bresler L, Ayav A et al (2005) Long-term results of Delorme's procedure and Orr-Loygue rectopexy to treat complete rectal prolapse. Dis Colon Rectum 48:1785–1790
16. Kim DS, Tsang CB, Wong WD et al (1999) Complete Rectal Prolapse: Evolution of Management and Results. Dis Colon Rectum 42:460–469
17. Agachan F, Reissman P, Pfeifer J et al (1997) Comparison of three perineal procedures for the treatment of rectal prolapse. South Med J 90:925–932
18. Prasad Ml, Pearl RK, Abcarian H et al (1986) Perineal proctectomy, posterior rectopexy, and postanal levator repair for the treatment of rectal prolapse. Diseases of the Colon and Rectum 29:547–552
19. Pescatori M, Interisano A et al (1998) Delorme's operation and sphincteroplasty for rectal prolapse and fecal incontinence. Int J Colorect Dis 13:223–227
20. Bachoo P, Brazelli M, Grant A (2000) Surgery for complete rectal prolapse in adults. Cochrane Database Syst Rev CD001758

14 Surgical Treatment of Rectal Prolapse: Rectopexy without Mesh

Roberto Bergamaschi, Michael Fealk

Introduction

More than 150 years have elapsed since the first report on full-thickness rectal prolapse (FTRP) surgery appeared in the literature [1]. Yet, no adequately powered randomized trials have been published on surgical treatment of FTRP. The title of this chapter emphasizes how rectopexy can be performed *without* a mesh rather than affirming that it can be done *with* sutures. This chapter represents a current opinion on the impact that suture rectopexy may have on the outcomes of care of FTRP; however, the chapter provides no systematic review of the evidence available in the literature. The objective is to present a concise insight on surgical technique, the authors' personal experience, and an overview of the literature dealing with this specific subject.

Surgical Technique

Rectal mobilization with suture rectopexy to repair FTRP is an abdominal procedure that can be performed via an open or laparoscopic approach. The procedure involves mobilization of the rectum followed by suture fixation of the rectum to the sacral promontory, restoring the anatomic position of the rectum. The goal of the procedure is to control the prolapse and prevent impaired evacuation.

Preoperative Preparation

The day prior to the planned surgical intervention, the patient should be limited to a clear diet. It is the authors' preference to administer a bowel preparation the day before surgery. The patient is instructed to take nothing by mouth as of midnight the night before surgery and to evacuate the rectum with an enema prior to traveling to the hospital.

Preoperatively, the patient should receive intravenous fluids, as the bowel preparation often contributes to dehydration. Antibiotics should be administered prior to the planned incision. The patient is identified, the proposed procedure is confirmed, and the patient is transported to the operation room.

Suture Rectopexy

General endotracheal anesthesia is administered by the anesthesiology department. After placement of a Foley catheter, the patient is positioned in the lithotomy position. If the rectum is prolapsed, it should be reduced prior to beginning the procedure. The patient is then prepped and draped in the usual sterile fashion. A lower midline incision from just below the umbilicus to the pubic tubercle is used for access. The opened peritoneum is secured to the fascia or the dermis with an 0-chromic suture to enhance exposure. It is the authors' practice to provide additional exposure with a Wexler retractor. The small bowel and omentum are retracted into the upper abdominal cavity.

A moist laparotomy pad is used to grasp and lift the rectosigmoid colon. We prefer a lateral to medial approach. Lateral attachments are taken down with electrocautery. The sigmoid mesentery is dissected away from the peritoneal reflection along the white line of Toldt. The dissection is kept close to the mesentery and directed toward the midline. Identification of the sigmoid fossa facilitates identification of the left ureter. The left ureter should be identified during the dissection.

Palpation of the iliac bifurcation as well as visualization of the gonadal vessels will facilitate this identification. The peritoneum should be opened into the pelvic sulcus toward the pouch of Douglas. This will define the extent of the lateral dissection.

Medial dissection is begun above the level of the sacral promontory. The peritoneum is divided at least 2 cm from the rectum in order to create peritoneal "wings" to be used for pexy. The peritoneum of the sigmoid mesentery is opened and connected with the lateral dissection just posterior to the inferior mesenteric pedicle, which is elevated as the rectosigmoid colon is maintained on stretch. The inferior mesenteric pedicle is palpable but will not be divided during this procedure. The medial peritoneal dissection is extended over the sacral promontory along the sulcus toward the pouch of Douglas to mirror the lateral dissection.

The posterior dissection is the most important portion of the procedure. At the level of the sacral promontory, the hypogastric nerves are amenable to injury. To avoid such an injury, the dissection is kept close to the fascia propria of the rectum. The sigmoid and rectum are continued to be lifted into the incision. Appropriate tension is of paramount importance. This dissection is often facilitated by the abnormal lack of fixation in this area that has contributed to the prolapse. The presacral fascia and hypogastric nerves should remain away from the area of dissection. As the dissection proceeds into the pelvis, the use of a St. Mark's retractor is helpful. It is important to be mindful of the presacral vessels as the dissection approaches the pelvic floor. As the levator ani muscles become visible/palpable, the rectum becomes parallel to the pelvic floor, and the angle of dissection should be adjusted to avoid injury to the presacral vessels. Difficult bleeding may occur if these vessels are inadvertently injured. The posterior dissection is completed to the level of the coccyx. The lateral dissection should spare the lateral stalks (ligaments). Attention to meticulous hemostasis facilitates the procedure. The rectum is lifted toward the incision, and a point is selected for the rectopexy. The rectum should not be placed on tension, but the prolapse defect should be reduced. Permanent silk sutures are secured to the right and left sacral promontory. The sites of sutures on the promontory are lateral to the hypogastric nerves and medial to the ureter on both sides of the rectum (Fig. 1) [2]. Attention to the position of the hypogastric nerves and the presacral vessels guides suture placement. The surgi-

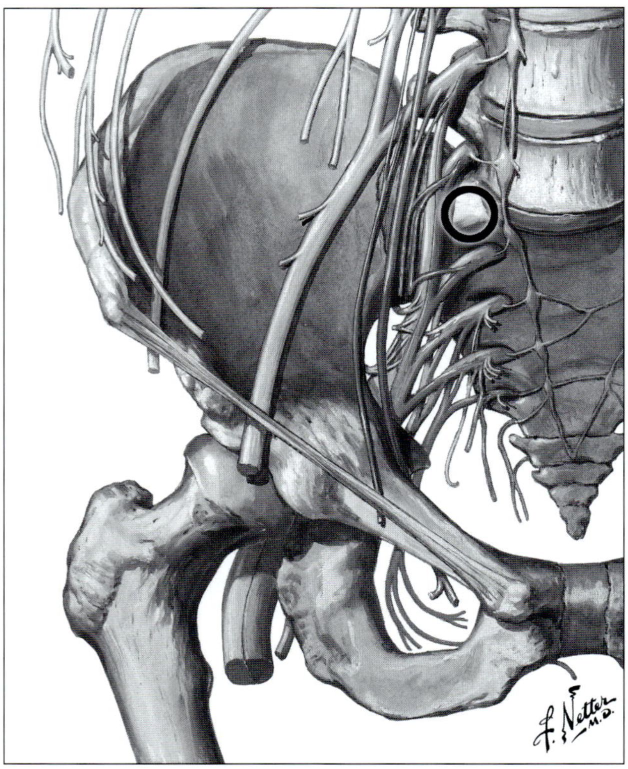

Fig. 1
Suture sites on the promontory are lateral to the hypogastric nerves and medial to the ureter on both sides of the rectum indicated by *circle*. Reprinted with permission from [2]

cal assistant maintains the anatomic position of the rectum while the surgeon secures the two previously placed sutures to the peritoneal wings.

Once the mobilization and rectopexy are complete, hemostasis should be reaffirmed. The pelvis is irrigated with saline. There should be no reason to place a drain in the pelvis. The peritoneum is approximated anteriorly with a running 0-chromic suture. The fascia is then closed in a running fashion, and the skin edges are approximated with interrupted 2-0 nylon sutures with vertical mattress-type stitches. The wound is cleaned and dressed, and the patient is extubated and taken to recovery. The Foley catheter should be left in place, but the oral–gastric tube may be discontinued.

Postoperative Considerations

Postoperatively, the usual considerations are addressed. Early activity and incentive spirometry are encouraged. Pain is initially controlled with intravenous narcotics and ketorolac. Diet is advanced with return of bowel function, and the intravenous narcotics are transitioned to oral formulations. The Foley catheter can be removed on the first postoperative day unless other comorbidities are present.

Upon discharge, the patient is instructed to avoid heavy lifting. Dietary goals should be addressed. Avoidance of constipation or overly loose stool should be discussed. The patient should be seen in the office within 1–2 weeks of discharge. Continued follow-up will assist the surgeon in his or her evaluation of the success of the repair.

Authors' Personal Experience

Treatment Algorithm

Patients with FTRP are a heterogeneous group with a variety of additional symptoms. Hence, a single treatment would not be appropriate [3], and treatment options should be selected. The first step of the algorithm is to evaluate the risk of death for a specific individual undergoing surgery. This evaluation should be based on the colorectal Physiologic and Operative Severity Score for the enUMeration of Mortality and Morbidity (POSSUM) score [4] rather than on the American Society of Anesthesiologists (ASA) score. Actually, the colorectal POSSUM score can be quickly evaluated online [5] by entering four physiological and four operative data points. If the patient is unfit for abdominal surgery in general anesthesia, a perineal procedure in spinal anesthesia should be offered. All patients fit for general anesthesia should be offered an abdominal procedure regardless of chronological age. One exception to this rule is the occasional male patient with true FTRP. The risk of iatrogenic hypogastric nerve injury and resulting impotence in abdominal surgery should be thoroughly explained to male patients. The advantages and disadvantages of perineal procedures must be considered individually on a case-by-case basis. There are four risk areas of autonomic nerve damage during rectal dissection [6]. Damage to the sympathetic nerves may occur while dissecting the inferior mesenteric artery and during posterior rectal mobilization at the promontory close to the hypogastric nerves. Damage to the parasympathetic nerves may occur during lateral stalk dissection of the rectum and the anterior rectal mobilization from the seminal vesicles and prostate.

The second step of the algorithm is to evaluate which abdominal procedure is most suitable for the patient. The two abdominal procedures to be considered are suture rectopexy or sigmoid resection. Sigmoid resection is beneficial in patients with documented constipation that is supported by clustering of radiopaque markers in the sigmoid colon on colon transit study. Sigmoid resection should be strictly avoided in patients with incontinence. If resection is indicated, the superior rectal artery should be spared [7]. Preserving blood supply to a long rectal stump may, in fact, minimize the risk of anastomotic leak. Avoiding dissection of the inferior mesenteric artery is particularly relevant in male patients undergoing resection for rectal prolapse due to potential damage to the sympathetic nerves.

Results

Outcomes for patients who underwent rectopexy for FTRP between 1992 and 2002 were reviewed. Rectal prolapse was defined as external FTRP. Recurrence was defined as the occurrence of FTRP after surgery. Rectopexy consisted of mobilization

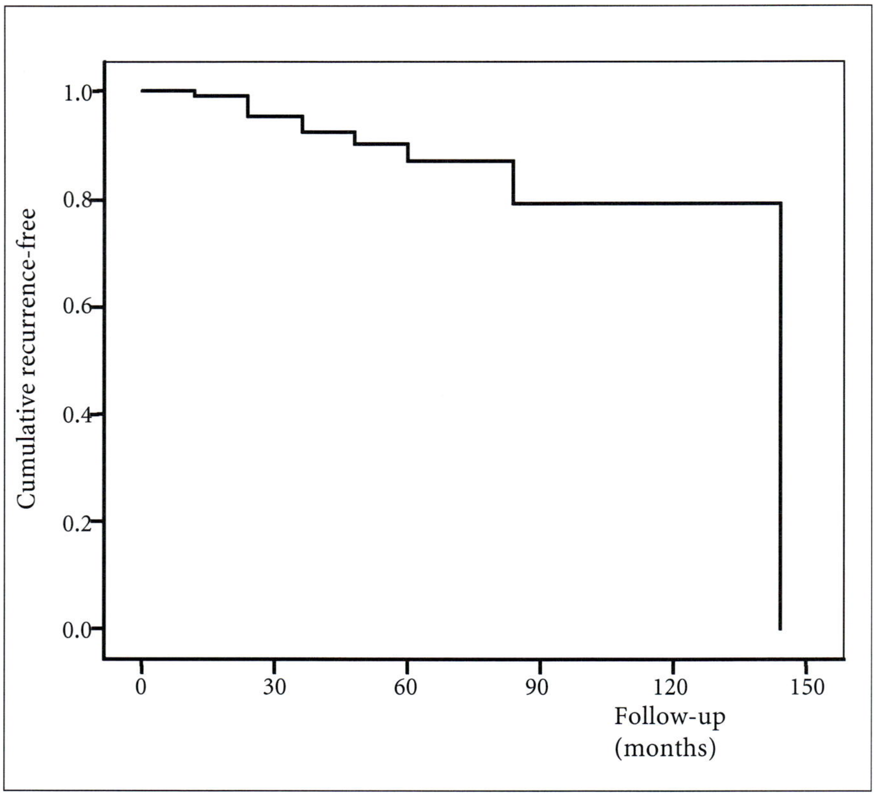

Fig. 2
Recurrence-free rates comparing suture rectopexy

of the rectum and suture rectopexy. There were 179 patients, with a median age of 62 (range 15–93) years. There were 154 females and 25 males. One hundred and thirty-eight patients underwent rectopexy, whereas 41 patients had a resection in addition to rectopexy. There were no deaths. Thirty-day complications occurred in seven patients (4%) and included pneumonia (n=1), urinary tract infection (n=2), urinary retention (n=1), wound infection (n=1), and left ureter partial injury (n=1). Seven patients (3.9%) were lost to follow-up; 172 patients (96%) were available at a median follow-up of 15.5 (range 1–132) months, and ten patients had a recurrence (5.8%) (Fig. 2).

Overview of the Literature

Controversies have not yet been resolved as to which step of the abdominal surgery for FTRP contributes the most to the containment of recurrence rates. Although the addition of rectopexy to mobilization of the rectum is supposed to decrease recurrences, there is presently no evidence to support this claim [8]. Moreover, the additional rectopexy may have disadvantages, including added operating time, foreign material implant, bleeding from sacral veins, and nerve injury of the presacral plexus. On the other hand, literature data on rectal mobilization only (without rectopexy) are very limited as long as data on resection are not taken into account. A series of 13 patients undergoing rectal mobilization only for FTRP had a 15% recurrence rate during a median follow-up of 1.09 (range 0.39–1.88) years [9]. Furthermore, published recurrence rates are often unreliable. In a recent meta-analysis on individual patient data, published recurrence rates differed by as much as 47% from recurrence rates re-estimated by actuarial analysis [10]. Therefore, a randomized controlled trial has been started to evaluate whether the addition of rectopexy to mobilization of the rectum significantly decreases recurrence rates. At the writing of this chapter, 193 of 251 patients were enrolled (personal communication).

Suture rectopexy was first described by Daher Cutait in 1959 [11]. The rationale of using sutures has been to keep the rectum in its new position to allow its eventual fixation to the sacrum by scar tissue [12]. A few technical details about the surgical technique of suture rectopexy require particular attention: Most authors would suture the posterior mesorectum to the presacral fascia [12–14]. Others would also include a partial thickness of the posterior rectum [12]. We prefer to suture the right and left peritoneal flaps to the presacral fascia. We agree with some authors [14] that the sutures may be placed on the sacral promontory. The exact location on the promontory is lateral to the hypogastric nerves and medial to the ureter on both sides of the rectum (Fig. 1). Alternative sites on the sacrum below the promontory have been suggested (Fig. 3). Most authors would agree that two sutures are adequate [12, 14].

We concur with the literature suggesting that rectopexy is as effective with sutures as with mesh [7, 15, 16]. A multicenter pooled analysis of 643 patients showed no difference in recurrence rates between suture rectopexy and mesh rectopexy [16] (Fig. 4). This leads to the question of whether mesh should be used at all, as it may increase postoperative constipation rates, and also carries the potential risk of infection [17].

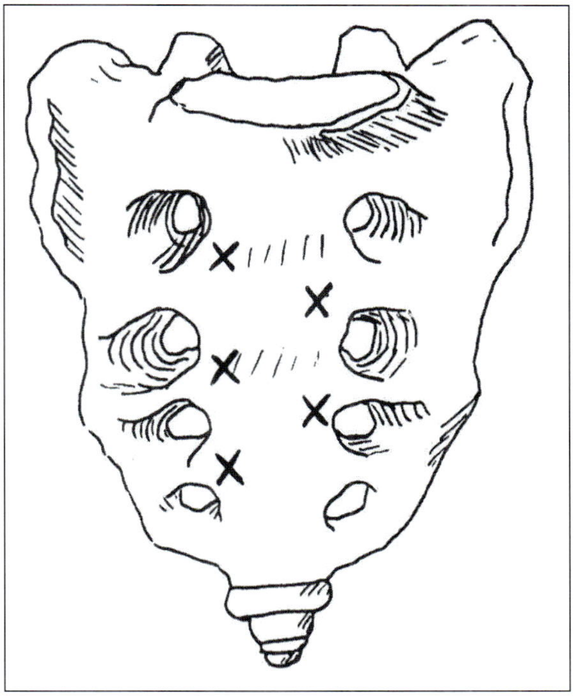

Fig. 3
Schematic diagram of the sacrum with the suture sites indicated with crosses. Reprinted with permission from [13]

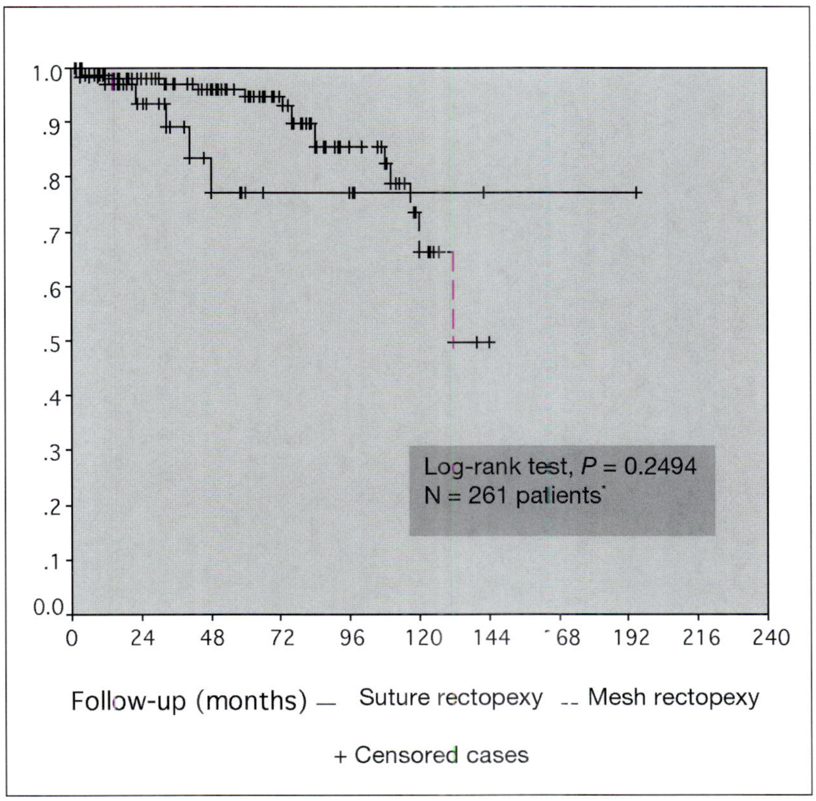

Fig. 4
Recurrence-free rates comparing suture rectopexy to mesh rectopexy. Reprinted with permission from [16]

References

1. Madoff RD, Mellgren A (1999) One hundred years of rectal prolapse surgery. Dis Colon Rectum 42:441–450
2. Frank H. Netter, Netter Images, http://www.netterimages.com
3. Brown AJ, Anderson JH (2004) Strategy for selection of type of operation for rectal prolapse based on clinical criteria. Dis Colon Rectum 47:103–107
4. Vather R, Zargar-Shoshtari K, Adegbola S, Hill AG (2006) Comparison of the possum, P-POSSUM and Cr-POSSUM scoring systems as predictors of postoperative mortality in patients undergoing major colorectal surgery. ANZ J Surg 76:812–816
5. Risk Prediction in Surgery (2007). http://www.riskprediction.org.uk/index-cr.php. Cited 21 May 2007
6. Lindsey I, Mortensen NJ (2002) Iatrogenic impotence and rectal dissection. Br J Surg 89:1493–1494
7. Bergamaschi R, Lovvik K, Marvik R (2003) Preserving the superior rectal artery in laparoscopic sigmoid resection for complete rectal prolapse. Surg Laparosc Endosc Percutan Tech 13:374–376
8. Bachoo P, Brazzelli M, Grant A (2000) Surgery for complete rectal prolapse in adults. Cochrane Database Syst Rev 2:CD001758
9. Nelson R, Spitz J, Pearl RK, Abcarian H (2001) What role does full rectal mobilization alone play in the treatment of rectal prolapse? Tech Coloproctol 5:33–35
10. DiGiuro G, Ignjatovic D, Brogger J, Bergamaschi R Rectal Prolapse Recurrence Study Group (2006) How accurate are published recurrence rates after rectal prolapse surgery? A meta-analysis of individual patient data. Am J Surg 191:773–778
11. Cutait D (1959) Sacro-promontory fixation of the rectum for complete prolapse. J R Soc Med 52(Suppl):105
12. Khanna AK, Misra MK, Kumar K (1996) Simplified sutured sacral rectopexy for complete rectal prolapse in adults. Eur J Surg 162:143–146
13. Graf W, Stefansson T, Arvidsson D, Pahlman L (1995) Laparoscopic suture rectopexy. Dis Colon Rectum 38:211–212
14. Heah SM, Hartley JE, Hurley J et al (2000) Laparoscopic suture rectopexy without resection is effective treatment for full-thickness rectal prolapse. Dis Colon Rectum 43:638–643
15. Duthie GS, Bartolo DC (1992) Abdominal rectopexy for rectal prolapse: a comparison of techniques. Br J Surg 79:107–113
16. Raftopoulos Y, Senagore AJ, Di Giuro G, Bergamaschi R (2005) Rectal Prolapse Recurrence Study Group. Recurrence rates after abdominal surgery for complete rectal prolapse: a multicenter pooled analysis of 643 individual patient data. Dis Colon Rectum 48:1200–1206
17. Sayfan J, Pinho M, Alexander-Williams J, Keighley MR (1990) Sutured posterior abdominal rectopexy with sigmoidectomy compared with Marlex rectopexy for rectal prolapse. Br J Surg 7:143–145

15 Mesh Rectopexy: The Wells Technique

Andrew P. Zbar

Introduction

Rectal prolapse as a clinical entity is still relatively poorly characterised [1], with a comparatively poor understanding of its complex physiology and pathogenesis [2–5]. It is well recognised that as more than 120 different types of surgical procedures have been described (and championed) for its treatment, there is currently no definitive surgical operation that suits all cases and is associated with an acceptably low recurrence rate [6, 7]. In part, the operative approach is a measure of our understanding of the pathophysiology of the prolapse as well as an appreciation of the relative perioperative risk to patients many, of whom are elderly women. In the first instance, abdominal surgery aims to correct some of the attendant pathology, such as the deep peritoneal cul-de-sac, the enlarged levator hiatus and the attenuated rectal fixation. In the second instance, the decision is one between a perineal and an abdominal approach, which is somewhat dependent upon the extent of the prolapse, patient comorbidity and clinical presentation (associated constipation/incontinence). This latter point may in part be answered by the ongoing UK Prolapse Surgery: Perineal or Rectopexy (PROSPER) trial [8], although it is unlikely that this study will be truly randomised in an environment where perineal rectosigmoidectomy is uncommonly practised and where there will be limited prospective data pertaining to postoperative functional outcome. The move towards a selected laparoscopic rectopexy approach has somewhat broadened the use of abdominal rectopexy in some cases in which it previously may have been precluded by virtue of attendant comorbidity [9].

The abdominal approach in nonrandomised studies is generally accepted as being associated with lower full-thickness recurrence rates when compared with a range of perineal procedures [10, 11], although this has not yet been subjected to a prospective, randomised analysis [12, 13]. In the abdominal approach, prolapse control is achieved by plication of the rectal redundancy with presacral fixation. This can be achieved with or without prosthetic material, open or laparoscopic and with or without sigmoid resection. This operative strategy may or may not have an effect on postoperative continence and reported evacuatory difficulty, which in part has to do with the amount of rectal dissection (lateral ligament division or not) [14], the compliance of a neorectum if established [15, 16], postoperative pelvic sepsis [17] and the complex physiology and integrity of the sphincter apparatus when untreated prolapse is prolonged [2, 18–20].

Rationale for Wells and Wells Modified Rectopexy: Current Controversies

The original description by Wells in 1959 was of utilisation of a full rectal mobilisation with the insertion of prosthetic Ivalon (polyvinyl alcohol) sponge [21]. This approach (and prosthetic) became particularly popular in the UK and Australia as a posterior mesh rectopexy with sacral mesh fixation with acceptably low mortality and recurrence rates, which were less than 5% overall [22–24].

Technical Aspects of the Procedure and Complications

We routinely prepare the bowel and use three doses of a second-generation cephalosporin and metronidazole for this procedure. The rectum may be adequately approached through a Pfannenstiel incision, as the sigmoid is redundant, with the use either of general or epidural anaesthesia. Rectal mobilisation is carried out in the standard manner, extending to the level of the pelvic floor, with close dissection of the rectum at the level of the lateral ligaments, which we routinely proceed beyond. This is most easily performed in the mesorectal plane as for a nerve-preserving total mesorectal excision (TME). Anterior dissection is carried out through the fascia of Denonvilliers, although anterior dissection of the rectum is currently limited in its extent. In the Wells procedure, mesh is employed to the midsacrum with suturing to the presacral space by the use typically of four sutures of 2/0 Prolene. Great care must be made not to injure the presacral veins, which may be very troublesome and which may require a sterilised thumbtack or a muscle plug for tamponade[25–27]. This is best achieved by a midline suture to the presacral fascia, placing the other end of a double-needled suture into the mesorectum. In the Wells procedure, an adequate rectal window is provided by a <270° loose wrap, which admits the finger alongside the rectum between the viscus and the mesh. Latterly, we have only employed suture rectopexy after full rectal mobilisation by suturing the straightened rectum on the stretch to the lumbosacral fascia, taking care to avoid any middle sacral artery that may be present. This has avoided the problem of presacral haemorrhage. The pelvis is routinely drained. We have not employed ancillary procedures such as levator hiatus repair [24, 28]. In our opinion, variations in approach towards standard abdominal rectopexy should be considered for repair in men where full rectal dissection can be difficult. Where this is contemplated, a more limited anterior and lateral dissection is used, with nerve preservation if the patient is young because of the real risk of postoperative erectile dysfunction [29, 30]. The Wells procedure and nerve-preserving sutured sacrorectopexy are shown in Figures 1–3 [31]. If a resection rectopexy is to be employed, our current policy is not to use mesh, and the vasculature is ligated close to the sigmoid mesocolon so that should recurrence occur, it can be adequately treated by perineal rectosigmoidectomy in selected cases.

A specific concern regarding Ivalon sponge was the risk of deep-seated pelvic infection (2–16% of rectopexy cases), which tended to occur within the first 3 months following rectopexy, necessitating a

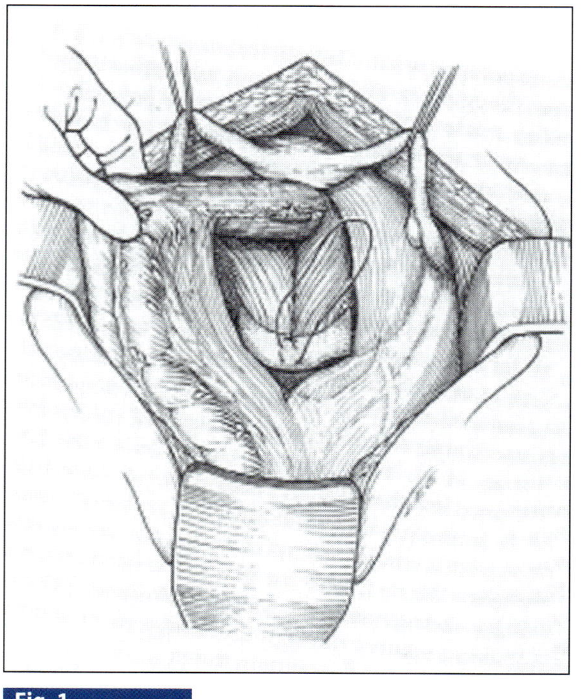

Fig. 1

Wells presacral mesh fixation. Reprinted from [31], with permission from Elsevier

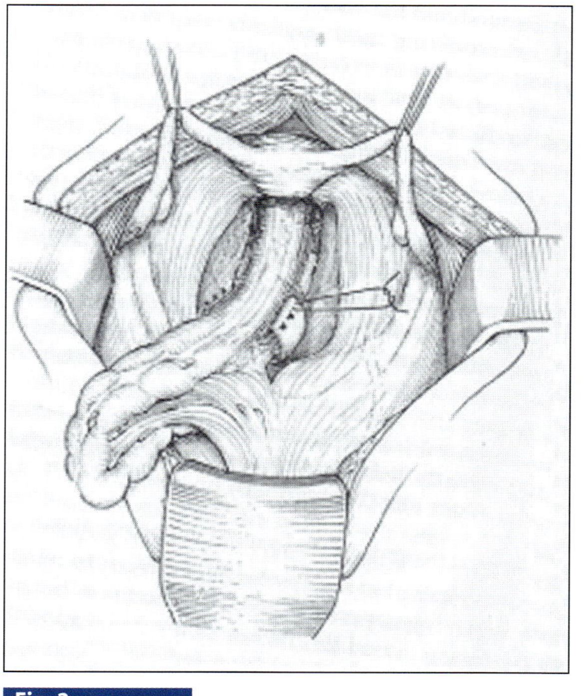

Fig. 2

Loose rectal wrap (<270° in rectal encirclement). Reprinted from [31], with permission from Elsevier generally difficult mesh removal procedure, although prolapse recurrence after mesh removal was uncommon [17, 32, 33]. This postoperative problem led to variant prosthetic use employing the same Wells-style technique of posterior rectopexy but using Marlex (knitted polypropylene) [34] Gore-Tex (Micromesh PTFE) [35], lyophilised dura [36], nylon strips [37], Teflon [38] and absorbable polyglycolic or polyglactin mesh [39, 40]. Each alternative mesh implant showed a generally lower severe pelvic sepsis rate [41–43]. Serious sepsis, which is uncommon using these alternative meshes, is significantly increased in resection rectopexy when compared with rectopexy alone [44, 45]. When prosthetic material is employed, Teflon (which is not widely available) holds sutures relatively well [46, 47], with Ivalon sponge becoming very hard to handle when wet and holding sutures comparatively poorly [22, 44, 48–51].

In the early days of mesh rectopexy, functional assessment showed an overall improvement in continence from 3% to 40% [52], an effect that appears independent of the level of rectal dissection (above or below the lateral ligaments), as well as whether the posterior Wells rectopexy or the complete Ripstein wrap is utilised [53]. Duration of procidentia, age at operation and length of incontinence history prior to rectopexy have not been shown to correlate with postoperative functional outcome when mesh rectopexy is employed [54].

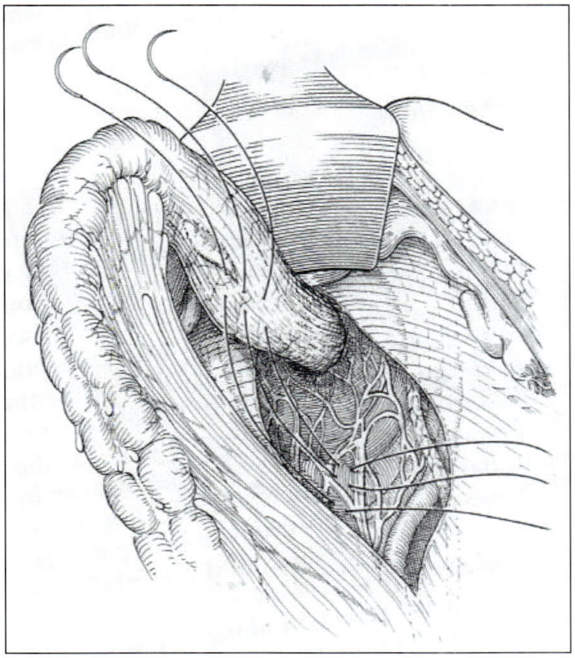

Fig. 3
Autonomic nerve-preserving sacrorectopexy (mesorectum not shown). Reprinted from [31], with permission from Elsevier

Despite an overall improvement in continence in many cases, there is a reported incidence of troublesome evacuatory difficulty following mesh rectopexy, some of which has been equated with distal lateral ligament division, a procedure that has been reported as a functional trade-off for reduced recurrence [55]. Despite the controversy in total mesorectal excision of the existence of a definitive lateral ligament [56, 57], the point is taken that the extent of rectal mobilisation may result in functional problems in rectal evacuation, probably consequent upon a local autonomic neuropathy independent of whether a neorectum is constructed with mesh in situ [58]. This more predictably occurs in patients presenting with rectal prolapse with incontinence [59] and may in part also result from an evacuatory block induced by the mobilisation (regardless of whether mesh is utilised) consequent upon a change in image-demonstrated rectal wall thickness and contour following extensive rectal dissection [52].

These effects appear not to be reflected in any demonstrable changes in rectal compliance following rectopexy [60], although studies of this type are somewhat limited. Rectal sensitivity in constipated postoperative cases after a Wells rectopexy with lateral ligament division is significantly dulled in comparison with patients undergoing a Ripstein procedure without lateral ligament division, an effect that can persist for more than a year following surgery [61, 62]. Concerns regarding the Ripstein procedure of the anterior sling versus the Wells operation of posterior partial fixation stem from reports that the Ripstein procedure has been associated with delayed fistula formation and perirectal stenosis in as much as 7% of cases [63, 64]. There are also concerns that in both prosthetic operations, retraction or poor fixation of the mesh may result in recurrence. This suggests that it is more the adequacy and security of the rectosacral fixation rather than the prosthetic that is of prime surgical importance [65]. Although some authors have found that rectoanal inhibition during rectal distension is similar before surgery in rectal prolapse patients when compared with age-matched controls [66], our group and others have shown that there is an exaggerated area under the inhibitory curve and a more rapid recovery of the rectoanal inhibitory reflex (RAIR), which mimics that of patients presenting with faecal incontinence from other causes [67–69]. We have previously suggested that a markedly attenuated RAIR in patients presenting with incontinence and full-thickness rectal prolapse may represent a contraindication to a perineal procedure, although this remains to be substantiated [70].

Some of these effects are clearly related to the radicality of rectal dissection, even in the absence of construction of a neorectum, where comparative studies assessing absorbable mesh rectopexy with resection rectopexy (the Frykman–Goldberg procedure) [71–73] in all patients presenting with rectal prolapse showed no difference in recurrence but substantially less constipation and less delayed colonic transit in the sigmoidectomy group [58, 73]. Sigmoidectomy combined with rectopexy has become the procedure of choice in patients presenting with significant preoperative constipation and a redundant sigmoid colon [74], although this has more often been performed as a suture rectopexy without mesh deployment [75]. A few studies have combined mesh rectopexy with resection, where Lechaux and colleagues have shown in a small selected study that this approach is safe, particularly in young patients [76].

Given these caveats, the need for mesh has been questioned by those believing that sutured rectopexy alone (or in combination with sigmoidectomy) is able to provide all the advantages of extensive rectal dissection with rectosacral fixation but without the disadvantages of the presence of a foreign body. Following the original descriptive report of this operation by Cutait in 1959 [77], there does not presently appear to be any clear evidence to the contrary that the use of a foreign material evokes any greater fibrotic response than sutured rectopexy alone [63]. This simpler approach has been shown to be safe [78, 79], with the same reservations regarding the role of sigmoidectomy as discussed above for those patients in whom mesh is employed. However, there is some evidence to suggest that female patients presenting with incontinence and prolapse have no improvement of incontinence where sutured rectopexy alone is used [80]. Alternatives to these approaches include the use of anterior resection alone, which-although familiar as a procedure to all colorectal surgeons-has a less predictable effect on postoperative continence [81]. Others have advocated as part of abdominal rectopexy omental support below the sacral fixation to avoid the use of mesh [82] as well as a combined nonmesh rectosacrocolpopexy for patients presenting with a simultaneous rectal and vaginal vault prolapse following hysterectomy [83–85].

Laparoscopic Wells-Style Rectopexy

The laparoscopic approach reproduces the open abdominal operation but with substantially less morbidity (and mortality), approaching that achieved with perineal procedures in elderly frail patients. The standard contraindications to laparoscopic access apply, and the proposed advantages of these approaches are those of other laparoscopic procedures, including shorter hospital stay, improved cosmesis and less postoperative pain. The laparoscopic procedures are identical to those employed open, although there is a greater trend towards extensive rectal dissection with simple suture rectopexy [86–88]. Laparoscopic-assisted resection, however, is a safe procedure in patients presenting with significant preoperative constipation [89] and is performed in association with a Pfannenstiel incision for specimen delivery and for access to any troublesome presacral veins should bleeding occur. Extraction via a left lower quadrant or umbilical incision can permit a wholly laparoscopic anastomosis to be performed [90]. Variants of laparoscopic rectopexy have been compared in randomised studies with the matched open rectopexy approach [91–93], which has shown a mortality varying between 0% and 3% and a recurrence rate equivalent to that of open procedures variably, reported at between 0% and 10% overall [94–96] after both medium-term follow-up out to 3 years [97, 98] or in one study by Kariv and colleagues, with long-term follow-up out to 60 months [99]. This latter study showed equivalent results between open and laparoscopic surgery in which the latter employed equal randomisation between suture and suture/resection rectopexy.

Functional outcomes for patients appear in both nonrandomised institutional [86–89, 95] and randomised [91–94, 99] studies to be equivalent with those of similar open surgeries. Summary of these studies shows overall improvement in faecal incontinence in up to three quarters of patients [86, 100] and a reduced incidence of troublesome constipation after resection when performed as a laparoscopic-assisted procedure [101]. In this latter study by Benoist and colleagues, the addition of laparoscopic-assisted resection was safe; however, the use of mesh insertion laparoscopically in a small number of cases conferred no advantage over simple suture rectopexy [101]. A recent meta-analysis combining data from six studies comparing laparoscopic with open rectopexy by Purkayastha et al. [102] showed that the laparoscopic approach took longer to perform, although there was an average of 3.5 fewer hospital stay days in the laparoscopic group, with a similar morbidity between the groups. Recurrence rates were equivalent, although in general, the follow-up periods were short, ranging from 12–31 months. Modifications of these laparoscopic approaches have included the use of sutureless stapled techniques for promontory fixation [103], limited spike mesh fixation [104], harmonic scalpel rectal dissection with endosuture fixation [105], DaVinci robotic-assisted rectopexy and resection rectopexy [106] and ventral-nerve-sparing rectopexy as a laparoscopic alternative for rectal prolapse presenting with severe constipation [107, 108]. In general, all procedures that have been described for open surgery have been adapted to the laparoscopic approach, with equivalent mortality and morbidity and similar functional effects and recurrence rates, although with substantially reduced hospital stay when laparoscopy is employed [109, 110]. The present accreditation process for laparoscopic surgeons training in rectal surgery is still nonuniform, but for the surgeon interested in this approach, rectal prolapse is an ideal starting point to acquire laparoscopic rectal dissection expertise given the relative width of the pelvis and the attenuation of the rectal structures.

Conclusion

Although the Wells procedure (as originally described) is safe and successful in terms of improvement of bowel function and acceptably low recurrence rates on prolonged follow-up, there seems little to commend the routine use of mesh (even when absorbable) over simple suture rectopexy after full rectal mobilisation. The extent of rectal dissection (whether or not to divide the lateral ligaments) seems moot if significant constipation is a preoperative symptom with inherently slow colonic transit, where a resection rectopexy is advocated in accordance with the recommendations of Frykman and Goldberg. Moreover, there would seem minimal advantage in laparoscopic-guided surgery (either over open surgery or between laparoscopic-assisted procedures), as the open procedure can be performed under spinal anaesthesia, with equivalent perioperative mortality and morbidity in selected cases to the laparoscopic surgeries so far reported [111]. Cost–benefit analysis for the laparoscopic approach is currently lacking, with the likelihood that short-term costs will be higher than with open procedures. A definitive comment concerning longer-term cost–benefit is difficult to predict, as the late recurrence rates are unknown, as are the readmission rates from adhesive obstruction. The operative decision by the colorectal surgeon will be based individually on preoperative extent of constipation, damage to the anal sphincter induced by prolonged untreated full-thickness prolapse, overall performance status of the patient and list of their comorbidities, patient gender, any significant prior history of pelvic surgery or sepsis that may preclude a laparoscopic approach, body habitus, patient/surgeon preferences and operative expertise. The call for controlled randomised surgical trials has been made extensively in the literature for the treatment of full-thickness rectal prolapse. However, given the average surgical volume even in experienced and active colorectal units, many of the important questions that might reasonably be expected to influence the operative procedure may well still be unable to be answered by such trials.

References

1. Pescatori M, Quondamcarlo C (1999) A new grading of rectal internal mucosal prolapse and its correlation with diagnosis and treatment. Int J Colorect Dis 14:245–249
2. Zbar AP, Takashima S, Hasegawa T, Kitabayashi K (2002) Perineal rectosigmoidectomy (Altemeier's procedure): a review of physiology, technique and outcome. Tech Coloproctol 6:109–116

3. Moschcowitz AV (1912) The pathogenesis, anatomy and cure of prolapse of the rectum. Surg Gynecol Obstet 15:7–21
4. Broden B, Snellman B (1968) Procidentia of the rectum studied by cineradiography. Dis Colon Rectum 11:330–347
5. Pantowitz D, Levine E (1975) The mechanism of rectal prolapse. S Afr J Surg 13:53–56
6. Jacobs LK, Lin YJ, Orkin BA (1997) The best operation for rectal prolapse. Surg Clin N Am 77:49–70
7. Steele SR, Goetz LH, Minami S et al (2006) Management of recurrent rectal prolapse: surgical approach influences outcome. Dis Colon Rectum 49:440–445
8. PROSPER – (PROlapse Surgery: PErineal or Rectopexy) Randomised Trial of Rectal Prolapse Surgery. http://www.prosper.bham.ac.uk. Cited 2 Jul 2007
9. Himpens J, Cadiere GB, Bruyns J, Vertruyen M (1999) laparoscopic rectopexy according to Wells. Surg Endosc 13:139–141
10. Aitola PT, Hiltunen KM, Matikainen MJ (1999) Functional results of operative treatment of rectal prolapse over an 11-year period: emphasis on transabdominal approach. Dis Colon Rectum 42:655–660
11. Raftopoulos Y, Senagore AJ, Di Giuro G, Bergamaschi R (2005) Rectal Prolapse Recurrence Study Group. Dis Colon Rectum 48:1200–1206
12. Bachoo P, Brazzelli M, Grant A (2000) Surgery for complete rectal prolapse in adults. Cochrane Database Syst Rev CD001758
13. Madiba TE, Baig MK, Wexner SD (2005) Surgical management of rectal prolapse. Arch Surg 140:63–73
14. Speakman CT, Madden MV, Nicholls RJ, Kamm MA (1991) Lateral ligament division during rectopexy causes constipation but prevents recurrence: results of a prospective randomized study. Br J Surg 78:1431–1433
15. Solla JA, Rothenberger DA, Goldberg SM (1989) Colonic resection in the treatment of complete rectal prolapse. Neth J Surg 41:132–135
16. Cirocco WC, Brown AC (1993) Anterior resection for the treatment of rectal prolapse: a 20-year experience. Am Surg 59:265–269
17. Ross AH, Thompson JP (1989) Management of infection after prosthetic abdominal rectopexy (Wells procedure). Br J Surg 76:610–612
18. Yoshioka K, Hyland G, Keighley MRB (1989) Anorectal function after abdominal rectopexy: parameters of predictive value in identifying return of continence. Br J Surg 76:63–64
19. Sainio AP, Voutilainen PR, Husa AT (1991) Recovery of anal sphincter function following transabdominal repair of rectal prolapse: cause of improved continence? Dis Colon Rectum 34:816–821
20. Hiltunen KM, Matikainen M (1992) Improvement of continence after abdominal rectopexy for rectal prolapse. Int J Colorect Dis 7:8–10
21. Wells C (1959) New operation for rectal prolapse. Proc R Soc Med 52:602–603
22. Morgan CN, Porter NH, Klugman DJ (1972) Ivalon sponge in repair of complete rectal prolapse. Br J Surg 59:841–846
23. Boutsis C, Ellis H (1974) The Ivalon-sponge-wrap operation for rectal prolapse: an experience of 26 patients. Dis Colon Rectum 17:21–37
24. Mann CV, Hoffman C (1988) Complete rectal prolapse: the anatomical and functional results of treatment by an extended abdominal rectopexy. Br J Surg 75:34–37
25. Lucarotti ME, Armstrong CP, Bartolo DCC (1991) Control of presacral bleeding in rectal surgery. Ann Roy Coll Surg Engl 73:289–190
26. Stolfi VM, Missom JW, Lavery IC et al (1992) Newly designed occluder pin for presacral hemorrhage. Dis Colon Rectum 35:166–169
27. Arnaud JP, Tuech JJ, Pessaux P (2000) Management of presacral venous bleeding with the use of thumbtacks. Dig Surg 17:651–652
28. Graham RR (1942) The operative repair of massive rectal prolapse. Ann Surg 115:1007–1012
29. Abou-Enein A (1978) Prolapse of the rectum in young men: treatment with a modified Roscoe Graham operation. Dis Colon Rectum 22:117–119
30. Aluwihare AP (1987) Rectal prolapse in young adults. Ann Acad Med Singapore 16:527–528
31. Keighley MRB, Williams NS (1993) Surgery of the anus, rectum and colon. WB Saunders, London, pp. 710–711
32. Lake SP, Hancock BD, Lewis AA (1984) Management of pelvic sepsis after Ivalon rectopexy. Dis Colon Rectum 27:589–590
33. Wedell J, Schlageter M, Meier zu Eissen P et al (1987) Die problematiek der pelvinen sepsis nach rectopexie mittels kunstoff unde ihre behandlung. Chirurg 58:423–427
34. Keighley MR, Fielding JW, Alexander-Williams J (1983) Results of Marlex mesh abdominal rectopexy for rectal prolapse in 100 consecutive patients. Br J Surg 70:229–232
35. Cicconi M, Romanelli P, Cardelli M et al (2003) Abdominal Wells rectopexy with patch micromesh PTFE (Goretex). G Chir 24:46–52
36. Schwemmel K, Hunger J (1973) Der ano-rektale Prolaps. Dtsch Med Wochenschr 98:1125–1129
37. Loygue J, Nordllinger B, Malafosse M et al (1984) Rectopexy to the promontory for the treatment of rectal prolapse: report of 257 cases. Dis Colon Rectum 27:356–359
38. Kuijpers JHC, De Morree H (1988) Towards a selection of the most appropriate procedure in the treatment of complete rectal prolapse. Dis Colon Rectum 31:355–357
39. Arndt M, Pircher W (1988) Absorbable mesh in the treatment of rectal prolapse. Int J Colorect Dis 3:141–143
40. Winde G, Reers B, Nottberg H et al (1993) Clinical and functional results of abdominal rectopexy with absorbable mesh-graft for treatment of complete rectal prolapse. Eur J Surg 159:301–305
41. Detry RJ, Vanheuverzwijn R, Mahieu P, Kestens PJ (1984) The use of prosthetic material in rectopexies. Int Surg 69:301–304
42. Athanasiadis S, Weyand G, Heiligers J et al (1996) The risk of infection of three synthetic materials used in rectopexy with or without colonic resection for rectal prolapse. Int J Colorect Dis 11:42–44
43. Galili Y, Rabau M (1997) Comparison of polyglycolic acid and polypropylene mesh for rectopexy in the treatment of rectal prolapse. Eur J Surg 163:445–448
44. Penfold JC, Hawley PR (1972) Experiences of Ivalon sponge implant for complete rectal prolapse at St.

Mark's Hospital. Br J Surg 59:846–848
45. Novell JR, Osborne MJ, Winslet MC, Lewis AA (1994) Prospective randomized trial of Ivalon sponge versus sutured rectopexy for full-thickness rectal prolapse. Br J Surg 81:904–906
46. Jurgeleit HC, Corman ML, Coller JA, Veidenheimer MC (1975) Procidentia of the rectum. Teflon sling repair of rectal prolapse. Lahey Clinic experience. Dis Colon Rectum 18:464–467
47. Lescher TJ, Corman ML, Coller J, Veidenheimer MC (1979) Management of late complications of Teflon sling repair for rectal prolapse. Dis Colon Rectum 23:445–467
48. Anderson JR, Kinninmonth AWG, Smith AR (1981) Polyvinyl alcohol sponge rectopexy for complete rectal prolapse. J Royal Coll Surg Edinb 26:292–294
49. Anderson JR, Wilson BG, Parks TG (1984) Complete rectal prolapse: the results of Ivalon sponge rectopexy. Postgrad Med J 60:411–414
50. Atkinson KG, Taylor DC (1984) Wells procedure for complete rectal prolapse: a ten year experience. Dis Colon rectum 27:96–98
51. Boulos PB, Stryker SJ, Nichols RJ (1984) The long-term results of polyvinyl alcohol, (Ivalon) sponge for rectal prolapse in young patients. Br J Surg 71:213–214
52. Allen-Mersh TG, Turner MJ, Mann CV (1990) Effect of abdominal Ivalon rectopexy on bowel habit and rectal wall. Dis Colon Rectum 33:550–553
53. Scaglia M, Fasth S, Hallgren T et al (1994) Abdominal rectopexy for rectal prolapse. Influence of surgical technique on functional outcome. Dis Colon Rectum 37:805–813
54. Winde G, Reers B, Holzgreve A et al (1993) Clinical and functional results of abdominal rectopexy using different fixation principles. Langenbecks Arch Chir 378:86–91
55. Mollen RM, Kuijpers HC, van Hoek F (2000) Effects of rectal mobilization and lateral ligaments division on colonic and anorectal function. Dis Colon Rectum 43:1283–1287
56. Pak-art R, Tansatit T, Mingmalairaks C et al (2005) The location and contents of the lateral ligaments of the rectum: a study in human soft cadavers. Dis Colon Rectum 48:1941–1944
57. Nano M, Lanfranco G, Dal Corso H et al (2000) The lateral ligaments of the rectum: myth or reality? Chir Ital 52:313–321
58. Sayfan J, Pinho M, Alexander-Williams J, Keighley MRB (1990) Sutured posterior abdominal rectopexy with sigmoidectomy compared with Marlex rectopexy. Br J Surg 77:143–145
59. Roig JV, Buch E, Alos R et al (1998) Anorectal function in patients with complete rectal prolapse. Differences between continent and incontinent individuals. Rev Esp Enferm Dig 90:794–805
60. Scaglia M, Delaini GG, Ribero F et al (1993) Variations in rectal capacity and compliance after abdominal rectopexy. Chir Ital 45:189–197
61. Scaglia M, Comotti F, Fornari M (1992) The functional and manometric-volumetric results following abdominal rectopexy for total rectal prolapse. Chir Ital 44:257–272
62. Scaglia M, Fasth S, Hallgren T (1994) Abdominal rectopexy for rectal prolapse. Influence of surgical technique on functional outcome. Dis Colon Rectum 37:805–813
63. Kuijpers HC (1992) Treatment of complete rectal prolapse: to narrow, to wrap, to suspend, to fix, to encircle, to plicate or to resect? World J Surg 16:826–830
64. Schultz I, Mellgren A. Dolk A et al (2000) Long-term results and functional outcome after Ripstein rectopexy. Dis Colon Rectum 43:35–43
65. Blatchford GJ, Perry RE, Thorson AG, Christensen MA (1989) Rectal prolapse: rational therapy without foreign material. Neth J Surg 41:126–128
66. Scaglia M, Delaini GG, Ribero F et al (1993) Evaluation of the sphincter function and rectal sensitivity in rectal prolapse associated with fecal incontinence. Chir Ital 45:124–131
67. Zbar AP, Aslam M, Gold DM et al (1998) Parameters of the rectoanal inhibitory reflex in patients with idiopathic fecal incontinence and chronic constipation. Dis Colon Rectum 41:200–208
68. Zbar AP, Aslam M, Hider A et al (1998) Comparison of vector volume manometry with conventional manometry in anorectal dysfunction. Techn Coloproctol 2:84–90
69. Kaur G, Gardiner A, Duthie GS (2002) Rectoanal reflex parameters in incontinence and constipation. Dis Colon Rectum 45:928–933
70. Zbar AP, Jonnalagadda R (2003) Parameters of the rectoanal inhibitory reflex in different anorectal disorders. Dis Colon Rectum 46:557–558
71. Frykman HM (1955) Abdominal proctopexy and primary sigmoid resection for rectal procidentia. Am J Surg 90:780–789
72. Frykman HM, Goldberg SM (1969) The surgical treatment of rectal procidentia. Surg Gynecol Obstet 129:1225–1230
73. Luukkonen P, Mikkonen U, Jarvinen H (1992) Abdominal rectopexy with sigmoidectomy vs. rectopexy alone for rectal prolapse: a prospective, randomized study. Int J Colorect Dis 7:219–222
74. Azimuddin K, Khuchandani IT, Rosen L et al (2001) Rectal prolapse: a search for the best operation. Am Surg 67:622–627
75. Huber FT, Stein H, Siewert JR (1995) Functional results after treatment of rectal prolapse with rectopexy and sigmoid resection. World J Surg 19:138–143
76. Lechaux JP, Atienza P, Goasguen N et al (2001) Prosthetic rectopexy to the pelvic floor and sigmoidectomy for rectal prolapse. Am J Surg 182:465–469
77. Cutait D (1959) Sacro-promontory fixation of the rectum for complete rectal prolapse. Proc Roy Soc Med 52(Suppl):105
78. Carter AE (1983) Rectosacral suture fixation for complete rectal prolapse in the elderly, the frail and the demented. Br J Surg 70:522–523
79. Ejerblad S, Krause U (1988) Repair of rectal prolapse by rectosacral suture fixation. Acta Chir Scand 154:103–105
80. Briel JW, Schouten WR, Boerma O (1997) Long-term results of suture rectopexy in patients with fecal incontinence associated with incomplete rectal prolapse. Dis Colon Rectum 40:1228–1232
81. Schlinkert RT, Beart RW, Wolff BG, Pemberton JH (1985) Anterior resection for complete rectal prolapse. Dis Colon Rectum 28:409–412

82. Di Giorgio A, Biacchi D, Sibio S et al (2005) Abdominal rectopexy for complete rectal prolapse: preliminary results of a new technique. Int J Colorect Dis 20:180–189
83. Zhioua F, Ferchiou M, Pira JM et al (1993) Uterine fixation to the promontory and the Orr–Loygue operation in the association of genital prolapse and rectal prolapse. Rev Fr Gynecol Obstet 88:277–281
84. Dekal A, Rabinerson D, Rafael ZB et al (2000) Concurrent genital and rectal prolapse: two pathologies – one joint operation. BJOG 107:125–129
85. Collopy BT, Barham KA (2002) Abdominal colporectopexy with pelvic cul-de-sac closure. Dis Colon Rectum 45:522–529
86. Kessler H, Jerby BL, Milssom JW (1999) Successful treatment of rectal prolapse by laparoscopic suture rectopexy. Surg Endosc 13:858–861
87. Kellokumpu IH, Virozen J, Scheinin T (2000) Laparoscopic repair of rectal prolapse: a prospective study evaluating surgical outcome and changes in symptoms and bowel function. Surg Endosc 14:634–640
88. Heah SM, Hartley J, Hurley J et al (2000) Laparoscopic suture rectopexy without resection is effective treatment for full-thickness rectal prolapse. Dis Colon Rectum 43:638–643
89. Sezai D, Demirbas S, Akin L et al (2005) The impact of laparoscopic resection rectopexy in patients with total rectal prolapse. Mil Med 170:743–747
90. Akbari RP, Read TE (2006) Laparoscopic rectal surgery: rectal cancer, pelvic pouch surgery and rectal prolapse. Surg Clin N Am 86:899–914
91. Boccasanta P, Venturi M, Reitano MC et al (1999) Laparotomic vs. laparoscopic rectopexy in complete rectal prolapse. Dig Surg 16:415–419
92. Solomon MJ, Young CJ, Eyers AA, Roberts RA (2002) Randomised clinical trial of laparoscopic versus open abdominal rectopexy for rectal prolapse. Br J Surg 89:35–39
93. Kairaluoma MV, Viljakka MT, Kellokumpu IH (2003) Open vs. laparoscopic surgery for rectal prolapse: a case-controlled study assessing short-term outcome. Dis Colon Rectum 46:353–360
94. Baker R, Senagore AJ, Luchtefeld MA (1995) Laparoscopic assisted vs. open resection: rectopexy offers excellent results. Dis Colon Rectum 38:199–201
95. Rose J, Schneider C, Scheidbach H et al (2002) Laparoscopic treatment of rectal prolapse: experience gained in a prospective multicenter study. Langenbecks Arch Surg 387:130–137
96. Demirbas S, Ogun I, Celenk T et al (2004) Early outcomes of laparoscopic procedures performed on military personnel with total rectal prolapse and follow-up. Surg Laparosc Endosc Percutan Techn 14:194–200
97. Stevenson AR, Stitz RW, Lumley JW (1998) Laparoscopic assisted resection rectopexy for rectal prolapse: early and medium follow-up. Dis Colon Rectum 41:46–54
98. Lechaux D, Trebuchet G, Siproudhis L, Campion JP (2005) Laparosocopic rectopexy for full-thickness rectal prolapse: a single-institution retrospective study evaluating surgical outcome. Surg Endosc 19:514–518
99. Kariv Y, Delaney CP, Casillas S et al (2006) Long-term outcome after laparoscopic and open surgery for rectal prolapse: a case-controlled study. Surg Endosc 20:35–42
100. Auguste T, Dubreuil A, Bost R et al (2006) Technical and functional results after laparoscopic rectopexy to the promontory for complete rectal prolapse. Prospective study in 54 consecutive patients. Gastroenterol Clin Biol 30:659–663
101. Benoist S, Taffinder N, Gould S et al (2001) Functional results two years after laparoscopic rectopexy. Am J Surg 182:168–173
102. Purkayastha S, Tekkis P, Athanasiou T et al (2005) A comparison of open vs. laparoscopic abdominal rectopexy for full-thickness rectal prolapse: a meta-analysis. Dis Colon Rectum 48:1930–1934
103. Darzi A, Henry MM, Guillou PJ et al (1995) Stapled laparoscopic rectopexy for rectal prolapse. Surg Endosc 9:301–303
104. Solomon MJ, Eyers AA (1996) Laparoscopic rectopexy using mesh fixation with a spiked chromium staple. Dis Colon Rectum 39:279–284
105. Tsugawa K, Sue K, Koyanagi N et al (2002) laparoscopic rectopexy for recurrent rectal prolapse: a safe and simple procedure without a mesh prosthesis. Hepatogastroenterology 49:1549–1551
106. Ayav A, Bresler L, Hubert J et al (2005) Robotic-assisted pelvic organ prolapse surgery. Surg Endosc 19:1200–1203
107. D'Hoore A, Cadoni R, Penninckx F (2004) Long-term outcome of laparoscopic ventral rectopexy for total rectal prolapse. Br J Surg 91:1500–1505
108. D'Hoore A, Penninckx F (2006) Laparoscopic ventral recto(colpo)pexy for rectal prolapse: surgical technique and outcome for 109 patients. Surg Endosc [Epub ahead of print].
109. Himpens J, Cadiere GB, Bruyns J, Vertruyen M (1999) Laparoscopic rectopexy according to Wells. Surg Endosc 13:139–141
110. Senagore AJ (2003) Management of rectal prolapse: the role of laparoscopic approaches. Semin Laparosc Surg 10:197–202
111. Madbouly KM, Senagore AJ, Delaney CP et al (2003) Clinically based management of rectal prolapse. Surg Endosc 17:99–103

16 Rectopexy with Mesh According to the Ripstein Technique

Vance Sohn, Scott R. Steele, Anders Mellgren

Introduction

Full-thickness external rectal prolapse is a distressing condition for both the patient and surgeon. In addition to its unsightly and at times alarming appearance, rectal prolapse may cause progressive symptoms that affect both patients' overall medical health as well as quality of life. This is distinct from internal rectal prolapse (also known as hidden or occult intussusception) in which the prolapse contains the full thickness of the rectal wall but the intussusception does not extend beyond the anal verge. Symptoms in the latter patients range from an asymptomatic finding in up to 40% of women on defecography to overt defecation dysfunction with obstructive symptoms. In contrast, full external prolapse occurs when the rectum descends beyond the anal verge, manifesting as concentric rings of rectal mucosa to the examiner. Varying degrees exist, as the prolapse may progress from initial reduction with standing or cessation of straining, to full-thickness prolapse with even minimal activity, and finally, in certain cases, to continual prolapse. As time passes, chronic prolapse through the sphincter complex, along with the presence of concomitant pelvic floor dysfunction, leads to problems with both continence and symptoms of constipation from outlet obstruction.

With more than 130 different procedures [1] described for the surgical management of rectal prolapse, it is not surprising that many authors disagree about proper management. More accurately, this highlights the fact that no perfect option exists for all patients. Factors to consider in selecting the ideal therapeutic approach include the patient's age and health, overall functional status, and the potential benefits and risks of a given surgical technique. In general, transperineal procedures are reserved for older patients and those with comorbid conditions who would gain the most benefit from a less morbid operation, shorter length of hospital stay, and faster recovery. Unfortunately, these perineal repairs are not as durable as transabdominal procedures, with a higher recurrence rate of 16–40%, depending on the particular procedure and follow-up time [2]. This is most evident in young patients who would otherwise outlive their repair [3]. Other factors also play a role in selecting the optimal approach, such as the young man with the potential risk of sexual dysfunction from autonomic nerve damage during pelvic dissection with an abdominal procedure versus the increased risk of recurrence with transperineal techniques. Although there are both subtle and not so subtle differences among the numerous repairs, the general principles of evaluation and treatment of rectal prolapse remain the same. In this chapter, we focus specifically on one of the more commonly performed abdominal procedures-the Ripstein rectopexy.

Background and Technical Aspects of the Ripstein Repair

Since its initial description by Charles Ripstein [4] in 1952, the Ripstein repair has undergone significant modifications as technology and better understanding of the pathophysiology of rectal prolapse have improved various aspects of the case. Synthetic mesh has replaced the originally described fascia lata graft, and laparoscopic approaches are commonly performed in place of the initially described open repair. However, the fundamental aspect of the procedure remains true today-restoring the normal posterior curve of the rectum in the hollow of the sacrum with attachment fixation to the sacral promontory.

Initial preparations for a Ripstein repair consist of bowel preparation, often limited to enemas on the morning of surgery (depending upon physician preference). Preoperative intravenous antibiotics are routinely given and timed for adequate concentration during the initial skin incision. In the operating theater, patients are positioned in the modified lithotomy position. Placing the patient in this position is invaluable, as it provides access to the anus and rectum as well as ideal positioning for retraction of the bladder, prostate, or vagina. Both surgeon and assistant should wear headlight devices to facilitate visualization during pelvic dissection. Ureteral stents may be helpful, especially in the patient with prior pelvic surgery or multiple adhesive disease, but are not routinely necessary.

A midline incision from umbilicus to pubis or a lower transverse incision provides adequate exposure for treating most patients. After placement of self-retaining retractors, the small bowel is displaced superiorly, and focus is directed toward the pelvis. The endpoints of rectal mobilization vary based on the position of dissection of the rectum. Posterior mobilization is carried down to the level of the coccyx. Contrary to the original description by Ripstein, emphasis is placed on preservation of the hypogastric nerves and the lateral rectal stalks near the pelvic floor, thus the preference of many surgeons to minimize all lateral dissection. Unintentional division of the hypogastric nerves typically occurs at the level of the inferior mesenteric artery takeoff or at the level of the sacral promontory and results in continence problems for both bowel and bladder, as well as sexual dysfunction. Although division of the lateral stalks has been shown to lower recurrence [5], its effect on postoperative function is more debatable. Some authors have shown a worsening of constipation [6], although other studies have found no change in postoperative functional outcome [7]. Proper identification of the avascular presacral plane is aided by application of forward traction on the rectum. Dissection is continued to the level of the coccyx posteriorly, keeping in mind that failure to recognize the anterior curve in the coccyx may result in injury to the presacral veins. Extending dissection to the tip of the coccyx ensures adequate length to suture the mesh to the presacral fascia at the sacral promontory. Anterior mobilization of the rectum begins with dissection between the anterior aspect of the rectum and the posterior aspect of the anterior pelvic structures. Dissection can be facilitated by a constant traction/countertraction presence between the rectum and the anterior organs. In addition, working from the posterior to lateral and finally anterior direction allows a more accurate assessment of the proper fascial plane of dissection. This anterior mobilization is carried caudally approximately 2–3 cm into the rectovaginal or rectovesicular septum. The anterior and posterior dissection planes can then be joined by dividing the interposing peritoneum according to surgeon preference.

Once fully mobilized, a rectangular-shaped piece of mesh is placed over the lower rectum. The mesh should lie over the rectum approximately 4–5 cm below the sacral promontory on the anterior aspect of the rectum and be secured to the presacral fascia (Figs. 1 and 2) [8]. In order to distribute tension evenly across the rectum and to more securely suture the mesh, suture placement is divided into left and right sides and performed in sequential order. Three 2-0 Prolene interrupted sutures are first placed on the right margin of the mesh and secured to the ipsilateral presacral fascia. The same technique is repeated on the contralateral side to ultimately result in an anteriorly

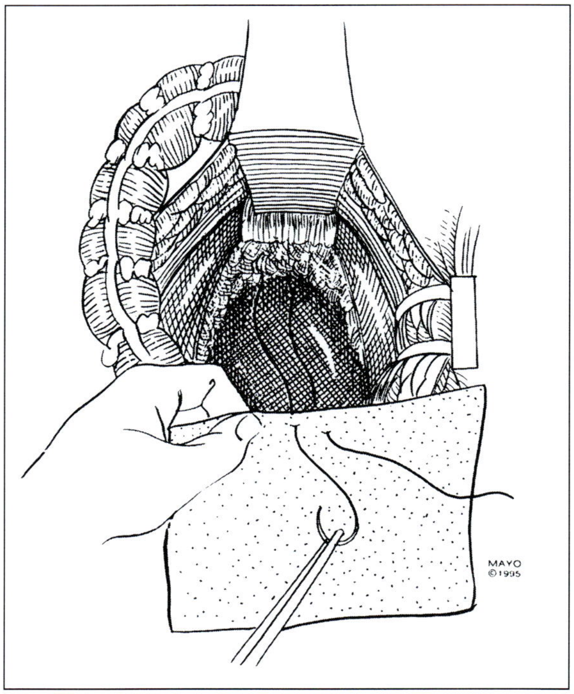

Fig. 1
Suturing the mesh to the sacrum. Reprinted from [8], with permission from Elsevier

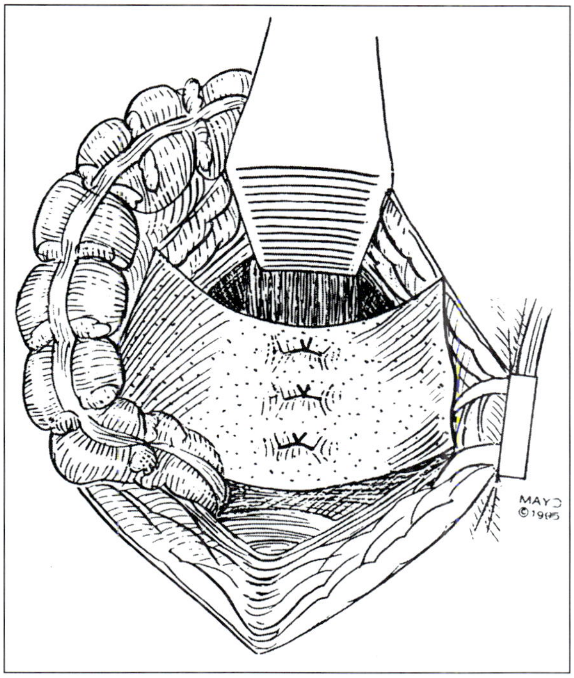

Fig. 2
Completed mesh to the sacrum. Reprinted from [8], with permission from Elsevier

mesh-wrapped rectum. The rectum is then pulled posterior toward the sacrum and superiorly to reduce redundancy (Fig. 3). Prior to tying the sutures, the tension on the rectum is inspected by having an assistant retract on the sutures while the surgeon places three to four fingers between the rectum and sacrum. Aggressive or tight wrapping should be avoided, as this may lead to constriction of the rectal vault with subsequent luminal narrowing. Once these sutures are secured under the proper tension, some surgeons prefer to place additional proximal and distal sutures along the margins of the mesh to prevent migration of the rectum underneath the mesh. The peritoneum is then closed, and an extraperitoneal drain may be placed in the presacral space and brought out through a separate stab incision along the abdominal wall. Finally, once hemostasis is adequate, the abdominal wall is closed in layers.

The typical postoperative course includes early ambulation and initiation of enteral feeding, as indicated. The bladder catheter may be removed immediately postoperatively. Patients are normally discharged in 48–72 h, with clinic follow-up in 7–10 days. The drain is removed either on a standard postoperative day or based on amount of effluent over a 24-h period. Dietary management, including increased fiber and fluid intake, should be continued to help avoid bowel dysfunction.

Perhaps the most significant shift in surgical technique is the application of laparoscopy for the treatment of rectal prolapse. While not yet in widespread use, laparoscopic Ripstein repair has been described and appears to have acceptable early re-

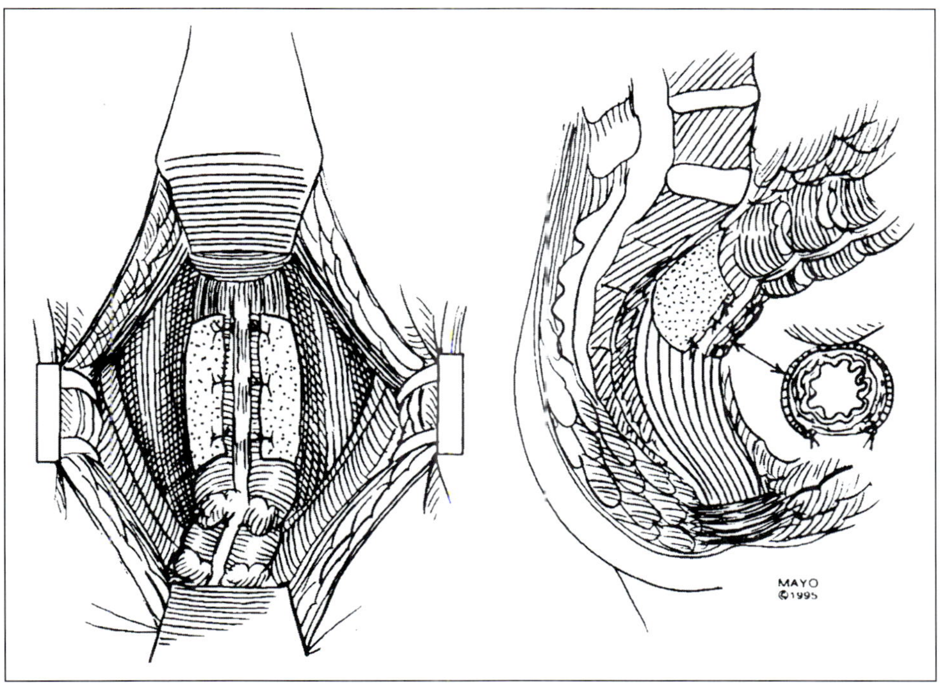

Fig. 3
Mesh affixed to bowel and completed rectopexy. Reprinted from [8], with permission from Elsevier

sults (see below). Preoperative preparation of the patient is similar to that of the open procedure. After bowel preparation, appropriate antibiotics, and urinary bladder catheterization, the patient is placed in the modified lithotomy position. Pneumoperitoneum to 12 mmHg can be obtained by either a Veress needle or an open cannula technique based on the surgeon's preference. If an open technique is used, this should be the supraumbilical 10-mm port. The remaining three trocars consist of two 5-mm ports placed in the right and left lower quadrants and a 12-mm trocar in the right iliac fossa, which will accommodate all laparoscopic stapling and tacking devices. Then, similar to the open procedure, exposure is obtained with displacement of small bowel and the often redundant sigmoid out of the pouch of Douglas.

Dissection with monopolar electrocautery begins anteriorly and ends approximately 2–5 cm below the peritoneal reflection. Posteriorly, dissection to the level of the levator complex is initiated, with the aid of the assistant retracting the rectum anteriorly. Again, the lateral ligaments are preserved. Upon complete mobilization of the rectum, the mesh is introduced via the lateral 12-mm port under direct vision. Just as in the open procedure, mesh is secured to the sacral promontory with either a tacking device or laparoscopic sutures. Drains are routinely placed, trocars are removed under direct vision, and the appropriate fascial closures performed. Similar variations of this laparoscopic procedure include the use of two separate pieces of mesh secured independently [9] or suture rectopexy [10, 11] in which each lateral rectal wall is secured to the presacral fascia.

Rectal Prolapse: Diagnosis and Evaluation

As the Ripstein repair is a transabdominal approach, patients undergoing consideration for this repair should be medically fit and able to tolerate a laparotomy. Primary indications for repair are symptomatic rectal prolapse, including presence of a mass, fecal incontinence, or constipation. Many authors claim that the mere presence of rectal prolapse is an indication for surgical repair, mostly due to the likely eventual progression of symptoms and risk of incarceration; yet, this is debatable. In internal or hidden intussusception, it is less well accepted as to whether or not rectopexy will help symptoms. In general, we define rectal intussusception as circumferential descent of the entire thickness of the rectal wall up to but not past the anal verge, and it is most often diagnosed by defecography. On the other hand, rectal prolapse refers to the full-circumferential descent of the rectal wall beyond the anal verge and is readily identifiable to the examining physician.

A detailed medical history is vital when evaluating patients with rectal prolapse. As a part of this, a thorough review of bowel habits is essential, as more than one-half of patients have coexisting incontinence [12, 13] and, to a slightly lesser degree, constipation. Upon presentation, patients frequently report not only a rectal mass or protrusion but give a history of abdominal discomfort and mucus discharge associated with altered bowel habits. Many patients will also strain to initiate or complete defecation, experience incomplete evacuation, or require digital maneuvers to aid with defecation. This may be secondary to the rectal prolapse itself or pelvic floor dysfunction associated with either anatomical defects (rectocele, cystocele, enterocele) or functional abnormalities such as paradoxical or nonrelaxing puborectalis.

In addition to a general physical examination, digital rectal examination can detect the presence of attenuated sphincter tone and masses and assess for concomitant pelvic floor pathology, as stated above. The patient should be asked to both tighten the anal sphincter as well as "bear down" as a simulation of defecation in order to assess proper contraction and relaxation of pelvic floor muscles. The perineum is assessed for associated increased perineal descent or bulge indicative of pelvic floor laxity that is often times seen with increasing age, multiparity, or prior pelvic floor surgery. Examination of the vaginal vault can also be helpful in identifying concomitant pelvic floor abnormalities and providing insight into the general support of the endopelvic fascia.

A detailed review of both prescription and over-the-counter medications can often identify common causes of constipation. Additionally, patients should be queried about diet and intake of fluids and fibers. Finally, laboratory evaluation should include thyroid function test, chemistry panel, calcium, and blood glucose to evaluate for associated diseases such as diabetes, hypothyroidism, and metabolic deficiencies.

Most patients should undergo a colonoscopy

to rule out an associated malignancy, especially those with no prior history of screening or patients with risk factors for colorectal cancer. Patients who complain of severe constipation with prolonged periods between bowel movements may also need to undergo a transit study. In selected patients, the dynamics of rectal evacuation can be studied with defecography. At this examination, the rectum is filled with contrast, and for women, the use of vaginal contrast enhances the possibility of visualizing abnormalities such as an enterocele or rectocele. Contrast agents include either a contrast medium gel or a tampon soaked with contrast medium. Gel is preferable, as a tampon might obscure important diagnostic information. Intraperitoneal contrast can enhance visualization of some findings [14]. In addition to rectal prolapse, abnormal rectal emptying, nonrelaxing pelvic floor, internal rectal prolapse, external rectal prolapse, enterocele, and rectocele can be seen on defecography [15].

Personal Experience

Prior to embarking on surgery, patients should be thoroughly counseled as to the expected outcomes. In general, bowel habits improve following prolapse repair. Yet, patients with a predominant symptom of constipation in addition to rectal prolapse need to be especially aware of the potential for worsening of symptoms following the Ripstein rectopexy. In a study of 30 patients, we found whole-gut transit time to be prolonged following the Ripstein repair. Compared with four out of 30 patients with prolonged transit time preoperatively, 13 out of 30 had abnormal postoperative retention of transit markers distributed in the left or rectosigmoid colon or both. There was no significant difference in the number of markers retained postoperatively between patients with rectal prolapse and those with rectal intussusception [16]. Despite overall improvement in continence, preoperative anorectal physiology studies have been unable to accurately predict which patients will have success [17]. We found continence improvement secondary to a postoperative rise in maximum resting pressure after 6 months, although squeeze pressure has been shown to not change, indicating that the internal anal sphincter may recover some function [18].

Long-term success with the Ripstein repair for patients with rectal prolapse is possible. Recently, we reviewed our institutional experience on 112 patients [19], including 69 with rectal prolapse and 43 with internal intussusception, over nearly two decades. With almost 6 years of follow-up, there were no perioperative deaths, although early (<30 days) and late (>30 days) complications were common. The majority of the 33% early complication rate was due to minor complications such as urinary tract, wound, or respiratory infections. However, significant problems requiring intervention included presacral hemorrhaging, fecal impaction requiring subtotal colectomy with ileorectal anastomosis, and obstructive hydronephrosis requiring reexploration. Of delayed complications, small-bowel obstruction, rectovaginal fistula, and severe constipation requiring hospitalization were the most common. In this series, only one patient had rectal prolapse recurrence, and no patients who underwent the procedure for internal intussusception developed prolapse. Overall, although incontinence did improve, patients continued to have problems with both constipation and incontinence. This is not surprising, as chronic prolapse of the rectum through the sphincters often leads to irreversible damage that has lasting effects on overall bowel function despite surgical correction.

Surgeons should also be aware of associated pelvic floor findings that may need to be addressed at the time of surgery. Concomitant pelvic floor pathology such as enteroceles or rectoceles can also be present in up to 50% of patients with rectal prolapse or internal intussusception [20]. Enteroceles are often found in older multiparous women, usually associated with a history of hysterectomy. Enteroceles can also be present in men and are most reliably diagnosed during defecography when bowel is seen within the rectal intussusception or the rectal prolapse. Therefore, surgical correction in this subset of patients can simultaneously address the coexistent enterocele and rectal pathology. In a study of 22 patients [21], we found that continence was universally improved; however, functional improvements in emptying difficulties were more varied. An equal percentage of patients demonstrated improved emptying, no change, or worse emptying after the procedure. However, there were no recurrences of enterocele, prolapse, or intussusception at follow-up. Based on these results, concomitant enteroceles can be repaired with the Ripstein technique alone, with associated improvement in 15 of 16 patients with incontinence [22]. Yet, the patient should again be counseled that correction of the anatomical defect may not necessarily lead to symptom relief.

Outcomes Following the Ripstein Repair

Functional Outcome

As previously stated, a well-described complication of the Ripstein repair is postoperative constipation, sometimes severe enough to require reoperation. The exact etiology of persistent or new onset constipation remains elusive. Not surprisingly, the surgical literature is replete with authors reporting worsening constipation postoperatively [23], whereas others have found constipation unchanged [24] or even decreased [25, 26]. Regardless, clinically significant severe postoperative constipation ranges from 15% to 71% despite careful patient selection. Ultimately, if patients manifest symptoms from severe constipation, a subtotal colectomy with ileorectal anastomosis may be warranted [27]. It is important, however, for the surgeon to attempt to document slow-transit constipation with functional studies such as sitz marker examination prior to embarking on an operation to attempt to avoid this problem.

Patients with constipation suffer primarily from rectal emptying difficulties, with the average number of bowel movements uniformly decreasing after surgery. Multiple theories have attempted to answer these questions and assess specific patient characteristics that may predict postoperative constipation. The first attributes the constipation to fecal impaction at the level of the narrow net. This may be a result of a technical error in which the mesh is secured too tightly to the rectum, thereby creating a mechanical outlet resistance. This theory was supported by a study by Gordon and Hoexter [28] published in 1978 in which complication rates from the Ripstein procedure were found to be higher for surgeons performing fewer than 20 cases per year. The most common complication related to inexperience was that of the sling being placed too snugly.

Another possible explanation for postoperative constipation may be attributable to the often redundant sigmoid colon kinking at the proximal rectum, again resulting in increased outlet resistance. One prospective study [29] tested this theory by randomizing patients to rectopexy alone versus rectopexy with sigmoidectomy. Although not using the Ripstein technique, they found that in patients undergoing rectopexy alone, constipation was more common, most likely from decreased rectal compliance. To counter this, the abdominal rectopexy with sigmoid resection (Frykman-Goldberg procedure) was developed for patients with rectal prolapse with a large redundant sigmoid colon and predominant constipation [30]. Finally, rectal stump denervation by lateral rectal stalk division may contribute to postoperative constipation. Speakman et al. [31] compared rectopexy with and without lateral ligament division and found that division increased constipation frequency.

Functional studies performed on patients with postoperative constipation have led to better insight into whole-gut and anorectal motility dysfunction. As previously mentioned, transit studies using retention markers demonstrated an increase in whole-gut transit after Ripstein rectopexy [32, 33]. Whereas the exact mechanism behind this delay is unknown, this delay may simply be an exacerbation of a preexisting but subclinical motility disorder. Additionally, paradoxical puborectalis reaction and concomitant outlet obstructions such as rectoceles or enteroceles have been implicated [34]. If these patients are properly identified preoperatively, a better functional result may be obtained by performing repair of the associated pelvic floor pathology alone or in conjunction with biofeedback [35, 36].

Whereas postoperative constipation may be worsened after a Ripstein repair, studies have consistently found that continence is improved after surgery for both rectal prolapse and intussusception [37–40]. Postoperative anorectal manometry has demonstrated an increase in maximal resting pressure associated with improved continence for patients undergoing the repair for prolapse [41]. This improvement in pressure is an indication of internal sphincter recovery after the mesh rectopexy. Curiously, although patients undergoing the same procedure for rectal intussusception had improved continence, there were no associated improvements in anorectal pressures.

Ripstein Rectopexy for Internal Intussusception

Once believed to be a precursor of rectal prolapse, internal rectal intussusception is a common finding in asymptomatic individuals [42] and rarely progresses to rectal prolapse [43]. Symptomatic patients with intussusception report difficulties in rectal emptying as well as anal incontinence and/or anal pain [44]. Whereas the advantages of repair are clear for prolapse, the indication for surgery in a patient with internal rectal intussusception continues to be a matter of debate, as surgery has not produced reliable postoperative improvements [45, 46]. The main indication for surgical correction for internal intussusception should be fecal incontinence of no known cause.

In our series [47] of 43 patients with intussusception undergoing the Ripstein procedure between 1980 and 1996, the main indication for surgery was fecal incontinence of no known cause ($n = 25$). Of those available for long-term follow-up, two patients underwent a sigmoid colostomy, the first for persistent incontinence and the second for persistent perineal pain associated with constipation. Overall, there was a significant increase in emptying difficulties when compared with preoperative evaluation. Improvements in continence, anal pain, rectal bleeding, and tenesmus were also identified when compared with preoperative evaluation. When queried as part of the follow-up evaluation, 70% of patients were satisfied with the procedure, with 73% reporting they would recommend this procedure to their friends. Thus, whereas continence may improve, increased postoperative constipation is possible, and the procedure should not be undertaken lightly in patients complaining only of constipation associated with internal intussusception.

Laparoscopic Ripstein Repair

Laparoscopy, with its more tolerable physiologic impact, may allow more patients to undergo a transabdominal rather than a transperineal repair for rectal prolapse. Whether this leads to better long-term results has been the focus of several studies [48]. As in the open technique, various laparoscopic variants to the mesh rectopexy are being performed. D'Hoore et al. [49] report a laparoscopic ventral rectopexy in which lateral mobilization of the rectum is altogether avoided. Mesh is sutured to the ventral aspect of the distal rectum and then to the lateral borders of the proximal rectum. Although theirs was a small series of 42 patients, there was acceptable improvement in continence. Of concern were the two cases of recurrence (5%) early on in the laparoscopic experience. This recurrence highlights the fact that as more surgeons attempt laparoscopy, a learning curve, similar to that extensively studied for laparoscopic cholecystectomy, may be required before optimal results are achieved. Yet, there is nothing to suggest that with further experience, results with the laparoscopic approach should mimic if not improve the open experience. Ashari et al. [50], in their series of 117 patients undergoing a laparoscopic resection rectopexy, had comparable mortality (0.9%) and morbidity (9%) rates to open procedures. With a 2.5% recurrent rectal prolapse rate and a 69% improvement in bowel frequency, this procedure appears promising.

Recurrent Rectal Prolapse

Data surrounding Ripstein repair for the patient with recurrent rectal prolapse is minimal. Hool et al. [51], in a study of 24 patients over a 30-year period at the Cleveland Clinic, found that the majority of recurrences were secondary to technical reasons. In their study of 29 patients, 18 had undergone a Ripstein procedure, with mesh failure as the most common identifiable reason for failure. They identified technical factors such as poor mesh placement, mesh pulling away from the sacrum, and too tight of a wrap as reasons for failure. The median time to recurrence was 2 years, with approximately one third of patients developing a recurrence within 7 months of the original operation. This highlights the particular attention that needs to be placed on proper mesh fixation and orientation to help ensure a successful outcome.

Complications

As evidenced from our own series, Ripstein rectopexy can be performed with minimal mortality and reasonable morbidity. Tjandra et al. [52] reviewed the Cleveland Clinic experience over 30 years of 142 patients undergoing a Ripstein procedure. In their series, the mortality rate was 0.6%, recurrent rectal prolapse occurred in 7%, and the complication rate was 27%. Functionally, whereas continence improved, 33% of patients suffered from constipation postoperatively.

Potential complications from this repair include small- or large-bowel obstruction, ureteral injury or fibrosis, recurrent prolapse, rectovaginal fistula, and fecal impaction. Other potential long-term complications from the Ripstein repair include intractable constipation, fecal incontinence, and recurrence. Additionally, mesh erosion through the rectum has been reported up to 6 years after the sentinel procedure [53]. Although this occurrence is rare, mesh migration may be corrected without further surgical intervention.

Conclusion

The Ripstein repair is a safe procedure indicated for rectal prolapse and in a few selected patients with symptomatic internal rectal intussusception. Long-term data demonstrate the reliability of this repair, with low recurrence rates, acceptable complication profile, and consistent improvement in fecal incontinence. The main functional disadvantage of this procedure is the variable decrement in postoperative constipation, occasionally severe enough to require further surgical intervention. Whereas specific patient characteristics that predict postoperative constipation has yet to be elucidated, caution should be exercised when considering this procedure for patients with constipation associated with internal rectal intussusception. As laparoscopic instrumentation, technique, and skills evolve, both laparoscopic and open Ripstein repair will likely find a continued place in the armamentarium of surgeons caring for patients with prolapse.

References

1. Karulf RE, Madoff RD, Goldberg SM (2001) Rectal prolapse. Curr Probl Surg 38:771–832
2. Azimuddin K, Khubchandani IT, Rosen L et al (2001) Rectal prolapse: a search for the "best" operation. Am Surg 67:622–627
3. Kim DS, Tsang CB, Wong WD et al (1999) Complete rectal prolapse: evolution of management and results. Dis Colon Rectum 42:460–466
4. Ripstein CB (1952) Treatment of massive rectal prolapse. Am J Surg 83:68–71
5. Speakman CT, Madden MV, Nicholls RJ et al (1991) Lateral ligament division during rectopexy causes constipation but prevents recurrence: results of a prospective randomized study. Br J Surg 78:1431–1433
6. Scaglia M, Fasth S, Hallgren T et al (1994) Abdominal rectopexy for rectal prolapse. Influence of surgical technique on functional outcome. Dis Colon Rectum 37:805–813
7. Mollen RM, Kuijpers JH, van Hoek F (2000) Effects of rectal mobilization and lateral ligaments division on colonic and anorectal function. Dis Colon Rectum 43:1283–1287
8. Pemberton JH (1996) Rectal prolapse. In: Keighley MRB et al (eds) Atlas of colorectal surgery. Churchill Livingstone, New York, pp. 157–158
9. Lechaux D, Trebuchet G, Siproudhis L et al (2005) Laparoscopic rectopexy for full-thickness rectal prolapse: a single-institution retrospective study evaluating surgical outcome. Surg Endosc 19:514–518
10. Bruch HP, Herold A, Schiedeck T et al (1999) Laparoscopic surgery for rectal prolapse and outlet obstruction. Dis Colon Rectum 42:1189–1194
11. Heah SM, Hartley JE, Hurley J et al (2000) Laparoscopic suture rectopexy without resection is effective treatment for full-thickness rectal prolapse. Dis Colon Rectum 43:638–643
12. Hiltunen KM, Matikainen M, Auvinen O et al (1986) Clinical and manometric evaluation of anal sphincter function in patients with rectal prolapse. Am J Surg 151:489–492
13. Keighley MR, Fielding JW, Alexander-Williams J (1983) Results of Marlex mesh abdominal rectopexy for rectal prolapse in 100 consecutive patients. Br J Surg 70:229–232
14. Bremmer S, Ahlback SO, Uden R et al (1995) Simultaneous defecography and peritoneography in defecation disorders. Dis Colon Rectum 38:969–973
15. Mellgren A, Johansson C, Dolk A et al (1994) Enterocele demonstrated by defaecography is associated with other pelvic floor disorders. Int J Colorectal Dis 9:121–124
16. Schultz I, Mellgren A, Oberg M et al (1999) Whole gut transit is prolonged after Ripstein rectopexy. Eur J Surg 165:242–247
17. Schultz I, Mellgren A, Nilsson BY et al (1998) Preoperative electrophysiologic assessment cannot predict continence after rectopexy. Dis Colon Rectum 41:1392–1398

18. Schultz I, Mellgren A, Dolk A et al (1996) Continence is improved after the Ripstein rectopexy. Different mechanisms in rectal prolapse and rectal intussusception? Dis Colon Rectum 39:300–306
19. Schultz I, Mellgren A, Dolk A et al (2000) Long-term results and functional outcome after Ripstein rectopexy. Dis Colon Rectum 43:35–43
20. Dippolito A, Esser S, Reed J III (2005) Anterior modification of Delorme procedure provides equivalent results to Delorme procedure in treatment of rectal outlet obstruction. Curr Surg 62:609–612
21. Mellgren A, Dolk A, Johansson C et al (1994) Enterocele is correctable using the Ripstein rectopexy. Dis Colon Rectum 37:800–804
22. Mellgren A, Dolk A, Johansson C et al (1994) Enterocele is correctable using the Ripstein rectopexy. Dis Colon Rectum 37:800–804
23. Holmstrom B, Broden G, Dolk A (1986) Results of the Ripstein operation in the treatment of rectal prolapse and internal rectal procidentia. Dis Colon Rectum 29:845–848
24. Tjandra JJ, Fazio VW, Church JM et al (1993) Ripstein procedure is an effective treatment for rectal prolapse without constipation. Dis Colon Rectum 36:501–507
25. Roberts PL, Schoetz DJ Jr, Coller JA et al (1988) Ripstein procedure. Lahey Clinic experience: 1963–1985. Arch Surg 123:554–557
26. Winde G, Reers B, Nottberg H et al (1993) Clinical and functional results of abdominal rectopexy with absorbable mesh-graft for treatment of complete rectal prolapse. Eur J Surg 159:301–305
27. Lahr SJ, Lahr CJ, Srinivasan A et al (1999) Operative management of severe constipation. Am Surg 65:1117–1121
28. Gordon PH, Hoexter B (1978) Complications of the Ripstein procedure. Dis Colon Rectum 21:277–280
29. McKee RF, Lauder JC, Poon FW et al (1992) A prospective randomized study of abdominal rectopexy with and without sigmoidectomy in rectal prolapse. Surg Gynecol Obstet 174:145–148
30. Kim DS, Tsang CB, Wong WD et al (1999) Complete rectal prolapse: evolution of management and results. Dis Colon Rectum 42:460–466
31. Speakman CT, Madden MV, Nicholls RJ et al (1991) Lateral ligament division during rectopexy causes constipation but prevents recurrence: results of a prospective randomized study. Br J Surg 78:1431–1433
32. Dolk A, Broden G, Holmstrom B et al (1990) Slow transit of the colon associated with severe constipation after the Ripstein operation. A clinical and physiologic study. Dis Colon Rectum 33:786–790
33. Schultz I, Mellgren A, Oberg M et al (1999) Whole gut transit is prolonged after Ripstein rectopexy. Eur J Surg 165:242–247
34. Dolk A, Broden G, Holmstrom B et al (1990) Slow transit of the colon associated with severe constipation after the Ripstein operation. A clinical and physiologic study. Dis Colon Rectum 33:786–790
35. Ko CY, Tong J, Lehman RE et al (1997) Biofeedback is effective therapy for fecal incontinence and constipation. Arch Surg 132:829–833
36. Van OM, Pelckmans P (2006) Biofeedback is superior to laxatives for normal transit constipation due to pelvic floor dyssynergia. Gastroenterology 131:333–334
37. Launer DP, Fazio VW, Weakley FL et al (1982) The Ripstein procedure: a 16-year experience. Dis Colon Rectum 25:41–45
38. Roberts PL, Schoetz DJ Jr, Coller JA et al (1988) Ripstein procedure. Lahey Clinic experience: 1963–1985. Arch Surg 123:554–557
39. Tjandra JJ, Fazio VW, Church JM et al (1993) Ripstein procedure is an effective treatment for rectal prolapse without constipation. Dis Colon Rectum 36:501–507
40. Winde G, Reers B, Nottberg H et al (1993) Clinical and functional results of abdominal rectopexy with absorbable mesh-graft for treatment of complete rectal prolapse. Eur J Surg 159:301–305
41. Schultz I, Mellgren A, Dolk A et al (1996) Continence is improved after the Ripstein rectopexy. Different mechanisms in rectal prolapse and rectal intussusception? Dis Colon Rectum 39:300–306
42 Goei R, van EJ, Schouten H et al (1989) Anorectal function: defecographic measurement in asymptomatic subjects. Radiology 173:137–141
43. Mellgren A, Schultz I, Johansson C et al (1997) Internal rectal intussusception seldom develops into total rectal prolapse. Dis Colon Rectum 40:817–820
44 Ihre T, Seligson U (1975) Intussusception of the rectum-internal procidentia: treatment and results in 90 patients. Dis Colon Rectum 18:391–396
45. Christiansen J, Zhu BW, Rasmussen OO et al (1992) Internal rectal intussusception: results of surgical repair. Dis Colon Rectum 35:1026–1028
46. Johansson C, Ihre T, Ahlback SO (1985) Disturbances in the defecation mechanism with special reference to intussusception of the rectum (internal procidentia). Dis Colon Rectum 28:920–924
47. Schultz I, Mellgren A, Dolk A et al (2000) Long-term results and functional outcome after Ripstein rectopexy. Dis Colon Rectum 43:35–43
48. Kusminsky RE, Tiley EH, Boland JP (1992) Laparoscopic Ripstein procedure. Surg Laparosc Endosc 2:346–347
49. D'Hoore A, Cadoni R, Penninckx F (2004) Long-term outcome of laparoscopic ventral rectopexy for total rectal prolapse. Br J Surg 91:1500–1505
50. Ashari LH, Lumley JW, Stevenson AR et al (2005) Laparoscopically-assisted resection rectopexy for rectal prolapse: ten years' experience. Dis Colon Rectum 48:982–987
51. Hool GR, Hull TL, Fazio VW (1997) Surgical treatment of recurrent complete rectal prolapse: a thirty-year experience. Dis Colon Rectum 40:270–272
51. Launer DP, Fazio VW, Weakley FL et al (1982) The Ripstein procedure: a 16-year experience. Dis Colon Rectum 25:41-45
52. Tjandra JJ, Fazio VW, Church JM et al (1993) Ripstein procedure is an effective treatment for rectal prolapse without constipation. Dis Colon Rectum 36:501–507
53. Karagulle E, Yildirim E, Turk E et al (2006) Mesh invasion of the rectum: an unusual late complication of rectal prolapse repair. Int J Colorectal Dis 21:724–727

17 Rectopexy with Mesh: The Orr–Loygue Technique

Aldo Infantino, Roberto Bellomo, Domenico Del Ciampo

Introduction

Rectal prolapse is a very disabling disease, and although its etiopathogenesis has not yet been well established, it is frequently associated with other abnormalities, including patulous anus, levator ani muscle diastasis, mesorectum elongation, deep pouch of Douglas, redundant rectosigmoid and increased width of the retrorectal space. The term complete rectal prolapse (CRP) is used for intussusception of the entire rectum outside the anal canal, which may be temporary or, more rarely, permanent. Rectoanal intussusception (RAI) is a partial or total rectal invagination without protrusion from the anus. However, although RAI may be strongly suggested by the patient's symptoms and suspected at clinical examination, and its demonstration at dynamic proctography is easy, its clinical implications are difficult to evaluate, as radiological images suggesting RAI may be found even in healthy subjects [1]. The interpretation of radiological images is, however, still controversial [2]. Ischaemia of the prolapsed mucosa and local trauma from self-digiting have been cited as possible causes of solitary rectal ulcer in 6–39% of cases [3]. The hypothesis that mucosal prolapse, solitary rectal ulcer and internal rectal intussusception are conditions leading to CRP [4] has not been confirmed [5–7].

Functional disturbances associated with rectal prolapse may include faecal incontinence (FI) and/or obstructed defecation. FI is present in 30–80% of patients with CRP [8] and also in up to 44% [9] of those with RAI. The incidence of FI increases with age [10]. Numerous authors support the hypothesis that sphincter muscle weakness is caused by a rectal prolapse itself, chronic mechanical stretching, chronic internal sphincter activity inhibition and coexisting pelvic floor neuropathy. Obstructed defecation syndrome (ODS) is often characterised by strenuous effort to expel stools, feeling of incomplete evacuation, rectal tenesmus and repeated call to toilet, digitation and the necessity of enemas and/or suppositories [11]. It is related to multiple alterations, variously associated and in different degrees, of pelvic and perineal organs: rectocele, rectal occult mucosal or full-thickness prolapse, and enterocele; and it is often associated with synchronous anatomic alterations of the anterior perineum: uterine, vaginal and bladder prolapses [12]. A unique pathophysiologic theory has been suggested but not yet demonstrated [13]. As a consequence of the variability of the affected organs, there is great difficulty in reaching a diagnosis, and the management and treatment of ODS is, to date, far from being standardised.

Treatment

There is strong agreement that surgery is the treatment of choice for CRP, whereas bowel retraining (i.e. high-fibre diet, bulk laxatives, avoidance of straining and digitation and pelvic floor exercises) must be considered as the first approach for rectal intussusception and solitary rectal ulcer, with surgery being considered only if conservative therapy fails.

The first decision to be made in surgical treatment is whether an abdominal or a perineal approach should be used. Abdominal rectopexy is considered more aggressive, although with the advent of laparoscopy, this is no longer the case. Nevertheless, it is commonly held that the perineal approach should be reserved for severely debilitated, frail or very elderly patients. Most of the literature seems to assert that the benefits of the abdominal approach consist principally in the reduced occurrence of relapses and in better functional results. In case of CRP, abdominal techniques have the advantage of incurring a lower recurrence rate [14, 15] and are associated with a higher rate of improvement in FI than are perineal techniques [16–20]. Many options have been proposed: whether or not to use mesh to fix the rectum to the sacrum; anterior (Ripstein technique) or posterior (Wells or Orr–Loygue) technique; rectopexy with or without sigmoid resection; absorbable or nonabsorbable mesh.

Orr [21] proposed fixing the rectum, after complete isolation of the organ, to the sacral promontory using two strips of muscular fascia sutured distally to the lateral sides of the rectum and proximally to the presacral fascia. Loygue [22] modified the technique using two synthetic meshes 3 cm large sutured to the anterolateral side of the lower extraperitoneal rectum with four or five nonabsorbable sutures. Avoiding tension, the two meshes are sutured to the sacral promontory 2–3 cm apart, taking care not to damaging the neurovascular pedicles.

A modified Orr–Loygue technique has been used in our surgical unit, using a video-laparoscopic approach whenever possible:

1. The rectum is isolated posteriorly, not to the levator muscle, but to the level of the lateral ligaments, which are not sectioned. The hypogastric nerve is spared. Anteriorly, the pouch of Douglas is opened, and the posterior vaginal fornix or vaginal vault is exposed.
2. A polypropylene mesh 5 × 8 cm is modelled as a pantaloon.
3. The mesh is fixed between the promontory and the sacral hollow with clips and with two stitches to the anterolateral rectal wall. The distal two stitches, one for each mesh, suture the posterolateral fornix of the vagina, or the vaginal vault in case of previous hysterectomy. The contemporary colpopexy and closure of the rectovaginal space are useful if there is associated genital prolapse and enterocele.
4. Using a late absorbable suture, a purse-string plication of the deep pouch of Douglas is performed following Moschcowitz [23], preventing stenosis of the anterior rectal wall. The peritoneum is closed with a running late absorbable suture.
5. In the majority of cases, an abdominal drain is not positioned in the pelvis.

Personal Experience

In the last 10 years, 99 sacral rectopexies have been performed in the surgical unit of S. Vito al Tagliamento General Hospital using the modified Orr–Loygue technique: 77 patients for RAI (77.8%) and 22 for CRP (22.2%). Patients' mean age was 54.4 ± 13.8 (range 16–83) years, with a female to male ratio of 98/1. Seventy-two patients complained of symptoms of obstructed defecation resistant to conservative treatment and 15 of anal incontinence (15.1%). Of the latter, six had CRP and nine had RAI; in three cases of CRP and in five cases of RAI, constipation was associated with FI. All patients were studied with dynamic defecography except those with full FI. FI was scored using the Cleveland Clinic score described by Jorge and Wexner [24] and constipation by evaluating stool frequency and symptoms of disturbed evacuation.

The approach was laparotomic in eight cases, and laparoscopic in 91 cases with conversion into laparotomy in seven. The average length of operation was 129 ± 42 (range 70–255) min for laparoscopic rectopexy and 90 min for the laparotomic approach. Mean postoperative in-hospital stay was 4.4 ± 1.7 (range 2–10) days for the laparoscopic group and 11 ± 2 days for the laparotomic group. Length of follow-up was 33.5 ± 25.7 (range 5–106) months: 24.7 ± 13.1 for the CPR group and 37.3 ± 28.7 for the RAI group. Eight patients were lost to follow-up

The results showed improvement of the Cleveland Clinic score for FI from the preoperative 9.1 ± 5.4 (range 4–20) to 3.6 ± 6.0 [24] (range 0–20): 8/14 (57.1%) patients were cured (one was lost to follow-up), in five patients (35.7%) FI improved, and the only patient with severe incontinence (score 20) did not improve (7.4%) (Table 1). Of patients with RAI, 62 with obstructed defecation (eight were lost to follow-up) were interviewed: nine were cured, 33 improved, 13 were unchanged and seven described their condition as worse. Of the nine constipated patients with CRP, two were cured, six improved and only one got worse. Analysis of pre- and postoperative symptoms revealed better results than the referred satisfaction of each patient. The number of bowel movements was not modified by surgical procedure: 26.6 ± 157 (4–70) vs. 27.2 ± 12.3 (4–60), in pre- and postoperative periods, respectively.

Table 1. Modified Orr–Loygue sacral rectopexy: comparative functional results between complete rectal prolapse and rectoanal intussusception

	Complete rectal prolapse ($n = 22$)	**Rectoanal intussusception ($n = 77$)[a]**
Recurrence	0	0
Faecal incontinence: postoperative/preoperative	66%	25%[b]
Incontinence cured	33.3%	66.6%
Incontinence improved	66.6%	16.6%
Constipation: postoperative/preoperative	11%	85%
Constipation cured	22.2%	14.5%
Constipation improved	66.6%	53.2%
Induced constipation	1	1

[a] Eight patients lost to follow-up
[b] One patient lost to follow-up

In the CRP group there were no recurrences, but one patient developed a solitary rectal ulcer with RAI and was subsequently treated with a Frykman–Goldberg procedure [25]. In one patient, the mesh was removed due to chronic rectal pain. There was no mortality. Major postoperative morbidity consisted of a bladder perforation by a trocar and two laparoscopic intestinal perforations that were repaired during the operation.

Discussion

There is no clear answer as to the best technique related to functional outcome in rectal prolapse. Many authors have demonstrated a statistically significant improvement in constipation and incontinence after rectopexy and sigmoid resection, with a low complication rate [26–28]. An increase in mean anal resting and maximum pressures has been recorded, and improvement in continence has been found to be closely related to sphincter tone [28]. Improvement can be observed within 6 months after surgery [29].

The incidence of postoperative constipation in patients who undergo rectopexy with resection appears to be lower than in patients undergoing rectopexy without resection [26, 27, 30]. Authors who advocate sacral suture rectopexy affirm that perirectal fibrosis secondary to mesh placement can leave a less compliant rectum, resulting in urgency and incontinence. It has also been suggested that postoperative constipation may occur if there is mechanical obstruction due to angulation of the sigma on the rectum [31] or due to acquired sigmoid motility disturbances above the rectopexy [32]. Unfortunately, many studies are not comparable due to the different classifications used, the definitions of success and the often short follow-up. Constipation, mainly due to rectal denervation consequent to lateral ligament sectioning to achieve complete rectal mobilisation [33, 34], can, of course, counteract FI [35]. The Orr–Loygue technique should reduce these complications, particularly when avoiding extensive isolation of the rectum, as proposed by our group; no comparative studies have been published to confirm this hypothesis.

RAI is difficult to treat. For the initial approach, conservative treatment is mandatory: dietary advice, biofeedback and rehabilitation of the pelvic floor muscles can help reduce outlet obstruction and incontinence. Improvement in symptoms after rectopexy is achieved in two thirds of patients [36, 37]. In their retrospective study on 37 incontinent patients who underwent suture sacral rectopexy, Briel et al. demonstrated that after a long-term follow-up (median 67 months), only 38% of patients with RAI and FI were continent compared with 67% of patients with CRP. All men in both groups were cured [38]. Better results were reported by Ihre and Selingson [39], with continence being restored in 77% of patients. The transanal approach has been proposed in the treatment of rectal intussusception [40], and recently, positive results have been reported: among 20 operated patients, only 8.3% (1/12) still had FI, and 5% of patients with preoperative constipation had outlet obstruction after a follow-up of at least 6 months [41]. The negative predictive preoperative data were proximal internal prolapse with rectosacral separation at defecography, chronic diarrhoea, FI and major per-

Table 2. Surgical approach to outlet obstruction after failure of conservative treatment. Modified from [41]

Sarles:
Predominance of rectocele (distension) 2 cm
Prolapse 1–10 mm (prevalently mucosal and anterior)
Absence of rectoanal dyssynegy (?)
Absence of uterine or vaginal vault prolapse or enterocele
Delorme:
Predominance of rectal intussusception (>10 mm)
High operative risk
Absence of uterine or vaginal vault prolapse or enterocele
Male
Orr–Loygue:
Large rectosacral space
Enterocele
Descending perineum >9 cm during straining at defecography
Genital prolapse
Frykman–Goldberg:
Symptomatic sigmoid diverticular disease
Prevalent left colonic constipation

ineal descent (>9 cm) on straining [41], so that the indications to sacral rectopexy are limited (Table 2).

Ripstein rectopexy can be performed with low mortality and recurrence rates, but increased constipation is a problem with this procedure: the number of bowel movements per week significantly decreased postoperatively ($P < 0.001$) [42]. The Orr–Loygue technique seems superior to the Ripstein procedure for absence of stenosis and better rectal motility due to the free anterior wall. However, as stated, no comparative studies have been published. Good functional results in respect to published data have been obtained in our experience for shorter isolation of the rectum with preservation of lateral ligaments and small mesh size.

The sectioning of rectal lateral ligaments has been advocated as a cause of prolonged intestinal transit time [33, 34], even if this hypothesis has not been confirmed [43]; preservation of lateral ligaments is associated with an overall reduction of FI, and there is a tendency towards improvement in constipation [44].

The abdominal approach has a low complication rate, although femoral nerve damage has been described [45]. The laparoscopic approach [17, 46–49] has reopened the debate as to which is the best technique to use, mesh rectopexy, suture rectopexy or resection rectopexy, but there are no grounds for sustaining that final functional results can be modified because a different access route is used. Laparoscopic surgery is generally considered less traumatic than open techniques, so many indications to perform perineal repair of rectal prolapse can be reappraised: surgery under laparoscopic guidance is particularly suitable for elderly or frail patients [50].

The laparoscopic approach compared with the laparotomic approach has shown the following advantages: reduced postoperative pain, requiring only minimal use of analgesics; reduced surgical morbidity; only minor aesthetic damage; minimal recovery time; and earlier return to work [27, 51–53]. Results regarding the cure of a CRP are similar, however. Access via laparoscopy seems to have a low postoperative morbidity that ranges between 4% and 9%, a mortality of 0–3% and a recurrence rate in the range of 0–10% [44], but it requires a longer operative time, especially during the learning curve [54, 55]. Recent studies have confirmed that the retrospective [26, 56–58] or prospective comparison between the "open" technique and laparoscopy favours the latter. In addition, a study on economic impact demonstrated that laparoscopic rectopexy in comparison with the open procedure, other than giving better clinical results, costs less [59].

The role of the laparoscopic approach for treating rectal prolapse has been studied extensively since the end of the 1980s but only recently have comparative studies of laparotomy been conducted considering the different procedures (direct suture, mesh use and resection rectopexy). Constipation and symptoms of difficult evacuation were solved or alleviated in 70% of patients who underwent sacral rectopexy and in 64% of those who underwent colonic resection, both with a laparoscopic approach [51]. In a retrospective study comparing the use of mesh, direct suture and resection-rectopexy, the latter offered better functional results, in particular, for improvement in constipation. Mesh use did not seem to add any particular advantage [60], even considering the incidence of prolapse recurrence [61].

To avoid posterior dissection of the rectum, a possible cause of postoperative constipation due to autonomic nerve lesion, an alternative technique has recently been proposed that consists of a ventral rectopexy performed with the laparoscopic approach [62]. After a median follow-up of 61 months, 16/19 patients with obstructed defecation were asymptomatic, and continence improved significantly in 28/31 incontinent patients. However, two patients developed symptoms of constipation in the postoperative period [62]. Portier et al. [63] stressed a limited dissection of the rectum: in 73 patients after Orr–Loygue ventral rectopexy, they obtained a low recurrence rate (5.9%) in the total rectal prolapse group and none in the internal rectal prolapse group. FI and constipation were cured in 58.1% and 51.9% in the first group and 70.6% and 60% in the latter group, respectively, with patient satisfaction of 94.5%. Age had no influence on functional results, which did not differ between patients who were older or younger than 70 years [64].

The combined repair of anterior and posterior perineum is mandatory in order to avoid multiple operations with higher risk of complications [65]. In case of associated genital prolapse, uterine fixation to the promontory associated with Orr–Loygue was shown to be reliable, with a low complication rate and no recurrence at a follow-up of 20 months [66]. Eighty-nine patients underwent combined surgery, and 60 of them had a concurrent vaginal repair. Improvement occurred in all major symptoms, and for all patients, this operation provided considerable symptom relief, with no evidence of recurrence of rectal or vaginal vault prolapse at follow-up [67]. In cases of vaginal vault prolapse or enterocele, the associated abdominal colposacropexy with mesh has a cure rate of 90% and a risk of mesh erosion of 3.3% [68–70]. In our experience, no patients complained of relapse of rectal or vaginal prolapse at long-term follow-up.

Conclusion

We believe that functional results that are not always encouraging after sacral rectopexy (worse for RAI than for CRP) are probably not linked only to technique. In fact, the centrality of the problem is not exclusively mechanical but also – if not mostly – biological. This is confirmed by psychological involvement [71, 72] and also by global alteration of intestinal motility, not simply that limited to the function of the large bowel [73]. Motility alterations can at times be diagnosed with anorectal manometry. Rectal hyposensitivity and sensory threshold volumes elevated beyond the normal range have been found in 33% of patients with rectocele, in 40% with rectal intussusception, and in 53% with no mechanical obstruction evident on defecography [74]. This suggests that damage to the rectal wall can be associated with and not simply consequent to rectal intussusception.

In conclusion, if sacral rectopexy with mesh is proposed, the modified Orr–Loygue technique is advised because it is less aggressive and most effective for anatomical replacement and improvement of FI and ODS. If, indeed, there is no overwhelming clinical evidence that suggests one surgical procedure over another [75], the laparoscopic approach, once abdominal rectopexy is decided upon, seems to offer maximal chances of early recovery, minor incidence of morbidity and the possibility of simultaneously repairing some defects of the anterior perineum; moreover it is also less expensive.

References

1. Shorvon PJ, McHugh S, Diamant NE et al (1989) Defaecography in normal volunteers: results and implications. GUT 30:1737–1749
2. Mellgren A, Bremmer S, Johansson C et al (1994) Defecography. Results of investigations in 2816 patients. Dis Colon Rectum 37:1133–1141
3. Muller-Lissner SA, Bartolo DCC, Christiansen J et al (1998) Interobserver agreement in defecography – an international study. Zeit Gastroenterol 36: 273–279
4. Thompson H, Hill D (1980) Solitary rectal ulcer: always a self-induced conditions? Br J Surg 67:784–785
5. Sun WM, Read NW, Donnelly TC et al (1989) A common pathophysiology for full thickness rectal prolapse, anterior mucosal prolapse and solitary rectal ulcer. Br J Surg 76:290–295
6. Broden B, Snellman B (1968) Procidentia of the rectum studied with cinematography: a contribution to the discussion of causative mechanism. Dis Colon Rectum 11:330–347
7. Ihre T (1972) Internal procidentia of the rectum: treatment and results. Scand J Gastroenterol 7:643–646
8. Mellgren A, Schultz I, Johansson C, Dolk A (1997) Internal rectal intussusception seldom develops into total rectal prolapse. Dis Colon Rectum 40:817–820
9. Wassef R, Rothenberger DA, Goldberg SN (1986) Rectal prolapse. Curr Probl Surg 23:397–451
10. Ihre T (1990) Intussusception of the rectum and the solitary rectal ulcer syndrome. Ann Med 22:419–423
11. Keighley MR (1993) Rectal prolapse. In: Keighley MR, Williams NS (eds) Surgery of the anus, rectum and

colon. WB Saunders, London, 675–719
12. Thakar R, Stanton S (2002) Management of genital prolapse. BMJ 324:1258–1262
13. Petros P (2003) Changes in bladder neck geometry and closure pressure after midurethral anchoring suggest a musculoelastic mechanism activates closure. Neurourol Urodyn 22:191–197
14. Senagore AJ (2003) Management of rectal prolapse: the role of laparoscopic approaches. Semin Laparosc Surg 10:197–202
15. Solomon MJ, Young CJ, Eyers AA, Roberts RA (2002) Randomized clinical trial of laparoscopic versus open abdominal rectopexy for rectal prolapse. Br J Surg 89:35–39
16. Poen AC, deBrauw M, Felt-Bersma RJF, Cuesta MA (1996) Laparoscopic rectopexy for complete rectal prolapse: clinical outcome and anorectal function tests. Surg Endosc 10:904–908
17. Husa A, Sainio P, Von SK (1988) Abdominal rectopexy and sigmoid resection for rectal prolapse. Acta Chir Scand 154:221–224
18. Duthie GS, Bartolo DCC (1992) Abdominal rectopexy for rectal prolapse: a comparison of techniques. Br J Surg 79:107–113
19. Bartolo DCC (1996) Rectal prolapse. Br J Surg 833–835
20. Blatchford GJ, Perry RE, Thorson AG, Chiristensen MA (1989) Rectopexy without resection for rectal prolapse. Am J Surg 158:574–576
21. Orr TG (1947) A suspension operation for prolapse of the rectum. Ann Surg.126:833–337
22. Loygue J, Nordlinger B, Cunci O et al (1984) Rectopexy to the promontory for the treatment of rectal prolapse. Dis Colon Rectum 27: 356–359
23. Moschcowitz AW (1912) The pathogenesis, anatomy and cure of prolapse of the rectum. Surg Gynecol Obstet 15:7–21
24. Jorge JM, Wexner SD (1993) Etiology and management of fecal incontinence. Dis Colon Rectum 36: 77–97
25. Frykman HM, Goldberg SM (1969) The surgical treatment of rectal procidentia. Surg Gynecol Obstet 129:1225–1231
26. Jacobs LK, Lin YJ, Orkin BA (1997) The best operation for rectal prolapse. Surg Clin North Am 77:49–71
27. McKee RF, Lauder JC, Poon FW et al (1992) A prospective randomized study of abdominal rectopexy with and without sigmoidectomy in rectal prolapse. Surg Gynec Obstet 174:145–148
28. Huber FT, Stein H, Siewert JR (1995) Functional results after treatment of rectal prolapse with rectopexy and sigmoid resection. World J Surg 19:138–143
29. Schultz I, Mellgren A, Dolk A et al (1996) Continence is improved after the Ripstein rectopexy. Different mechanism in rectal prolapse and rectal intussusception? Dis Colon Rectum 39:300–306
30. Luukkonen P, Mikkonen U, Jarvinen H (1992) Abdominal rectopexy with sigmoidectomy vs rectopexy alone for rectal prolapse: a prospective, randomized study. Int J Colorectal Dis 7:219–222
31. McMahan JD, Ripstein CB (1987) Rectal prolapse: An update on the rectal sling procedure. Am J Surg 53:37–40
32. Siproudhis L, Ropert A, Gosselin A et al (1993) Constipation after rectopexy for rectal prolapse: where is the obstruction? Dig Dis Sci 38:1801–1808
33. Speakman CTM, Madden MV, Nicholls RJ, Kamm MA (1991) Lateral ligament division during rectopexy causes constipation but prevents recurrence: results of a prospective randomized study. Br J Surg 78:1431–1433
34. Scaglia M, Fasth S, Hallgren T et al (1994) Abdominal rectopexy for rectal prolapse. Influence of surgical technique on functional outcome. Dis Colon Rectum 37:805–813
35. Mann CV, Hoffman C (1988) Complete rectal prolapse: anatomical and functional results of treatment with extended abdominal rectopexy. Br J Surg 75: 34–37
36. Van Tets WF, Kuijpers JH (1995) Internal rectal intussusception – fact or fancy. Dis Colon Rectum 38: 1080–1083
37. Gemsenjager E (1996) Internal rectal prolapse: therapy out-come and current status. J Suisse Med 126:1377–1384
38. Briel JW, Schouten WR, Boerma MO (1997) Long-term results of suture rectopexy in patients with fecal incontinence associated with incomplete rectal prolapse. Dis Colon Rectum 40:1228–1232
39. Ihre T, Selingson U (1975) Intussusception of the rectum-internal procidentia: treatment and results in 90 patients. Dis Colon Rectum 18:391–396
40. Berman IR, Harris MS, Rabeler MB (1990) Delorme's transrectal excision for rectal prolapse: patients selection, technique, and three years follow-up. Dis Colon Rectum 33:573–580
41. Sielzneff I, Malouf A, Cesari J et al (1999) Selection criteria for rectal prolapse repair by Delorme's transrectal excison. Dis Colon Rectum 42:367–373
42. Schultz I, Mellgren A, Dolk A et al (2000) Long-term results and functional outcome after Ripstein rectopexy. Dis Colon Rectum 43:35–43
43. Mollen RM, Kuijpers JH, van Hoek F (2000) Effects of rectal mobilization and lateral ligaments division on colonic and anorectal function. Dis Colon Rectum 43:1283–1287
44. Madiba TE, Baig MK, Wexner SD (2005) Surgical management of rectal prolapse. Arch Surg 140:63–73
45. Infantino A, Fardin P, Pirone E et al (1994) Femoral nerve damage after abdominal rectopexy. Int J Colorectal Dis 9:32–34
46. Kwok SPY, Cared DP, Lau WY, Li AKC (1994) Laparoscopic rectopexy. Dis Colon Rectum 37:947–948
47. Baker R, Senagore AJ, Luchtefeld MA (1995) Laparoscopic-assisted vs open resection: rectopexy offers excellent results. Dis Colon Rectum 38:199–201
48. Hartley J, Farouk R, Monson JRT (1996) Laparoscopic sutured rectopexy for full-thickness rectal prolapse. Min Invas Ther 5:540–542
49. Cuschieri M, Shimi SM, Vander Velpen G et al (1994) Laparoscopic prosthesis fixation rectopexy for complete rectal prolapse. Br J Surg 81:138–139
50. Reissman P, Agachan F, Wexner SD (1996) Outcome of laparoscopic colorectal surgery in older patients. Am Surg 62:1060–1063
51. Kellokumpu IH, Vironen J, Scheinin T (2000) Laparoscopic repair of rectal prolapse: a prospective study

evaluating surgical outcome and changes in symptoms and bowel function. Surg Endosc 14:634–640
52. Ratelle R, Vollant S, Péloquin AB, Gravel D (1994) Abdominal rectopexy (Orr-Loygue) in rectal prolapse: ceioscopic approach or conventional surgery. Ann Surg 48:679–684
53. Auguste T, Dubreuil A, Bost R et al (2006) Technical and functional results after laparoscopic rectopexy to the promontory for complete rectal prolapse. Prospective study in 54 consecutive patients. Gastroenterol Clin Biol 30:659–563
54. Kairaluoma MV, Viljakka MT, Kellokumpu IH (2003) Open vs. laparoscopic surgery for rectal prolapse: a case-controlled study assessing short-term outcome. Dis Colon Rectum 46:353–360
55. Ashari LH, Lumley JW, Stevenson AR, Stitz RW (2005) Laparoscopically-assisted resection rectopexy for rectal prolapse: ten years' experience. Dis Colon Rectum 48:982–987
56. Demirbas S, Akin ML, Kalemoglu M et al (2005) Comparison of laparoscopic and open surgery for total rectal prolapse. Surg Today 35:446–445
57. Lechaux D, Trebuchet G, Siproudhis L, Campion JP (2005) Laparoscopic rectopexy for full-thickness rectal prolapse: a single-institution retrospective study evaluating surgical outcome. Surg Endosc 19:514–518
58. Rose J, Schneider C, Scheidbach H et al (2002) Laparoscopic treatment of rectal prolapse: experience gained in a prospective multicenter study. Langenbecks Arch Surg 387:130–137
59. Salkeld G, Bagia M, Solomon M (2004) Economic impact of laparoscopic versus open abdominal rectopexy. Br J Surg 91:1188–1191
60. Benoist S, Taffinder N, Gould S et al (2001) Functional results two years after laparoscopic rectopexy. Am J Surg 182:168–173
61. Tsugawa K, Sue K, Koyanagi N et al (2002) Laparoscopic rectopexy for recurrent rectal prolapse: a safe and simple procedure without a mesh prosthesis. Hepatogastroenterology 49:1549–1551
62. D'Hoore A, Cadoni R, Penninckx F (2004) Long-term outcome of laparoscopic ventral rectopexy for total rectal prolapse. Br J Surg 91:1500–1505
63. Portier G, Iovino F, Lazorthes F (2006) Surgery for rectal prolapse: Orr-Loygue ventral rectopexy with limited dissection prevents postoperative-induced constipation without increasing recurrence. Dis Colon Rectum 49(8):1136–1140
64. Kaiwa Y, Kurokawa Y, Namiki K et al (2004) Outcome of laparoscopic rectopexy for complete rectal prolapse in patients older than 70 years versus younger patients. Surg Today 34:742–746
65. Nager CW, Kumar D, Kahn MA, Stanton SL (1997) Management of pelvic floor dysfunction. Lancet 350:1751
66. Zhioua F, Ferchiou M, Pira JM et al (1993) Uterine fixation to the promontory and the Orr-Loygue operation in associated genital and rectal prolapse. Rev Fr Gynecol Obstet 88(4):277–281
67. Collopy BT, Barham KA (2002) Abdominal colporectopexy with pelvic cul-de-sac closure. Dis Colon Rectum 45:522–526
68. Timmons MC, Addison WA, Addison SB, Cavenar MG (1992) Abdominal sacral colpopexy in 163 women with posthysterectomy vaginal vault prolapse and enterocele. Evolution of operative techniques. J Reprod Med 37:323–327
69. Fox SD, Stanton SL (2000) Vault prolapse and rectocele: assessment of repair using sacrocolpopexy with mesh interposition. Br J Obstet Gynecol 107:1371–1375
70. Visco AG, Weidner AC, Barber MD et al (2001) Vaginal mesh erosion after abdominal sacral colpopexy. Am J Obstet Gynecol 184:297–302
71. Wang J, Luo MH, Qi QH, Dong ZL (2003) Prospective study of biofeedback retraining in patients with chronic idiopathic functional constipation. World J Gastroenterol 9:2109–2113
72. Emmanuel AV, Mason HJ, Kamm MA (2001) Relationship between psychological state and level of activity of extrinsic gut innervation in patients with a functional gut disorder. Gut 49:209–213
73. Bassotti G, de Roberto G, Sediari L, Morelli A (2004) Colonic motility studies in severe chronic constipation: an organic approach to a functional problem. Tech Coloproctol 8:147–150
74. Gladman MA, Scott SM, Williams NS, Lunniss PJ (2003) Clinical and physiological findings, and possible aetiological factors of rectal hyposensitivity. Br J Surg 90:860–866
75. Bachoo P, Brazzelli M, Grant A (2000) Surgery for complete rectal prolapse in adults. Cochrane Database Syst Rev(2):CD001758

18 Rectopexy According to Frykman–Goldberg Technique

Gian Gaetano Delaini, Gianluca Colucci

"...... for his whoring bowels fell out by reason of the sickness day by day ......"
Old Testament: II Chronicles 21: 1–16
King James Version

Introduction

Rectal prolapse is defined as a full-thickness protrusion of the rectal wall through the anus that is also called procidentia. This disease has plagued human beings throughout history, as it was first described in the Eber papyrus (1500 BC). Hippocrates proposed the first treatment for rectal prolapse by hanging the patient upside down and vigourously shaking him [1]. It is extremely difficult to report the real incidence of this condition, as it has been generally underestimated. The risk factors, as described by Vongsangnak et al. [2], are chronic straining (due to long-standing constipation), prior surgery, neurological and mental illness and ageing. Even if in the past the disease was described as a condition especially affecting young men (as it seems to still be in developing countries), the female to male ratio is now 10:1 [3].

Considering gender, in women, the incidence of procidentia is rare under age 20 and increases gradually from the second decade, peaking in the seventh decade. In men, rectal prolapse is uncommon beyond the fourth decade. Previous pregnancies are not a significant factor in the development of rectal prolapse [4]; however, up to 60% of women with procidentia have a neurogenic weakness of the pelvic floor that is usually caused by childbirth [4]. This can also explain why faecal incontinence is less frequent in nulliparous women with rectal prolapse.

Background

Treatment of rectal prolapse, especially in extensive cases, had been extremely challenging. In 1902 in Vienna, von Eiselsberg [5] reported two cases treated by colopexy and primary resection. Even if von Eiselsberg had planned only a colopexy, he found the sigmoid colon was unusually long and feared that a volvulus might occur. Only one patient survived, but von Eiselsberg speculated that there was a role for this operation in the foreseeable future.

A cornerstone for the future development of abdominal surgery for rectal prolapse was the improvement of anatomical knowledge about this condition. In 1912, Moschcowitz [6] described three essential abnormalities of the pelvic floor in procidentia: (1) an abnormal deep cul-de-sac of Douglas, (2) the rectum must have weak and elongated suspensory ligaments in the pelvis and (3) a mobile redundant sigmoid colon with a long mesentery must be present to reach the deep pelvic floor. In 1939, Pemberton and Stalker [7] concluded that an abnormally loosely attached rectum was the most important factor in the development of a massive rectal prolapse and that prolapse could not develop if the organ was firmly fixed. They concluded that the complete posterior mobilisation of the rectum, its elevation and intra-abdominal fixation, along with raising the level of the pelvic floor, was the best treatment for procidentia. According to Moschcowitz's principles [6], in 1942, Graham et al. [8] thought that rectal procidentia repair could follow the same principles applied to all hernias. By thinking of the rectal prolapse as a "sliding hernia", they postulated peritoneal sac excision and closure of the defect in the pelvic floor by suturing the levator fascia anterior to the rectum.

Disagreeing with this approach, other surgeons, such as Bacon et al. [9] and Hayden [10], moved to the exteriorising resection. Even with slight differences, they accomplished elevation and shortening of the redundant bowel by firm fixation of the sigmoid colon to the anterior abdominal wall. Extraperitoneal closure of the colostomy was done later. Encouraged by the satisfactory results using the Block–Mikulicz technique, the next step was to try to avoid the temporary faecal fistula. In 1951, 50 years after von Eiselsberg, Stabins [11] treated a patient by laparotomy with division of the pelvic peritoneum to bring the prolapsed rectum up into the abdomen, and performed a primary resection and end-to-end anastomosis of the excess sigmoid colon. In 1955, Frykman [12] described a series of seven cases of abdominal proctopexy and primary resection with good overall results. In 1969, Frykman and Goldberg [13] described a series of 80 cases and published the classic description of their procedure: the Frykman–Goldberg technique.

In recent years, introduction of laparoscopic surgery has offered a minimally invasive approach to this operation [14–16]. The acceptance of laparoscopic techniques for diagnosis and therapy has opened a new debate about the safety and the efficacy of the laparoscopic versus the open approach [17, 18].

Surgical Technique

Open Surgery

All patients received a graduated compression stocking, subcutaneous heparin and short-term prophylaxis (single dose of cefotaxime within 30 min of the beginning of the operation). Even if there is much evidence about avoiding bowel preparation [19], many surgeons prefer to give a standard mechanical bowel preparation the day before surgery (2–3 l of polyethylene glycol) to avoid any faecal contamination of the abdominal cavity or abdominal wound. In case of laparoscopic surgery, the preparation is given 2 days before the procedure, and the patient has a light oral diet the day before the procedure to avoid small-bowel-loop distension. The benchmark for this procedure was described by Frykman and Goldberg in 1969 [13]. The operation is carried out under general anaesthesia. The patient is placed in a Trendelenburg position on the operating table using a bean-bag support device. Through a midline incision, the rectum is fully mobilised posteriorly down to the levator ani, preserving the blood supply. Since the introduction of the concept of mesorectum and "holy plane" [20], the dissection is no longer blunt but sharp, in order to preserve the pelvic autonomic nerves and to render the operation virtually bloodless. The pelvic peritoneum is opened in the retrovesical or retrouterine sulcus, and the dissection is carried out down to the prostate or low on the posterior vaginal wall. When the rectum is fully mobilised, the lateral rectal stalks become prominent. The freed rectum is pulled up into the abdomen, and the lateral ligaments are attached to the periosteum of the sacral promontory to hold the organ firmly by interrupted 2/0 nonabsorbable stitches. It is very important not to tie the knot before all the stitches are placed, as it must be ensured that the rectum has been elevated to its maximum extent. The cul-de-sac is obliterated by suturing the endopelvic fascia anterior to the rectum.

The sigmoid colon is then prepared for resection. The extension of the resection may greatly change. The anastomosis should not be under tension, but all redundant colon needs to be removed. The mesocolon and the blood vessel down to the superior haemorrhoidal artery are prepared, and the resection is performed. Any convenient site cranial to the promontory where the sutures are placed can be chosen. An end-to-end anastomosis is then performed. We prefer to use one layer of interrupted stitches with polyglycolic acid sutures (Fig. 1).

Laparoscopic Surgery

Careful attention should be paid to patient position. In order to improve vision within the operative field by displacing the small bowel loops, the operating table should have a range of tilt in every direction and be easily moved by remote control. As a maximum Trendelenburg position and right tilt could be necessary, the patient should be secured to the bed, and bilateral shoulder braces are needed. The patient's arms should be positioned and secured along the body. In order to avoid any nerve stretching or compression, it is preferable

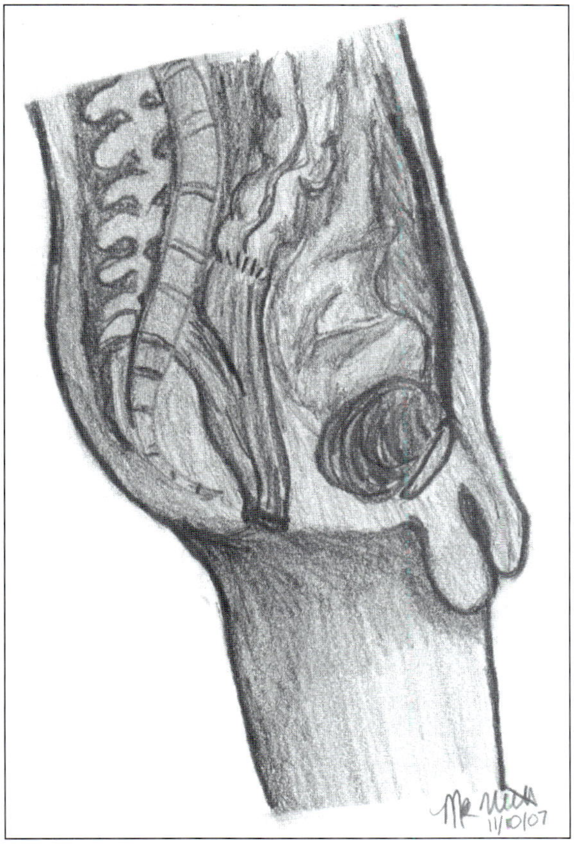

Fig. 1
Rectopexy according to Frykman–Goldberg technique

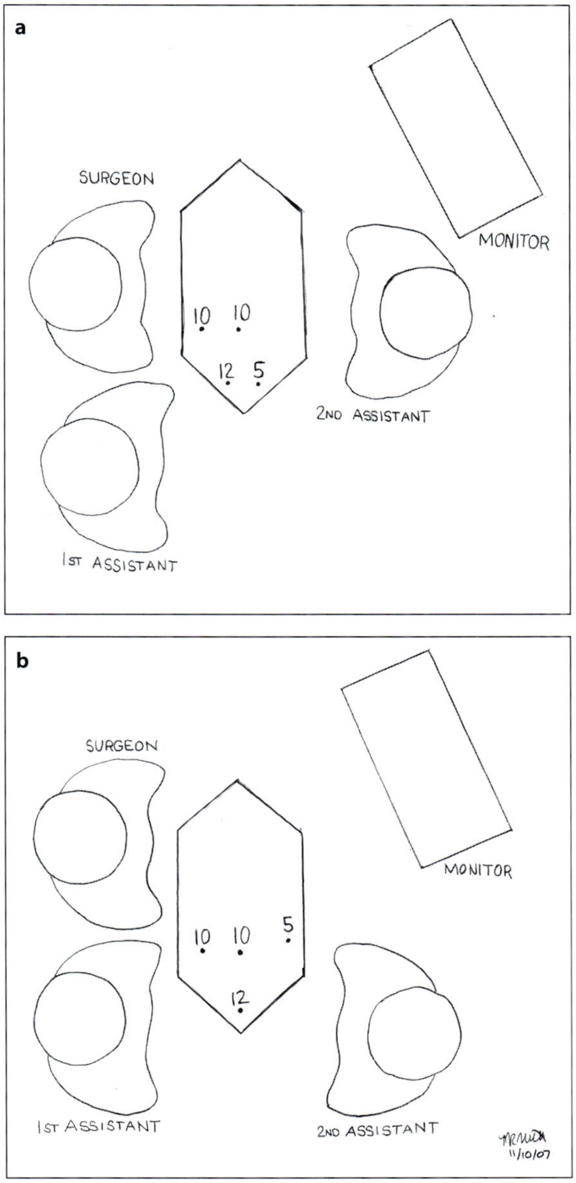

Fig. 2a,b
Operating room set-up. Note the different positions in **a** and **b** of trocars

to place and secure the patient on the bed when he or she is still awake and able to give feedback about the position. The use of foam or gel cushions is mandatory to prevent nerve damage.

Trocar positions are shown in Figure 2. They represent the two more common positions used by laparoscopic surgeons in pelvic surgery. The monitor should be placed on the patient's left, initially towards the head, but may be shifted towards the leg during the procedure. The are no strict rules about the operating-room setup but it is useful to create a routine in order to speed up the setup procedure and have a neat operating field without crossing leads and tubes. The pneumoperitoneum can be created by an open technique or using a Veress needle. The other trocars are placed under direct vision.

The steps are basically the same as those for the open procedure. In our experience, the use of the harmonic scalpel (Ligasure) makes the operation easier to perform and virtually bloodless, but coagulating shears could be used. The rectum is divided distally using an endoscopic stapler and extracted by a small transverse incision in the left iliac fossa. The proximal resection margin is transected with a purse-string device, and the detached anvil of the circular stapler is inserted and secured. The abdominal incision is closed, the pneumoperitoneum is recreated and the end-to-end anastomosis is made with the usual double-stapled technique.

The placement of stitches to secure the lateral ligaments to the periosteum can be very demanding. They can be tied intracorporeally or extracorporeally using an external slipknot. The authors think the use of two laparoscopic needle holders and the intracorporeal technique is the best way to perform this task and to allow more precise control of the tension created. We place 2/0 non-absorbable stitches (Ethibond). Care should be taken to avoid any unintentional lesions when the needle is introduced or moved around.

Robot-assisted Laparoscopic Approach

As already stated, pelvic surgery can be really demanding. The use of robot-assisted laparoscopy has already been explored in order to help overcome the lack of space and the need of still vision [21–24]. There is no reported series of patients submitted to resection rectopexy, but there are series of patients submitted to rectopexy only. The long learning curve, high costs and increase in operative time [25] have led to the use of these devices in a few centres only, and hopefully the good initial results will lead to widespread use of robot-assisted surgery in the foreseeable future.

In the experiences reported, the port position is slightly different to the conventional laparoscopic one in order to allow movement of the robotic arms. The other steps of the operation are virtually the same as the conventional laparoscopic approach.

Results

Resection and rectopexy seem to have a low recurrence rate (between 0% and 9% [26]), even though it has been observed that the recurrence rate reported in the literature seems to underestimate the real incidence of these events [27]. Mortality ranges from 0% to 2.1% [28]. Both constipation and incontinence seem to improve. Delaney [29] emphasised how constipation could balance incontinence and, for this reason, patients with preoperative diarrhoea and incontinence or normal function should not be offered a resection.

Comparing the use of mesh rectopexy versus resection and rectopexy, Kellokumpu et al. [30] demonstrated the latter have identical results but with a reduced incidence of constipation. Also, avoiding the use of foreign material reduces the danger of infection, which occurs in 2–16% of patients after surgery.

The laparoscopic approach seems to be safer compared with the open approach. The major advantages of laparoscopic colonic surgery are seen when large incisions can be avoided, thus reducing postoperative pain, allowing rapid return of bowel function [16], shortening hospital stays (4 days) and decreasing periods of disability. As for open surgery, the laparoscopic resection and pexy has a better outcome than does resection only [18, 29, 31–33].

Indications and Conclusions

In the armament of a colorectal surgeon, more than 100 operations are now available to treat rectal prolapse [34]. Unfortunately, the last word about which surgery is best for treating rectal prolapse is far from having been said. There is still a vigourous debate about which is the best approach for this condition [29, 35–47], and even if many algorithms have been written, the evaluation of patient condition and expectation and the surgeon's attitude still play a big role in the final decision-making process.

It has already been demonstrated that the perineal approach has fewer risks and complications. For these reasons, some authors believe it is more suitable for elderly patients [35, 36, 41]. Recently, Carpelan-Holmstrom et al. [48] challenged this point of view by presenting a cohort of 75 patients (half scored as American Society for Anesthesiologists III or IV), and they had excellent surgical outcomes after both simple rectopexy or rectopexy plus resection.

The higher rate of recurrence after the pelvic approach can obviously make the resection rectopexy the first choice in young patients with a longer life expectancy. Also, the incidence of diverticula increases with the age. The coexistence of diverticula and rectal prolapse could support the idea of "killing two birds with one stone" and guide the surgeon towards performing a resection rectopexy in the elderly [49]. In case of recurrence (after either the pelvic or abdominal approach), the abdominal approach seems to offer better results [50], even if the surgery can be more challenging due to the altered anatomy, especially if a laparoscopic approach is carried out.

In our experience, resection rectopexy seems to be a safe approach and could be offered to almost all patients affected by this condition. The laparoscopic approach is feasible and safe, with a faster recovery and return to home and work. New efforts are needed to shorten the steep learning curve and to create a combined, multidisciplinary approach between gynaecologist and urologist, as the laparoscopic abdominal approach offers the opportunity of simultaneous treatment of pelvic organ prolapse [21, 51].

References

1. Pemberton J, Swash M, Henry MM (2002) The pelvic floor: its function and disorder. W.B. Sauders, Philadelphia
2. Vongsangnak V, Varma JS, Smith AN (1985) Reappraisal of Thiersch's operation for complete rectal prolapse. J R Coll Surg Edinb 30:185–187
3. Watts JD, Rothenberger DA, Buls JG et al (1985) The management of procidentia. 30 years' experience. Dis Colon Rectum 28:96–102
4. Neill ME, Parks AG, Swash M (1981) Physiological studies of the anal sphincter musculature in faecal incontinence and rectal prolapse. Br J Surg 68:531–536
5. von Eiselsberg F (1902) Zur operativen behandlung grosser rectum-prolapse. Arch f Klin Chir 745
6. Moschcowitz A (1912) The pathogenesis, anatomy and care of prolapse of rectum. Surg Gynecol Obstet 15:7
7. Pemberton JD, Stalker LK (1939) Surgical treatment of complete rectal prolapse. Ann Surg 109:799–808
8. Graham W, Clegg JF, Taylor V (1984) Complete rectal prolapse: repair by a simple technique. Ann R Coll Surg Engl 66:87–89
9. Bacon HE, Burkett W, Sauer J (1950) Surgical management of rectal procidentia. South Surgeon 11:15
10. Hayden E (1947) Prolapse of the rectum. S Clin North Am 27:1062
11. Stabins SJ (1951) A new surgical procedure for complete rectal prolapse in the mentally ill patient; case report. Surgery 29:105–108
12. Frykman HM (1955) Abdominal proctopexy and primary sigmoid resection for rectal procidentia. Am J Surg 90:780–789
13. Frykman HM, Goldberg SM (1969) The surgical treatment of rectal procidentia. Surg Gynecol Obstet 129:1225–1230
14. Senagore AJ, Luchtefeld MA, Mackeigan JM, Mazier WP (1993) Open colectomy versus laparoscopic colectomy: are there differences? Am Surg 59:549–553
15. Sackier JM, Berci G, Hiatt JR, Hartunian S (1992) Laparoscopic abdominoperineal resection of the rectum. Br J Surg 79:1207–1208
16. Ballantyne GH (1992) Laparoscopically assisted anterior resection for rectal prolapse. Surg Laparosc Endosc 2:230–236
17. Baker R, Senagore AJ, Luchtefeld MA (1995) Laparoscopic-assisted vs. open resection. Rectopexy offers excellent results. Dis Colon Rectum 38:199–201
18. Johnson E, Stangeland A, Johannessen HO, Carlsen E (2007) Resection rectopexy for external rectal prolapse reduces constipation and anal incontinence. Scand J Surg 96:56–61
19. Guenaga K, Atallah AN, Castro AA et al (2005) Mechanical bowel preparation for elective colorectal surgery. Cochrane Database Syst Rev (1):CD001544
20. Heald R, Husband E, Rayall R (1982) The mesorectum in rectal cancer surgery – the clue to pelvic recurrence? Br J Surg 69:613–619
21. Novara G, Galfano A, Secco S (2007) Prolapse surgery: an update. Curr Opin Urol 17:237–241
22. Ayav A, Bresler L, Hubert J et al (2005) Robotic-assisted pelvic organ prolapse surgery. Surg Endosc 19:1200–1203
23. Ayav A, Bresler L, Brunaud L, Boissel P (2004) Early results of one-year robotic surgery using the Da Vinci system to perform advanced laparoscopic procedures. J Gastrointest Surg 8:720–726
24. Munz Y, Moorthy K, Kudchadkar R et al (2004) Robotic assisted rectopexy. Am J Surg 187:88–92
25. Heemskerk J, de Hoog DE, van Gemert WG et al (2007) Robot-assisted vs. conventional laparoscopic rectopexy for rectal prolapse: a comparative study on costs and time. Dis Colon Rectum (E-pub ahead of print)
26. Kim DS, Tsang CB, Wong WD (1999) Complete rectal prolapse: evolution of management and results. Dis Colon Rectum 42:460–466
27. DiGiuro G, Ignjatovic D, Brogger J, Bergamaschi R (2006) How accurate are published recurrence rates after rectal prolapse surgery? A meta-analysis of individual patient data. Am J Surg 191:773–778
28. Husa A, Sainio P, von SK (1988) Abdominal rectopexy and sigmoid resection (Frykman-Goldberg operation) for rectal prolapse. Acta Chir Scand 154:221–224
29. Delaney CP (2007) Laparoscopic management of rectal prolapse. J Gastrointest Surg 11:150–152
30. Kellokumpu IH, Vironen J, Scheinin T (2000) Laparoscopic repair of rectal prolapse: a prospective study evaluating surgical outcome and changes in symptoms and bowel function. Surg Endosc 14:634–640
31. Gurlich R, Sixta B, Drastich P et al [Laparoscopic rectopexis]. Rozhl Chir 85:233–235
32. Kariv Y, Delaney CP, Casillas S et al (2006) Long-term outcome after laparoscopic and open surgery for rectal prolapse: a case-control study. Surg Endosc

20:35–42
33. Sezai D, Demirbas S, Akin L (2005) The impact of laparoscopic resection rectopexy in patients with total rectal prolapse. Mil Med 170:743–747
34. Gourgiotis S, Baratsis S (2007) Rectal prolapse. Int J Colorectal Dis 22:231–243
35. Marderstein EL, Delaney CP (2007) Surgical management of rectal prolapse. Nat Clin Pract Gastroenterol Hepatol 4:552–561
36. Sailer M, Bonicke L, Petersen S (2007) [Surgical options in the treatment of rectal prolapse: indications, techniques and results]. Zentralbl Chir 132:350–357
37. Stein EA, Stein DE (2006) Rectal procidentia: diagnosis and management. Gastrointest Endosc Clin N Am 16:189–201
38. Munoz F, del Valle E, Rodriguez M, Zorrilla J (2005) [Rectal prolapse. Abdominal or perineal approach? Current situation]. Cir Esp 78(Suppl 3):50–58
39. Lechaux D, Trebuchet G, Siproudhis L, Campion JP (2005) Laparoscopic rectopexy for full-thickness rectal prolapse: a single-institution retrospective study evaluating surgical outcome. Surg Endosc 19:514–518
40. Chiu HH, Chen JB, Wang HM (2001) Surgical treatment for rectal prolapse. Zhonghua Yi Xue Za Zhi (Taipei) 64:95–100
41. Kellokumpu IH, Kairaluoma M (2001) Laparoscopic repair of rectal prolapse: surgical technique. Ann Chir Gynaecol 90:66–69
42. Madoff RD, Mellgren A (1999) One hundred years of rectal prolapse surgery. Dis Colon Rectum 42:441–450
43. Stevenson AR, Stitz RW, Lumley JW (1998) Laparoscopic-assisted resection-rectopexy for rectal prolapse: early and medium follow-up. Dis Colon Rectum 41:46–54
44. Hool GR, Hull TL, Fazio VW (1997) Surgical treatment of recurrent complete rectal prolapse: a thirty-year experience. Dis Colon Rectum 40:270–272
45. Jacobs LK, Lin YJ, Orkin BA (1997) The best operation for rectal prolapse. Surg Clin North Am 77:49–70
46. Penninckx F, D'Hoore A, Sohier S, Kerremans R (1997) Abdominal resection rectopexy versus Delorme's procedure for rectal prolapse: a predictable outcome. Int J Colorectal Dis 12:49–50
47. Kockerling F, Schneider C, Hohenberger W (1996) [Rectal prolapse—choice of procedure and minimally invasive possibilities]. Chirurg 67:471–482
48. Carpelan-Holmstrom M, Kruuna O, Scheinin T (2006) Laparoscopic rectal prolapse surgery combined with short hospital stay is safe in elderly and debilitated patients. Surg Endosc 20:1353–1359
49. Gaivoronskaia SS, Vasil'ev SV, Chaniia ZD et al (2007) [Potentialities of complex treatment of prolapse of the rectum]. Vestn Khir Im I I Grek 166:100–102
50. Steele SR, Goetz LH, Minami S et al (2006) Management of recurrent rectal prolapse: surgical approach influences outcome. Dis Colon Rectum 49:440–455
51. Verdaasdonk EG, Bueno de Mesquita JM, Stassen LP (2006) Laparoscopic rectovaginopexy for rectal prolapse. Tech Coloproctol 10:318–222

19 Laparoscopic Ventral Rectocolpopexy for Complex Rectogenital Prolapse

Andre D'Hoore, Freddy Penninckx

Introduction

Rectal prolapse is a full-thickness intussusception of the rectum. When the intussusception is still confined to the anal canal, it is referred to as internal prolapse. Once the prolapse protrudes beyond the anal verge, it is called a total rectal prolapse. Inevitably, a significant descensus of the posterior pelvic compartment will influence the static and dynamic stability of the other pelvic compartments (especially the middle compartment). The presence of an abnormally deep pouch of Douglas is a constant finding in total rectal prolapse. In the ageing woman, weakening of the pelvic floor and rectovaginal septum further contribute to the development of more complex pelvic organ prolapses.

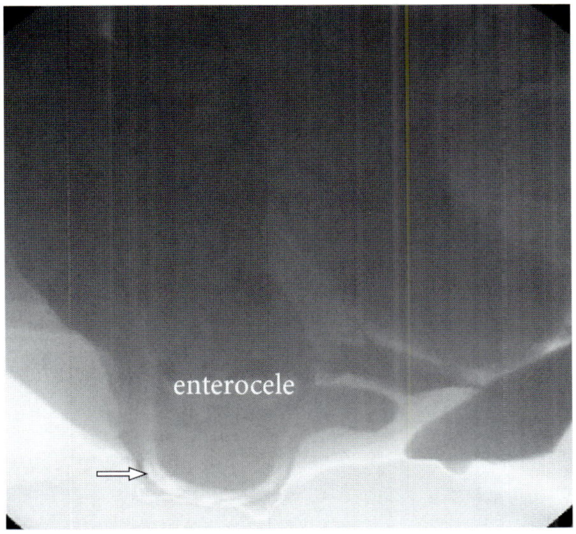

Fig. 1
Colpocystodefecogram at the end of straining. Note the intussusception of the rectum protruding through the anal ring (*arrow*) and the presence of a huge enterocele compressing the anal canal

The observation of Roscoe Graham that "major portion of the visible bulge occurs at the expense of the anterior rectal wall" [1] was later confirmed by Broden and Snellman in dynamic proctographic studies [2]. More recently, video colpocystodefecography [3] further enhanced the understanding of the anatomy of pelvic organ prolapse. An example of total rectal prolapse and huge enterocele is shown in Figure 1. Mellgren et al. [4] in a large defecography study in 2,816 patients showed that a grade III enterocele is present in up to 42% of patients with a total rectal prolapse. This emphasises the need to correct the descensus of the middle compartment along with the rectal prolapse. In classic rectopexy, obliteration of the pouch of Douglas is performed by adding serial purse-string sutures according to the Moschcowitz procedure [5], or by adding a second mesh to perform a mesh colpopexy.

Rationale for Laparoscopic Ventral Rectocolpopexy

Anatomical Considerations

Those radiological findings were the basis for the design of a new, modified rectal suspension technique. The so-called laparoscopic ventral rectocolpopexy (LVR) (Fig. 2) is, in essence, a combination of a modified Orr [6] technique and a sacral colpopexy. According to DeLancey [7], three different levels of vaginal support seem to play a role in the stability of the middle compartment: the cardinal uterosacral ligaments (level I), the rectovaginal septum (level II) and the perineal body (level III). In the LVR technique, suspension of the apex of the posterior vaginal fornix or vaginal vault can be performed to the same mesh (level I). The position of the mesh on the anterior aspect of

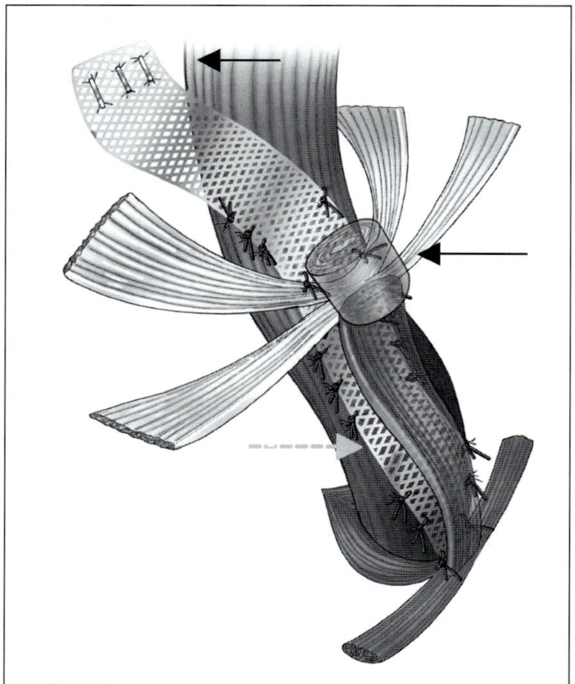

Fig. 2
Schematic representation of the laparoscopic ventral rectopexy: *upper arrow* promontory fixation; *middle arrow* colpopexy; *lower arrow* ventral rectopexy

the rectum reinforces the rectovaginal septum (level II).

Functional Considerations

Rectal prolapse surgery not only aims to restore anatomy but also to improve anorectal function. Postoperative constipation has been a constant concern after classic mesh rectopexy techniques. Extensive rectal mobilisation and the subsequent autonomic nerve damage (extrinsic sympathetic innervation S2–S4) may result in disturbed rectosigmoid motility [8]. In the presented LVR technique, dissection is restricted to the anterior aspect of the rectum and therefore limits the risk for autonomic nerve damage. Mesh position reinforces the rectovaginal septum, and the colpopexy allows correction of a concomitant prolapse of the middle compartment. Constipation, especially outlet delay constipation, is a common finding in patients with a total rectal prolapse.

A full-thickness intussusception of the rectum and/or an important enterocele can cause a mechanical outlet obstruction. In patients with a rectocele, descending perineum syndrome and total rectal prolapse and dissipation of the force vector at straining will further impede rectal emptying. In a long-term follow-up study [9] on functional outcome after LVR, postoperative constipation seemed to be avoidable in most patients. Furthermore, the surgery seemed to cure obstructed defecation, or at least attenuate related symptoms. LVR allows correction of combined prolapse of the posterior and middle compartments without extensive lateral dissection [10]. This mesh suspension technique impedes further intussusception of the rectum (and as such corrects the rectal prolapse).

Laparoscopic Approach

In a prospective study, Solomon et al. [11] demonstrated the superiority (perioperative morbidity, postoperative pain, hospital stay and costs) of a laparoscopic approach in prolapse surgery. LVR allows correction of rectal intussusception and prolapses of the middle pelvic compartment without extensive dissection.

Surgical Technique of Laparoscopic Ventral Rectocolpopexy

Patient Preparation and Installation

All patients receive limited bowel preparation (fleet enema, Fleet Pharmaceuticals, NV Wolf, Sint-Niklaas, Belgium) and a single dose of a broad-spectrum antibiotic. Thrombose prophylaxis using low-molecular-weight heparin is continued during hospital stay. Patients are placed on a mouldable "bean bag", allowing safe steep Trendelenburg position during the laparoscopic procedure. The patient is positioned in a modified lithotomy position with both arms along the body and is catheterised. The vagina is disinfected using a Betadine 10% solution.

After installation of a pneumoperitoneum, the camera port is introduced at the umbilicus. Three additional ports are inserted into the right flank (5 mm), the left iliac fossa (5 mm) and the right lower quadrant (12 mm). Routinely, a 30° optic is used to allow adequate visualisation in the rectovaginal septum. A temporary hysteropexy can be

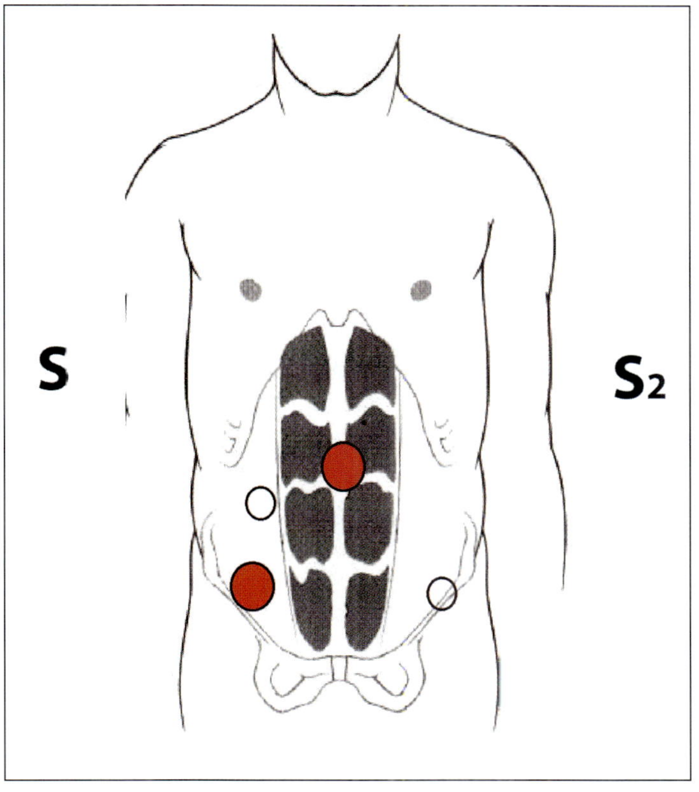

Fig. 3

Positioning of camera ports. *Red dots* represent 12-mm ports. *Open dots* represent the 5 mm ports. *S* surgeon, *S2* assistant surgeon

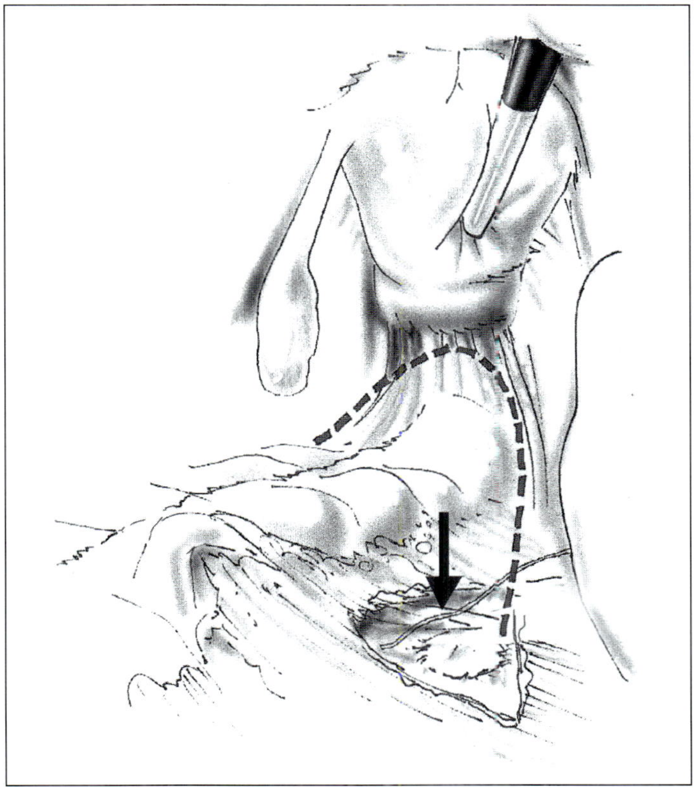

Fig. 4

The *dotted line* depicts the line of peritoneal incision. The course of the right hypogastric nerve (*arrow*) is also shown. Reprinted with permission from [10]

performed to enhance the pelvic view. The entire small bowel is retracted out of the pelvis. Figure 3 shows schematically the port position.

Peritoneal Incision and Sacral Promontory Dissection

The mesosigmoid is retracted to the left. A peritoneal incision is made over the sacral promontory and caudally extended along the rectum and over the deepest part of the pouch of Douglas (Fig. 4). Special care is taken to preserve the right hypogastric nerve. The sacral promontory should be sufficiently dissected to allow safe mesh fixation. Too medial a dissection must be avoided to safeguard the left iliac vein.

Opening the Rectovaginal Septum

The rectovaginal septum is opened after firm retraction of the deepest part of the fold of Douglas. Denonvilliers fascia is incised, and dissection is performed upon the anterior aspect of the rectum, leaving all fibrous tissue against the posterior vaginal wall. A redundant pouch of Douglas can be resected, but hemostasis has to be meticulous.

Mesh Fixation (Rectum – Promontory)

In all patients, a Marlex mesh (Bard, Crawley, UK) (trimmed approximately to 3 × 17 cm) has been used. The mesh is sutured to the ventral aspect of the distal rectum using nonabsorbable sutures (EthibondExcel 0; Ethicon, Johnson & Johnson, Brussels, Belgium). Extracorporeal suturing seems the most appropriate in the deepest part. Care should be taken that the mesh lies flat upon the rectum to avoid any mechanical erosion due to mesh kinking (Fig. 5). Those sutures will inhibit further rectal intussusception. The mesh is then fixed to the sacral promontory using either sutures or an endoscopic "tacker" device. No traction is exerted on the rectum, which remains in the sacrococcygeal hollow.

Colpopexy and Peritoneal Closure

The posterior vaginal apex (vaginal vault) is then elevated and sutured to the same strip of mesh. Two lateral sutures incorporate the (remainder of the) uterosacral ligament. More suturing is needed depending upon the degree of middle compartment prolapse. (Fig. 6). Preferentially, the sutures should not perforate the vaginal wall. The mesh can be left broader at that site to allow adequate vault suspension. This suturing restores level I (according to DeLancey [7]) support of the vagina. The lateral borders are closed over the mesh, elevating the neo-Douglas over the colpopexy. This manoeuvre is important to avoid any later small-bowel entrapment and/or erosion.

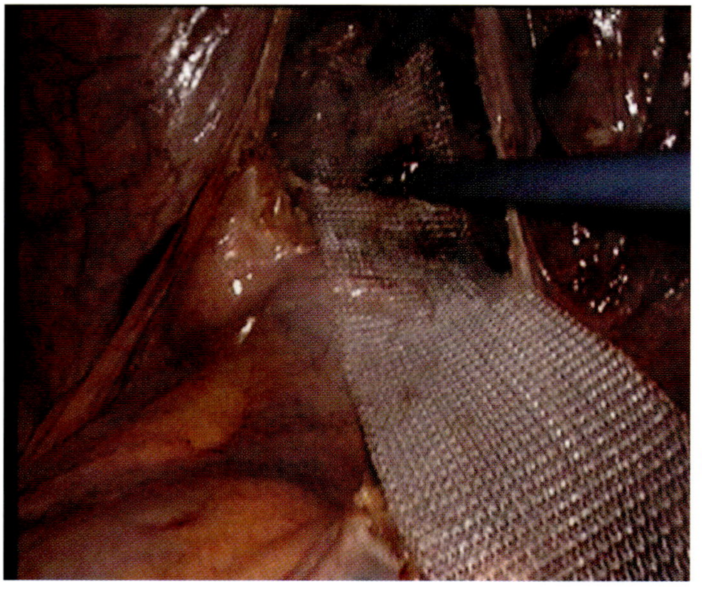

Fig. 5
Laparoscopic view of the position of the mesh strip upon the anterior aspect of the rectum (in the rectovaginal septum) slightly deviating to the right side of the sacral promontory

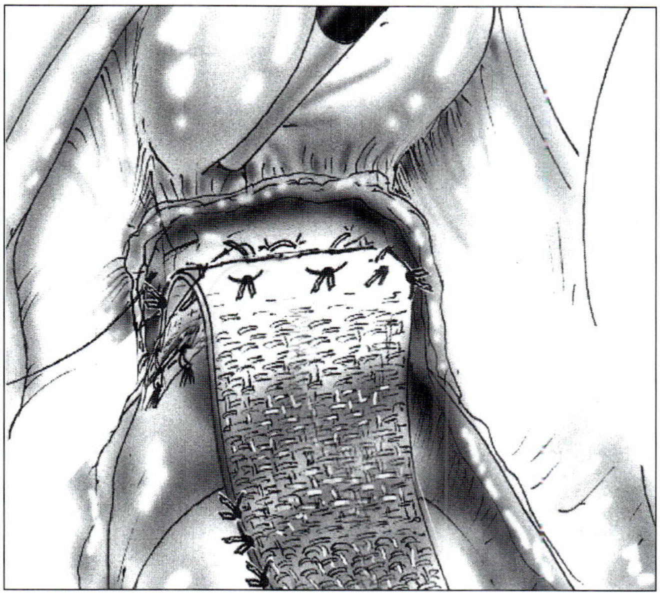

Fig. 6
Colpopexy to the same mesh as seen in Figure 5. Reprinted with permission from [10]

Perineotomy (Facultative)

It can be difficult to complete the rectovaginal septum dissection to the pelvic floor level. This manoeuvre is important in treating a complex rectocele. In that specific situation, the surgeon can decide to complete the laparoscopic dissection with a small perineotomy. The incision is made immediately dorsal to the vaginal orifice to open the perineal body. Dissection should be meticulous to avoid any perforation of the vagina or rectum. After perineotomy, this dissection joins the laparoscopic dissection plane, allowing mesh fixation in the deepest part of the rectovaginal septum and restoring the perineal body. A perineotomy, however, can be avoided in most patients with a total rectal prolapse.

Postoperative Treatment

No peritoneal drain is left in. The patient can resume oral intake the day of surgery. A fibre-enriched diet is prescribed. The urinary catheter is removed the following day, and mobilisation is started. According to clinical evolution, the patient can be discharged from day 1 on. Straining efforts and heavy lifting are discouraged for 4–6 weeks.

Outcome after Laparoscopic Ventral Rectocolpopexy

An overview of the different patient groups who underwent LVR at the University Hospital in Leuven is given in Table 1.

Table 1. Different patient cohorts treated with laparoscopic ventral rectocolpopexy

Indication	Period	F (n)	M (n)	Age (range)	Conv. [*n* (%)]	FU (months)	Rec *n* (%)	Erosion (*n*)
Total rectal prolapse [9]	1995–2004	100	9	49.3 (16–88)	4 (3.6)	73	5 (4.6)	–
Internal rectal prolapse	2001–2004	20	5	58.0 (30–81)	–	30	–	–
Complex rectocele (+ perineotomy)	2003–2006	57	–	58.0 (38–80)	–	24.2	NDA	1 (vagina)

F female, *M* male, *Conv.* conversion to laparotomy, *FU* follow-up, *Rec.* recurrence, *NDA* no data available

Conversion to Laparotomy

Although roughly 30% of all patients in our series had previous pelvic surgery, the need for conversion to laparotomy due to adhesions was very limited ($n = 2$). In one patient, acute bleeding from the left iliac vein occurred and mandated an emergent laparotomy to obtain hemostasis. Mesh fixation to the sacral promontory (in comparison with a posterior pelvic dissection and fixation to the presacral fascia) certainly reduces the risk for a cumbersome presacral haemorrhage.

Hospital Stay and Perioperative Morbidity

Over time, hospital stay decreased to a median of 4.2 (2–10) days, and perioperative morbidity was minor. No major septic complications (mesh infection, pelvic abscess) occurred.

Recurrences

One hundred and nine patients (nine men) underwent LVR for total rectal prolapse after a mean follow-up of 73 (12–100) months. Clinical recurrence was noted in five patients. Dehiscence of mesh fixation to the sacral promontory was noted in three patients. In one patient, a recurrent enterocele was diagnosed, and in another, incomplete reduction of the prolapse at the time of mesh fixation evidently resulted in a persistent prolapse. This recurrence rate of 4.6% is in line with reported recurrences of classic mesh repair. Longer follow-up seems necessary to allow a more complete picture of recurrence [12].

Mesh Erosion

In our total series of 172 female patients, only one mesh erosion to the vagina was noted (see Table 1). This patient underwent a combined approach (laparoscopic and perineotomy) for a grade III low rectocele and rectal intussusception. None of the patients with a total rectal prolapse have thus far developed mesh erosion. It therefore can be concluded that the use of polypropylene mesh on the anterior aspect of the rectum is safe. Dissection posterior to Denonvilliers fascia seems to offer protection from any vaginal erosion. The follow-up of the group of patients who underwent a combined perineotomy is short (24.2 months); no final conclusion for this subgroup therefore seems appropriate.

Functional Outcome

Incontinence

Faecal incontinence is a common clinical finding in patients with total rectal prolapse (especially in the aged patient). In our series, 74% of patients had some degree of incontinence. After LVR, a significant improvement occurred in 90% of patients. The mean Wexner incontinence score decreased significantly from 11.19 ± 7.3 SD before to 3.59 ± 6.1 SD after surgery. This finding is in agreement with results of classic rectopexy and reflects the importance of preserving the rectal ampulla.

Apposition of polypropylene mesh within the rectovaginal septum on the anterior aspect of the rectum induces fibrosis and could interfere with the distensibility of the rectum and rectal visceroperception. A subgroup of patients underwent extensive manometry and rectal barostat to evaluate remaining anorectal function. The rectal capacity remains unchanged after rectopexy. Only a limited change in the first part of the pressure/volume curve, resulting in an improved (earlier) perception of lower rectal volumes, was observed.

Constipation

In a long-term follow-up study of patients with total rectal prolapse, we reported a significant decrease in constipation [9]. Symptoms of obstructed defecation resolved in 16 of 19 patients, whereas only minor beneficial effect on slow-transit constipation was noted (Fig. 7).

Dyspareunia

Dyspareunia is of concern, especially after surgery to correct a rectocele. The position of the mesh posterior to the vagina and fixation of the vaginal vault to the mesh could induce dyspareunia. In three patients (3/55) in our series, postoperative dyspareunia was noted. Two patients mentioned worsening of preexisting dyspareunia. The patient with vaginal erosion evidently developed new-onset sexual dysfunction. On structural questioning in the group of patients treated for total or internal rectal prolapse, none mentioned dyspareunia or sexual dysfunction.

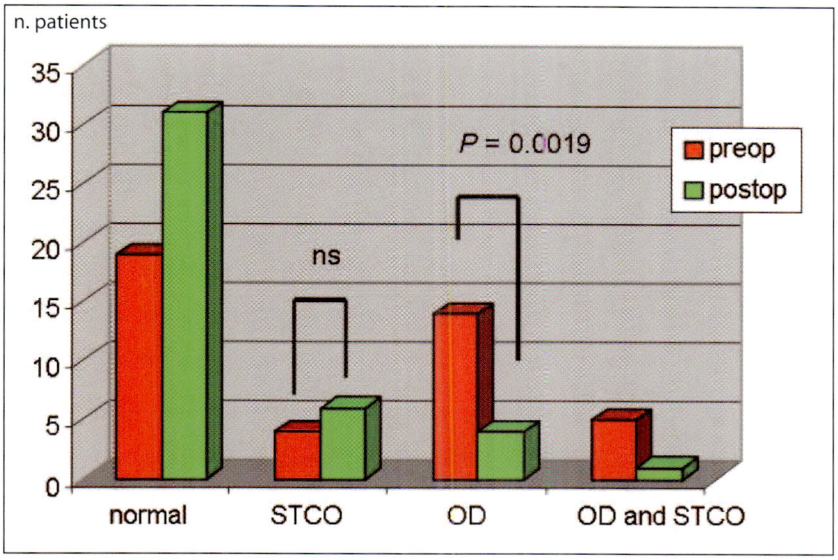

Fig. 7 Summary of findings as reported previously [9]. A significant reduction in patients with obstructed defecation is observed. LVR had no effect on the problem of slow transit constipation. *ns* not significant; *STCO* slow transit colonic obstipation; *OD* obstructed defecation (according to Rome II criteria)

Discussion

The above-mentioned results are a single-centre experience with a newly designed mesh rectopexy technique, and therefore, confirmation of these results is awaited. Recently, the Oxford experience (Radcliffe Hospital, Oxford, UK) was reported in 63 consecutive patients using the same LVR technique, resulting in a similar outcome [13]. Nevertheless, it seems appropriate to wait for longer follow-up and comparative data to allow final conclusions.

Conclusion

LVR is a safe and reliable new technique to correct rectal prolapse. The anatomical correction coincides with a significant improvement in rectal emptying in most patients. The technique is therefore appropriate in selected patients with internal rectal prolapse and therapy-resistant obstructed defecation. Adding a perineotomy to the laparoscopic dissection allows correcting complex rectoceles. The technique seems a valuable adjunct to the surgical armamentarium to treat complex prolapse of the posterior and middle pelvic compartment.

References

1. Graham RR (1985) The operative repair of massive rectal prolapse. Dis Colon Rectum 28:374–379
2. Broden B, Snellman B (1968) Procidentia of the rectum studied with cineradiography. A contribution to the discussion of causative mechanism. Dis Colon Rectum 11:330–347
3. Altringer WE, Saclarides TJ, Dominguez JM et al (1995) Four-contrast defecography: pelvic "floor-oscopy". Dis Colon Rectum 38:695–699
4. Mellgren A, Bremmer S, Johansson C et al (1994) Defecography: results of investigations in 2816 patients. Dis Colon Rectum 37:1133–1141
5. Moschconitz AW (1992) The pathogenesis, anatomy, and cure of prolapse of the rectum. Surg Gynecol Obstet 15:7–21
6. Orr TG (1947) A suspension operation for prolapse of the rectum. Ann Surg 126:833–840
7. DeLancey JO (1999) Structural anatomy of the posterior pelvic compartment and it relates to rectocele. Am J Obstet Gynecol 180:815–823
8. Speakman CTM, Madden MV, Nicholls RJ, Kamm MA (1991) Lateral ligament division during rectopexy causes constipation but prevents recurrence: results of a prospective randomized study. Br J Surg 78: 1431–1433
9. D'Hoore A, Cadoni R, Penninckx F (2004) The long-term outcome of laparoscopic ventral rectopexy for total rectal prolapse. Br J Surg 91:1500–1505
10. D'Hoore A, Penninckx F (2006) Laparoscopic ventral recto(colpo)pexy for rectal prolapse. Surgical tech-

nique and outcome for 109 patients. Surg Endosc 20:1919–1923

11. Solomon MJ, Young CJ, Eyers AA, Roberts RA (2002) Randomized controlled trial of laparoscopic versus abdominal rectopexy for rectal prolapse. Br J Surg 89:35–39
12. Raftopoulos Y, Senagore AJ, Di Giuro G, Bergamaschi R (2005) Rectal prolapse recurrence study group. Dis Colon Rectum 48:1200–1206
13. Collonson RJ, Boons P, Cunningham C, Lindsey I (2007) Laparoscopic anterior rectopexy: cures rectal prolapse and improves preop constipation without inducing new-onset constipation. ANZ J Surg 77:A28

20 Management of Rectal Prolapse: The Role of Laparoscopic Approaches

Dan R. Metcalf, Anthony J. Senagore

Introduction

Rectal prolapse has a profound effect on quality of life and has been associated with a multitude of surgical treatment options since its original description. It is defined as a full-thickness protrusion of the rectal wall through the anal sphincter. Clinical management is confounded by the fact that whereas 75% of patients with rectal prolapse experience problems with anal incontinence, 25–50% will have significant constipation [1–4]. Symptoms of anal incontinence may be due to acquired changes in bowel motility or a reduction in resting anal pressure as a result of continual activation of rectoanal inhibition [5–7]. Constipation in patients with rectal prolapse may be a consequence of slow colonic transit or an increase in external anal sphincter contractions [4, 8]. These symptoms have a significant influence on the choice of operative approach in the treatment of rectal prolapse. However, due to the variable results of operative approaches, it is unclear whether optimal treatment can be selected based on preoperative physiologic testing.

The primary objectives in surgical management of full-thickness rectal prolapse are to minimize operative risk, eliminate the external prolapse, improve continence and bowel function, and decrease the risk of recurrence. Surgical approaches are generally classified into two groups: perineal and transabdominal. Prior to the introduction of laparoscopic techniques, perineal repairs were considered ideal based on a perceived decrease in operative risk. The most prevalent of these repairs are perineal proctosigmoidectomy and the Delorme procedure. Although they are commonly performed in this often-elderly patient population, perineal approaches are associated with higher recurrence rates [9, 10]. Douard et al. [11] demonstrated higher complication rates in a recent evaluation of the Orr–Loygue procedure, which showed a 29% morbidity rate and a 6% reoperation rate. In a report by Watkins et al. [12], the modified Delorme procedure was even associated with a length of hospital stay averaging 4.9 postoperative days. For the most part, transabdominal approaches consist of either rectal mobilization in conjunction with some type of rectopexy, or sigmoid resection with suture rectopexy. Transabdominal approaches offer the benefits of preserving rectal reservoir function, lower recurrence rates, and improvement in symptoms with superior functional results [13–17]. Carpelan-Holmström et al. demonstrated in a recent report that laparoscopic rectal prolapse surgery can be a safe and effective option in patients with American Society for Anesthesiologists (ASA) scores of III and IV [18]. Prior to the advent of laparoscopic techniques, these patients would likely have undergone perineal approaches to repair their rectal prolapse.

First introduced by Berman in 1992, rectopexy without bowel resection was the initial approach to laparoscopic management of rectal prolapse [17]. The intent of a laparoscopic approach was to combine the attributes of lower surgical stress characteristics of the perineal approach with the durability achieved in the open abdominal approach to rectal prolapse repair. The decision to pursue a laparoscopic approach still involves the choices of whether or not to perform a sigmoid resection and whether suture or artificial material will be used for the rectopexy [19, 20].

As demonstrated by studies that compare the same approach for rectal prolapse using both laparoscopic and open techniques, laparoscopy offers benefits related to reduced postoperative pain, shorter length of stay, and earlier bowel function return [21–25]. A multicenter report from the German Study Group for Laparoscopic

Colorectal Surgery identified 150 patients with rectal prolapse managed laparoscopically [26]. Sigmoid resection with rectopexy was the procedure most commonly performed, with a conversion rate of only 5.3% and a severe complication rate of 3.3%. A recent prospective randomized trial by Solomon et al. utilized a clinical pathway for patients undergoing either an open or a laparoscopic posterior mesh rectopexy [27]. Laparoscopic patients experienced fewer significant respiratory complications, higher completion of the clinical pathway (75% vs. 37%), and significantly shorter hospital stay (3.9 days vs. 6.6 days). Kairaluoma et al. were able to demonstrate a similar advantage in length of stay and lower operative complications in a case-control study comparing laparoscopic resection with rectopexy or rectopexy alone to an open technique [28].

Nearly all of the open transabdominal procedures to repair rectal prolapse have been performed laparoscopically. At present, laparoscopic surgical procedures include suture and stapled rectopexy, posterior mesh rectopexy with artificial material, and sigmoid resection with or without suture rectopexy [29–32]. In addition, D'Hoore et al. described a novel technique of laparoscopic ventral rectopexy for total rectal prolapse, which avoids posterolateral rectal mobilization and involves the placement of mesh anterior to the rectum [33]. During this procedure, the dissection is limited to the anterior aspect of the rectum, therefore limiting the risk of autonomic nerve injury. Although the use of foreign material for rectopexy has the potential benefit of a greater degree of rectal fixation, there is a theoretically increased risk in the setting of an anastomotic leak after resection. Therefore, mesh rectopexy is not usually performed in conjunction with bowel resection. Suture rectopexy avoids this potential risk and is less technically demanding; however, there is potentially a higher recurrence rate and a comparable risk of postoperative constipation [31]. Both Wells posterior mesh rectopexy and Sudeck suture rectopexy offer the advantages of secure rectal fixation and low rates of recurrence. However, as a result of exaggeration and fixation of the sigmoid loop, both have the risk of new-onset postoperative constipation [29, 32]. The use of mesh fixation carries the risk of fibrotic bowel stricture with obstruction or mesh erosion [2, 7]. Resection rectopexy provides the lowest recurrence rates and minimizes the risk of postoperative constipation. Unfortunately, the likelihood of longer hospital stays and the risk of anastomotic leakage are higher with resection [2, 7].

We prefer to use either a laparoscopic Wells mesh rectopexy or sigmoid resection with suture rectopexy repair in the majority of patients with rectal prolapse. The selection criteria used to distinguish patients best served by a given procedure are demonstrated in Figure 1. All patients receive general anesthesia and are placed in the modified lithotomy position using Dan-Allen stirrups, providing leg abduction and limited hip flexion. An umbilical trocar (10 mm) is placed using an open technique, and pneumoperitoneum is maintained at 12 mmHg throughout the procedure. When performing a laparoscopic Wells procedure, two additional 5-mm trocars are used – one in the right iliac fossa lateral to the rectus sheath and another in the same line just above the level of the umbilicus. To allow the use of an endoscopic lin-

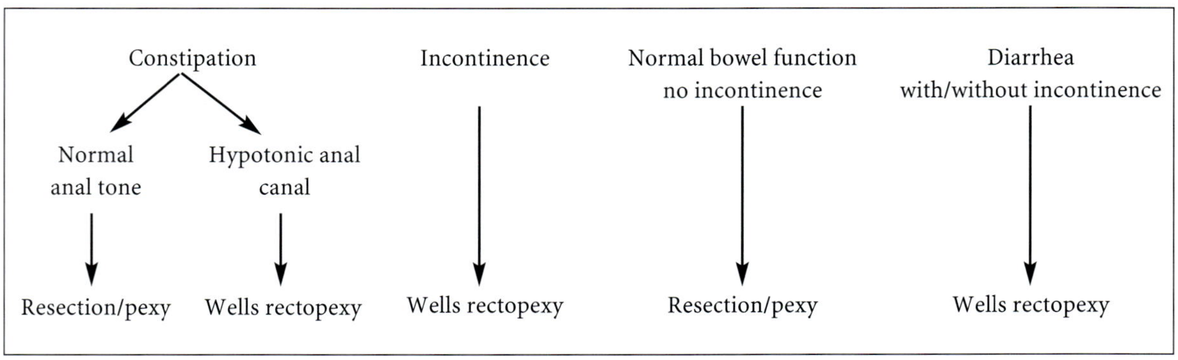

Fig. 1
Clinical algorithm for choosing a laparoscopic approach to rectal prolapse

ear stapler during laparoscopic resection rectopexy, a 12-mm trocar is used in the right iliac fossa location. A 5-mm trocar for the assistant is placed in the left iliac fossa in both procedures.

With both techniques, a medial approach is used to mobilize the rectum. The left ureter is identified posterior and lateral to the inferior mesenteric artery. After the retrorectal space is entered, the posterior 60% of the rectum is mobilized down to the pelvic floor. Both the hypogastric sympathetic plexus and the lateral stalks are preserved. The marginal artery is preserved in all patients. To allow for lateral fixation of the colon, limited mobilization of the left colon is performed. This in turn helps to support the prolapse repair.

When performing a laparoscopic Wells procedure, a 5 × 5-cm piece of polypropylene mesh (Atrium; Menlo Park, CA, USA) is inserted behind the mobilized rectum. The mesh is then cut to size and fixed to the sacral promontory using a hernia stapler (EndoUniversal; USSC). On either side of the rectum, two to three polypropylene sutures are placed to provide mesh attachment to the mesorectum posteriorly, avoiding mesh exposure in the pelvis. This approach provides excellent fixation while avoiding a potential site of adhesion formation if the mesh were exposed to small bowel. The pelvic peritoneum is not closed over the repair, and drains are not used.

In laparoscopic resection rectopexy procedures, rectosigmoid mobilization is performed using a similar technique. The peritonealized rectum is divided at the rectosigmoid junction using an endoscopic linear stapler. The sigmoidal branch vessels are divided, and the sigmoid colon is exteriorized through a 3- to 4-cm muscle-splitting incision at the left lower quadrant trocar site. The descending colon is divided extracorporeally, and a 29-mm stapler anvil is inserted and secured using a purse-string technique. The bowel is returned to the abdominal cavity, the fascia is closed, and pneumoperitoneum is reestablished. The circular stapler is inserted transanally to complete the anastomosis. Using two to four polypropylene sutures, the rectum is then secured high on the presacral fascia.

Choosing a laparoscopic technique to repair rectal prolapse using this clinically based algorithm has demonstrated successful resolution of the prolapse in all patients [34]. Longer operative times were observed in the resection group (128.5 ± 80.6 min vs. 69.9 ± 13.4 min), and although the hospital stay was low for both groups, the resection/rectopexy group had a slightly longer length of stay (3.6 ± 3.1 days vs. 2.2 ± 1.03 days). Using this algorithm, 80% of patients with preoperative incontinence achieved normal continence scores postoperatively. No recurrent prolapses were observed in either group, and no patients developed postoperative constipation. Constipation improved in 100% of patients who underwent a resection/rectopexy. We strongly believe there is a direct correlation between division of the lateral rectal ligaments with resultant parasympathetic denervation and postoperative evacuation problems. Zittel et al. reported persistent constipation in 18% of patients after resection/rectopexy [35]. In contrast, Bruch et al. [32] identified significant improvement in constipation after either resection/rectopexy or suture rectopexy when the lateral ligaments were preserved.

Conclusion

It is well established in the growing body of literature that the benefits of low recurrence rates and improved functional outcome can be safely achieved using laparoscopic surgical techniques to repair full-thickness rectal prolapse. Selecting an operative approach based on clinical criteria provides exceptional functional outcomes with regard to symptoms of constipation and incontinence. Adherence to such an algorithm can often negate the need for costly diagnostic tests prior to surgery. In addition, the practice of preserving the lateral rectal ligaments and avoiding injury to the hypogastric nerves is essential in order to obtain good functional outcomes.

References

1. Madden MV, Kamm MA, Nicholls RJ et al (1992) Abdominal rectopexy for complete rectal prolapse: prospective study evaluating changes in symptoms and anorectal function. Dis Colon Rectum 35:48–55
2. Keighley MRB, Fielding JWL, Alexander-Williams J (1983) Results of Marlex mesh abdominal rectopexy for rectal prolapse in 100 consecutive patients. Br J Surg 70:229–232
3. Madoff RD, Williams JG, Wong WD et al (1992) Long-term functional results of colon resection and rectopexy for overt rectal prolapse. Am J Gastroenterol 87:101–104
4. Metcalf AM, Loening-Baucke V (1988) Anorectal function and defecation dynamics in patients with rectal prolapse. Am J Surg 155:206–210
5. Keighley MRB, Shouler PJ (1984) Abnormalities of colonic function in patients with rectal prolapse and faecal incontinence. Br J Surg 71:892–895
6. Matheson DM, Keighley MRB (1981) Manometric evaluation of rectal prolapse and faecal incontinence. Gut 22:126–12
7. Gordon PH (1999) Rectal procidentia. In: Gordon PH, Nivatvongs S. Principles and practice of surgery for the colon, rectum, and anus. Quality Medical Publishers, St. Louis, pp. 503–540
8. Madoff RD (1992) Rectal prolapse and intussusception. In: Beck WE, Wexner SD, eds. Fundamentals of anorectal surgery. McGraw-Hill, New York, pp 89–103
9. Watts JD, Rothenberger DA, Buls JG et al (1985) The management of procidentia: thirty years' experience. Dis Colon Rectum 28:96–102
10. Eu K-W, Seow-Choen F (1997) Functional problems in adult rectal prolapse and controversies in surgical treatment. Br J Surg 84:904–911
11. Douard R, Frileux P, Brunel M et al (2003) Functional results after the Orr–Loygue transabdominal rectopexy for complete rectal prolapse. Dis Colon Rectum 46:1089–1096
12. Watkins BP, Landercasper J, Belzer E et al (2003) Long-term follow-up of the modified Delorme procedure for rectal prolapse. Arch Surg 138:498–503
13. Bartolo CC (1996) Rectal prolapse. Br J Surg 83:3–5
14. Duthie GS, Bartolo DC (1992) Abdominal rectopexy for rectal prolapse: a comparison of techniques. Br J Surg 79:107–113
15. Huber FT, Stein H, Siewert JR (1995) Functional results after treatment of rectal prolapse with rectopexy and sigmoid resection. World J Surg 19:138–143
16. Kimmins MH, Evetts BK, Isler J, Billingham R (2001) The Altemeier repair: outpatient treatment of rectal prolapse. Dis Colon Rectum 44:565–570
17. Berman IR (1992) Sutureless laparoscopic rectopexy for procidentia: technique and implications. Dis Colon Rectum 35:689–693
18. Carpelan-Holmström M, Kruuna O, Scheinin T (2006) Laparoscopic rectal prolapse surgery combined with short hospital stay is safe in elderly and debilitated patients. Surg Endosc 20:1353–1359
19. Cirocco WC, Brown AC (1993) Anterior resection for the treatment of rectal prolapse: a 20-year experience. Am Surg 59:265–269
20. Giordano P, Wexner SD (2001) The assessment of fecal incontinence in women. J Am Coll Surg 193(4): 397–406
21. Baker R, Senagore AJ, Luchtefeld M (1995) Laparoscopic-assisted vs. open resection: rectopexy offers excellent results. Dis Colon Rectum 38:199–201
22. Boccasanta P (1999) Laparotomic vs. laparoscopic rectopexy in complete rectal prolapse. Dig Surg 16(5):415–419
23. Boccasanta P, Rosati R, Venturi M et al (1998) Comparison of laparoscopic rectopexy with open technique in the treatment of complete rectal prolapse: clinical and functional results. Surg Laparosc Endosc 8(6):460–465
24. Kessler H, Jerby BL, Milsom JW (1999) Successful treatment of rectal prolapse by laparoscopic suture rectopexy. Surg Endosc 13:858–861
25. Darzi A, Henry MM, Guillou PJ et al (1995) Stapled laparoscopic rectopexy for rectal prolapse. Surg Endosc 9:301–303
26. Rose J, Schneider C, Scheidbach H et al (2002) Laparoscopic treatment of rectal prolapse: experience gained in a prospective multicenter study. Langebecks Arch Surg 387(3–4):130–137
27. Solomon MJ, Young CJ, Eyers AA, Roberts RA (2002) Randomized clinical trial of laparoscopic versus open abdominal rectopexy for rectal prolapse. Br J Surg 89:35–39
28. Kairaluoma MV, Viljakka MT, Kellokumpu IH (2003) Open vs. laparoscopic surgery for rectal prolapse. Dis Colon Rectum 46:355–360
29. Himpens J, Cadiere GB, Bruyns J, Vertruyen M (1999) Laparoscopic rectopexy according to Wells. Surg Endosc 13:139–141
30. Xynos E, Chrysos E, Tsiaoussis J et al (1999) Resection rectopexy for rectal prolapse: the laparoscopic approach. Surg Endosc 13:862–864
31. Heah SM, Hartley JE, Hurley J et al (2000) Laparoscopic suture rectopexy without resection is effective treatment for full-thickness rectal prolapse. Dis Colon Rectum 43(5):638–643
32. Bruch HP, Herold A, Schiedeck T, Schwandner O (1999) Laparoscopic surgery for rectal prolapse and outlet obstruction. Dis Colon Rectum 42:1189–1195
33. D'Hoore A, Cadoni R, Penninckx F (2004) Long-term outcome of laparoscopic ventral rectopexy for total rectal prolapse. Br J Surg 91:1500–1505
34. Madbouly KM, Senagore AJ, Delaney CP et al (2003) Clinically based management of rectal prolapse. Surg Endosc 17(1):99–103
35. Zittel TT, Manncke K, Haug S et al (2000) Functional results after laparoscopic rectopexy for rectal prolapse. J Gastrointest Surg 4(6):632–641

21 Surgery for Rectal Prolapse: Functional Outcome from the Abdominal Approach – An Overview

Lars Påhlman, Urban Karlbom

Introduction

In a long, historical perspective, local procedures for reduction of a rectal prolapse have dominated. The evolution of anaesthesia and better understanding of anatomy during nineteenth and twentieth centuries have made more invasive treatments possible.

Abdominal Surgery

The transabdominal approach for rectal prolapse surgery dates back approximately 100 years. In 1912, Moschcowitz described an abdominal operation for rectal prolapse based upon the theory that the prolapse was a form of sliding hernia and developed with the herniation of a deep pouch of Douglas [1]. Straining at defecation would promote further herniation. A possible mechanism of the increased straining could be the kinking of the rectosigmoid junction secondary to a redundant sigmoid colon. The proposed surgery was closure of the pouch of Douglas by several purse-string sutures. Due to the frequent recurrence of prolapse, this method is no longer used on its own. Another early clinical observation is that patients with a rectal prolapse have a weak pelvic floor, and this could be an important cause of the prolapse [2]. Consequently, a surgical repair of the pelvic floor has been tried as an anterior [3, 4] or posterior [5, 6] repair only and also as a combined anterior–posterior [7] repair. After the rectum has been totally mobilised, the edges of the levator ani and puborectalis muscles were sutured together in front or behind the rectum in order to strengthen the pelvic floor. The results in terms of recurrent prolapse after these procedures have varied from 8% to 50%. The combined abdominal and perineal procedure with anterior–posterior repair showed better results, with a 6% recurrence rate [7]. Abdominal pelvic floor repair and pouch of Douglas closure have also been used together, even in combination with other surgical techniques. Several other abdominal surgical techniques have been described but have not gained wide acceptance. Examples are suspension and suture fixation of the sigmoid colon to the anterior abdominal wall [8] and extraperitonealisation of the sigmoid colon [9].

Resection surgery for rectal prolapse includes sigmoid and anterior resection [10–12]. The potential advantage of a resection is a straight bowel course from the fixation at the level of the splenic flexure towards the rectum. Resection of a redundant sigmoid colon might by it self reduce some symptoms of associated constipation and straining. In the case of an anterior resection, mobilisation and construction of an anastomosis would create fibrosis and fixation in the pelvis. Although it has a relatively low prolapse recurrence rate [10–12], anterior resection is not frequently used. Reduction of the rectal capacity and a definite risk of anastomotic dehiscence of the low anastomosis are factors contributing to the choice of other methods by most surgeons.

The dominating technique in recent decades has been rectopexy. Either the prolapse is considered to be a sliding hernia or, as in later theories, progression of an internal rectal intussusception [13]; treatment with rectal fixation may apply to both theories. Many variations of details in the surgical procedure have been described, and there has been a definite development in the surgical technique during the last two decades (e.g. careful and sharp dissection in the mesorectal planes and attention to nerves). As there is no specimen retrieval, abdominal rectopexy is considered to be

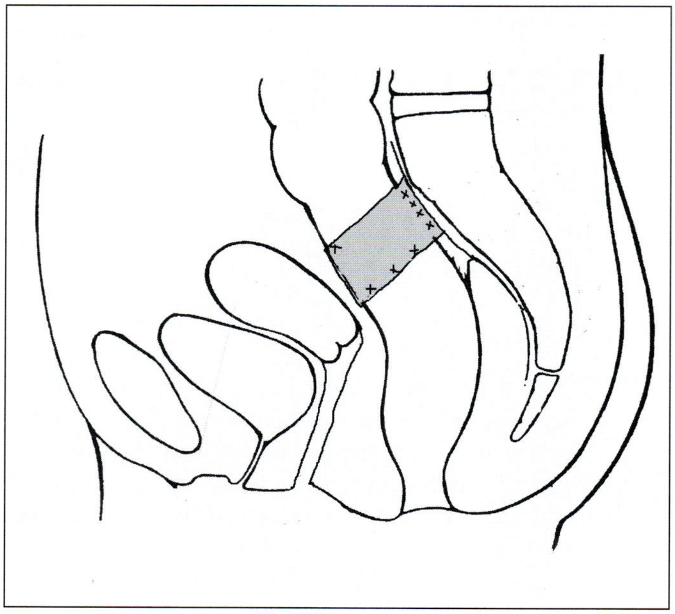

Fig. 1
Anterior rectopexy (Ripstein). The mesh encircles the rectum and is anchored posteriorly with sutures to the presacral fascia. Modified from [19], with permission from Elsevier

an operation well suited for laparoscopic surgery.

The surgical procedure, open or laparoscopic, begins with mobilisation of the rectum. The extent of the dissection varies a great deal in different series, from a complete circumferential mobilisation down to the pelvic floor [14] to minor anterior dissection [15]. Complete mobilisation most frequently includes dividing the so-called lateral ligaments. Although rectal mobilisation without separate fixation (natural scaring processes work as fixation) may be effective [16], most surgeons rely on some method of rectal fixation or suspension. Fixation may be anterior, anterolateral or posterior. Over time, suture and mesh materials have changed and parallel developments in other areas of surgery. Both nonabsorbable and absorbable sutures and meshes are now in use, without major differences in outcome.

In the literature, several types of operations have been named after surgeons. Although the procedures have developed since their original descriptions, some principles of these operations will be discussed. The Ripstein procedure [17, 18], anterior rectopexy, includes complete rectal mobilisation and rectal fixation with an encircling sling of polytef mesh (initially fascia lata, Figure 1) [19] to the sacrum. If the sling is constructed too tightly, there is a definite risk of stricture and faecal obstruction. Even if the sling initially is loose, reduced rectal expansion in that area and subsequent fibrosis in the rectal wall could induce or worsen constipation

In the Well's operation, the anterior part of the rectum is not incorporated in the fixation and is referred to as a posterior fixation method [20]. A polyvinyl alcohol sponge was initially used and sutured to the sacrum and the anterolateral aspect of the rectum after mobilisation (Fig. 2). The sponge (Ivalon) evoked a strong tissue response and fibrous reaction that secured the fixation. An increased risk of infection with the sponge led to the use of other materials [21–22].

The combination of rectopexy and sigmoid resection is often referred to as the Frykman–Goldberg operation [23, 24]. Full mobilisation of the rectum to the pelvic floor is followed by a sutured (nonabsorbable) rectopexy to the sacrum (Fig. 3) and then a resection of the redundant sigmoid colon. Mesh fixation is avoided because of the concomitant anastomosis and thus an increased risk of infection. The fixation between the presacral fascia and mesorectum/rectum can be done several ways: as single row with interrupted sutures in the midline, with double rows of interrupted sutures laterally, or as purse-string sutures. Mostly frequently, nonabsorbable sutures are used.

The Orr–Loygue procedure [25, 26] includes both a rectal suspension and a pouch of Douglas closure. The suspension is achieved with two nylon strips sutured to the low anterior and lateral

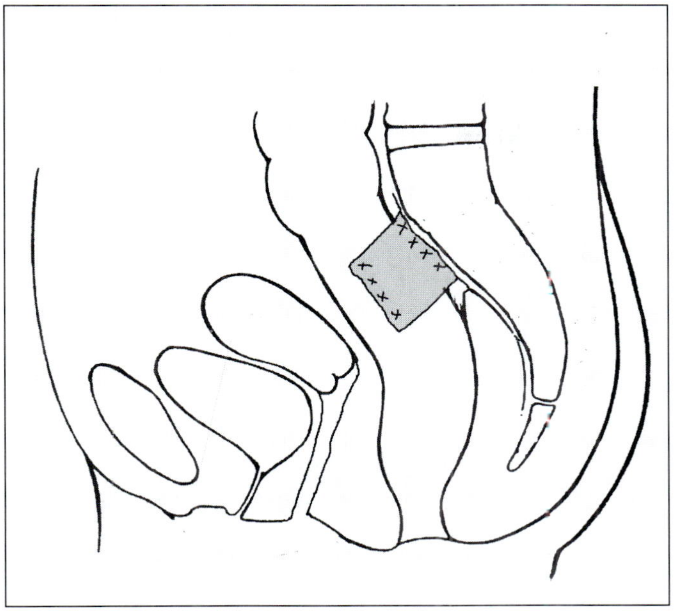

Fig. 2
Posterior rectopexy with mesh. The mesh is sutured to the presacral fascia and to the anterior–lateral parts of the rectum, leaving the anterior third of the circumference free. Modified from [19], with permission from Elsevier

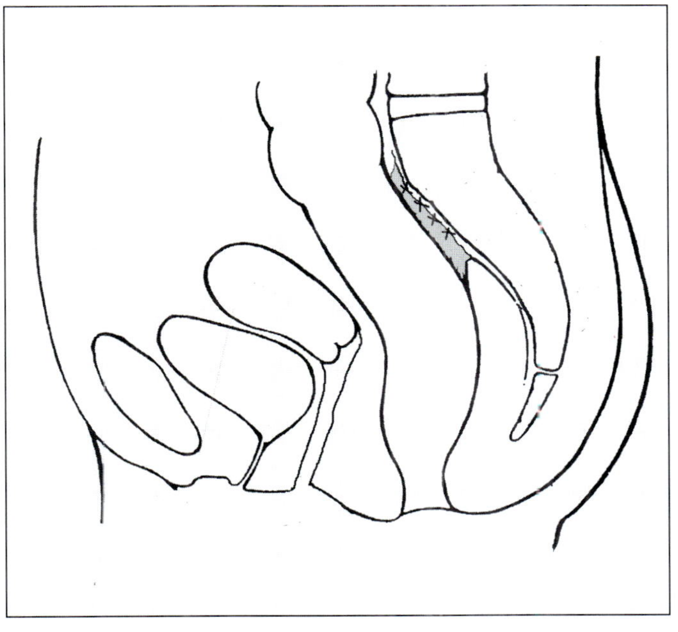

Fig. 3
Sutured rectopexy is a posterior fixation method in which the mesorectum is attached to the presacral fascia with interrupted sutures. Modified from [19], with permission from Elsevier

parts of rectum, which are then fixed to the promontory on each side of the rectum (Fig. 4). Rectal mobilisation is circumferential and as far down as possible but the lateral stalks are mostly preserved. The peritoneum is closed over the strips.

A combined rectopexy and colpopexy using one mesh with posterior rectal fixation and pouch of Douglas closure has been advocated for patients with vaginal-vault prolapse and rectal prolapse [27].

Laparoscopic Surgery

The evolution of laparoscopic surgery over the last 15 years shows that laparoscopic prolapse surgery for mobilisation, fixation and resection can

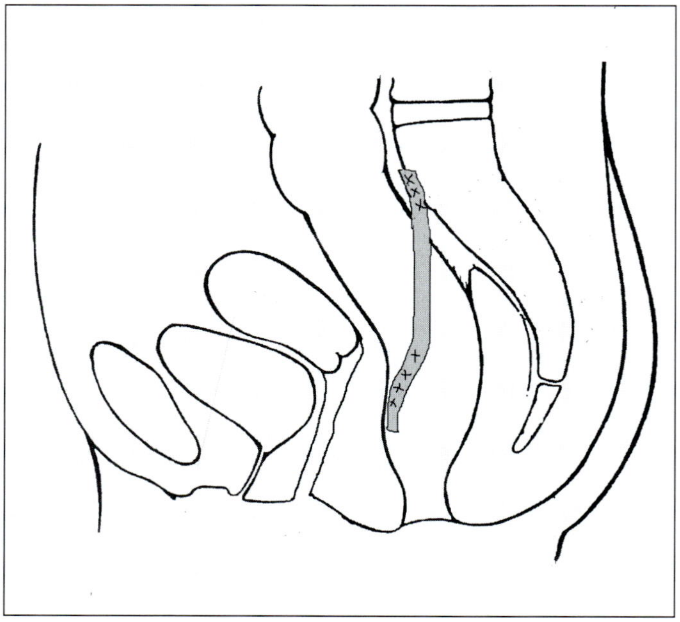

Fig. 4
Rectopexy according to Orr–Loygue, with bilateral strips of nylon sutured to the lower anterior and lateral part of rectum. The strips are then sutured to the level of the promontory. Modified from [19], with permission from Elsevier

be performed according to the principles of open surgery. The most common laparoscopic procedures are posterior mesh rectopexy and suture rectopexy. However, this development has brought some technique variations, such as the use of tackers and staplers [28, 29] for mesh and rectal fixation, which possibly makes these procedures easier and faster. Laparoscopic ventral rectopexy is a new approach that has recently been evaluated [30]. Rectal mobilisation is avoided in the posterior and lateral parts, and thus the main dissection is anteriorly in the pouch of Douglas. The rectum is suspended with mesh sutured to the low ventral part of rectum incorporating the vaginal fornices and then fixed to the promontory with staplers. A 3.6% recurrence rate with low morbidity was reported in 109 patients [30].

Although larger randomised studies regarding laparoscopic surgery are lacking, existing data regarding mortality and recurrence do not indicate any differences. The benefit of laparoscopic surgery is less surgical trauma and subsequently a smoother postoperative course as expressed in less pain, early return of gastrointestinal function and short hospital stay. Laparoscopic surgery has been considered safe even for the elderly and debilitated patient [31]. A meta-analysis of 195 patients in five comparative and one randomised studies showed significantly shorter hospital stay but longer operative time for the laparoscopic group [32]. In the randomised study by Salomon and colleagues [33], the postoperative immune and neuroendocrine response (C-reactive protein, cortisol, catecholamines) were lower in the laparoscopic group, as were cardiopulmonary complications. Mean hospital stay was 3.9 days compared with 6.6 days in an open approach. A separate cost-effectiveness analysis in this study showed an advantage for the laparoscopic group due to the shorter hospital stay [34]. With experience in enhanced postoperative rehabilitation programmes, the hospital stay for open surgery can be clearly shortened. Basse et al. reported a consecutive series of 31 patients with rectal prolapse having a posterior mesh rectopexy [including 14 patients in physical American Society of Anaesthesiologists (ASA) status 3–4], with a mean postoperative stay of 4.4 days [35]. Half of the patients were discharged after 2 days. On the other hand, the hospital stay following laparoscopic procedures can possibly be further shortened with the use of such fast-track programmes.

Authors' Choice of Surgery

The authors preferred surgical technique for rectal prolapse is a sutured rectopexy. This can be performed as an open [36, 37] or a laparoscopic

[38] procedure. The principles of dissection and posterior fixation are the same in both open and laparoscopic surgery. Preoperative bowel preparation has not been used in more recent years. All patients receive a preoperative oral prophylactic antibiotic regimen consisting of oral trimethoprim sulphate and metronidazole early on the day of surgery. For open surgery a lower midline incision is used, and in laparoscopic surgery four ports allow good access.

The pelvic peritoneum is incised on the right lateral side from above the promontory. The presacral space is opened just behind to the haemorrhoidal vessels, and care is taken to visualise and avoid the presacral nerves. Rectal mobilisation is advanced posteriorly in the avascular plane down to the tip of the coccyx. The lateral ligaments are always preserved, and there is no further dissection in the anterior and left aspect of the rectum. The rectum is then pulled straight and sutured to the sacrum, with the most cranial suture at promontory level. Four to five nonabsorbable (polypropylene) sutures are placed approximately 1 cm apart in the midline of the presacral fascia and through the midline of the mesorectum. No drains are used, and the peritoneal incision is left open.

In patients with constipation, a more extensive preoperative workup is performed, including physiological studies, defecography and colonic transit time. Constipated patients with a normal colonic transit time may be considered for concomitant sigmoid resection, whereas patients with diagnosed slow transit constipation are further investigated with segmental scintigraphic transit studies [39]. Most patients seem to have a motility disturbance in the left colon. These patients are offered an extended left-sided hemicolectomy with an anastomosis between the transverse colon and rectum at the promontory level [40]. Colectomy and ileorectal anastomosis is not performed primarily but may be considered later on for a few patients with disabling constipation. Before resection is considered, the symptoms of constipation must be carefully counterbalanced with symptoms of faecal incontinence.

Outcome of Abdominal Procedures

The main concerns in early studies were mortality, morbidity and recurrence rates. Although mortality has been reported to more than 4%, most modern studies do not show any mortality. Table 1 shows pooled data of selected studies regarding mortality and recurrences over a long time span [14, 15, 24, 26, 37, 41–83]. Most studies are retrospective, and there is incomplete follow-up for all patients. Moreover, there is always a problem with publication bias, as the worst series will never be reported. Recurrence rates are generally low for both open and laparoscopic abdominal surgery. Recurrence rates for open suture rectopexy generally range between 0% and 9% and for laparoscopic suture rectopexy between 0% and 7%. The corresponding figures for posterior mesh rectopexy and resection–suture rectopexy are of the same magnitude. Length of follow-up is shorter for the laparoscopic series, and that may influence

Table 1. Mortality and recurrence rates in pooled data of selected studies of open abdominal surgery for rectal prolapse

	Number	Mortality	Recurrence
Anterior rectopexy (Ripstein procedure) 1978–2000, 8 studies, 1 review [14, 41–48]	1,746	11 (0.6%)	61 (3.5%)
Posterior mesh rectopexy 1975–1999, 24 studies [14, 46, 49–70]	1,189 (Various types of mesh)	7 (0.6%)	32 (2.7%)
Posterior suture rectopexy 1971–1997, 11 studies [36, 37, 66, 71–78]	516	3 (0.6%)	17 (3.3%)
Resection rectopexy 1969–1998, 8 studies [24, 47, 67, 69, 79–82]	335	1 (0.3%)	2 (0.6%)
Orr–Loygue 1984–2006, 3 studies [15, 26, 83]	339	2 (0.6%)	16 (4.7%)

recurrence rates, as there are late recurrences [47]. Morbidity is 5–25% in modern series but may be considerably higher if minor complications are included and thus reach over 50%. Major procedure-related complications that are potentially lethal and may compromise the outcome include bleeding from presacral veins and pelvic sepsis. The latter may arise from an infected haematoma or an anastomotic leak but may in the long term also be secondary to mesh-migration rectal erosion. Pelvic infection in a mesh rectopexy may need urgent surgery to control sepsis. However, these more serious complications are few.

Functional Outcome

Both faecal incontinence and constipation are frequently associated with rectal prolapse. The incidence of preoperative symptoms varies a great deal between studies, and this may be secondary to case selection or symptom definition. The use of symptom grading or scaling in patients with incontinence makes for easier comparison between studies and techniques. In constipation the definitions are more diverse, even if symptoms related to the Rome criteria of functional constipation are better described in later years. Apart from curing the prolapse and its local symptoms, the aim of surgery is to restore physiology and function. Table 2 shows studies where preoperative and postoperative functional symptoms are reported [15, 37, 44, 47, 48, 66, 67, 70, 78, 82–93]. However, direct comparisons are difficult for the reasons mentioned above.

Incontinence

Associated incontinence is reported in 25–80% of patients. Anorectal physiology in these patients has shown several interesting findings. Whether they constitute a possible cause, contributing factor or a consequence of the prolapse is not clear. Patients with rectal prolapse are a heterogeneous group, and variations in findings are to be expected. Both anal resting and squeeze pressures are lower in patients with incontinence compared with continent prolapse patients [58, 94]. Anal pressure measurements may have some prognostic value, as patients with the lowest pressure have less chance to regain continence. Electromyographic signs of denervation in the external sphincter and puborectalis muscle and prolonged pudendal nerve latencies are also reported in incontinent patients [95], but the predictive value of preoperative neurophysiology is unclear [96, 97]. The prolapse itself may act as a cause of persistent rectoanal inhibition. High-pressure rectal waves in response to rectal distension will lead to a pressure overcoming the anal pressure and thus subsequent incontinence [98, 99]. Lower rectal sensory thresholds and adaptation to distension are found in some studies [96, 100]. Previous and recent studies of colon motility have also shown an increased motility in the sigmoid and descendent colon with increased luminal pressures [101, 102]. Thus, physiologic abnormalities have been identified at separate anatomic levels: in the left colon, rectum and at the anal level, including the sphincter complex.

Irrespective of the method of abdominal surgery, continence is improved for many patients, and the chance of improvement reaches 60–80%. Internal sphincter function recovery has been considered an important factor in restoring continence. Correspondingly, increased resting anal pressure and increased electromyographic activity of internal sphincter activity has been reported after correction of prolapse [99, 103, 104]. Farouk et al. [103] suggested the mechanism of improvement was that the persistent rectoanal inhibition is removed by rectal fixation. Several studies have also reported improved external sphincter function with increased squeeze pressure [82, 87, 105]. Improvement in sphincter function is usually seen within 3–6 months, although some further improvement may occur. Rectal mobilisation with subsequent scarring and fibrosis, as well as the fixation – especially in methods engaging the rectal wall – may affect function. Rectal-wall thickening after posterior mesh rectopexy is reported, and reduction of rectal compliance has also been noted [106, 107]. However, most studies do not find significant changes in these parameters. Brown et al. [108] investigated colonic motility before and after suture rectopexy and found a reduction of colonic pressure towards normality after surgery, but propulsive high-pressure waves were few (compared with controls) and unchanged postoperatively. Furthermore, six patients developed prolonged colonic transit time postoperatively.

Although data are not consistent, rectopexy probably improves incontinence by several differ-

Table 2. An overview of preoperative and postoperative faecal incontinence and constipation related to the type of abdominal surgery performed

Author	Number	Type	Follow-up (months)	Incontinence		Constipation	
				Preop	Postop	Preop	Postop
Open surgery							
Holmström et al. (1986) [44]	108	Ripstein	83	67%	28%	27%	43%
Tjandra et al. (1993) [47]	129	Ripstein	50	37%	19%	36%	33%
Schultz et al. (2000) [48]	69	Ripstein	82	56%	28%	43%	43%
Yoshioka et al. (1989) [84]	165	Posterior mesh	36	58%	16%	24%	44%
Madden et al. (1992) [85]	23	Posterior mesh	3	65%	26%	48%	52%
Aitola et al. (1999) [70]	96	Posterior mesh	78	49%	16%	32%	56%
Novell et al. (1994) [66]	32	Suture	47	31%	15%		31%
Graf et al. (1996) [37]	33	Suture	97	39%	27%	55%	60%
Khanna et al. (1996) [78]	65	Suture	65	25%	6%	9%	2%
Luukkonen et al. (1992) [67]	15	Suture/resection	–	50%	11%	28%	11%
Tjandra et al. (1993) [47]	18	Suture/resection	50	28%	17%	67%	11%
Huber et al. (1995) [82]	42	Suture/resection	54	67%	23%	44%	25%
Douard et al. (2003) [83]	31	Orr–Loygue	28	81%	51%	35%	48%
Portier et al. (2006) [16]	51	Orr–Loygue	–	61%	25%	53%	25%
Laparoscopic							
Himpens et al. (1999) [86]	37	Posterior mesh	26	32%	3%	6%	27%
Zittel et al. (2000) [87]	29	Posterior mesh	22	80%	55%	40%	50%
Benoist et al. (2001) [88]	14	Posterior mesh	47	43%	22%	36%	64%
Heah et al. (2000) [89]	25	Suture	26	60%	28%	36%	50%
Benoist et al. (2001) [88]	18	Suture	24	50%	19%	38%	62%
Kairaluoma et al. (2003) [90]	26	Suture	12	73%	15%	50%	27%
Benoist et al. (2001) [88]	16	Suture/resection	20	28%	17%	61%	11%
Kairaluoma et al. (2003) [90]	27	Suture/resection	12	56%	4%	74%	44%
Luai et al. (2005) [91]	77	Suture/resection	62	69%	26%	72%	36%
Kariv et al. (2006) [92]	23	Suture/resection	56	30%	13%	48%	26%
D'Hoore et al. (2004) [93]	42	Ventral mesh	61	74%	23%	55%	17%

ent mechanisms. For most incontinent patients with prolapse, a rectopexy seems sufficient as the primary operation. Further evaluation 6–12 months postoperatively may reveal some patients with the need for further treatment of incontinence.

Constipation

Rectal prolapse is associated with constipation in 15–65% of patients. Some of the possible mechanisms have already been outlined above, such as the redundant sigmoid colon as a cause of straining and the motility disturbances with few propulsive high-pressures contractions in the left colon. For some patients, this will be associated with prolonged gastrointestinal transit, which will not be cured by rectopexy. Regarding the prolapse as a consequence of constipation and straining, then all potential causes of outlet-obstruction constipation could play a part in the development of rectal prolapse. Diagnoses such as paradoxical puborectalis contraction and rectocele may be considered.

Constipation is thus common before surgery, but in some patients, symptoms deteriorate, and some develop de novo constipation postoperatively. This may be attributed to the surgical technique of rectal mobilisation and/or fixation. It is obvious that the original Ripstein operation caused constipation due to the fixation method itself, with the mesh encircling the rectum. Constipation related to the mesh was seen in 7–19% of patients [41, 43]. However, even with posterior fixation methods, postoperative constipation has remained a problem, which has brought the pelvic dissection into focus. The lateral ligaments, which are located posterior and laterally, contain nerves [109], including parasympathetic nerve fibres, to supply the rectum and left colon. A division of lateral fixation could thus denervate the rectum and left colon and thereby be a possible cause of postoperative constipation. The role of the lateral ligaments has been addressed in some studies: In a small, randomised study, Speakman et al. [110] found less constipation but a tendency towards more recurrences when the ligaments were preserved. Scaglia et al. [14] reported more constipation, reduced rectal capacity and increased sensory thresholds if the ligaments were divided, without differences in recurrence rates. Mollen et al. noted an increase in transit time irrespective of division of the lateral fixations, but a tendency towards decreased resting pressure and rectal compliance was found in the group with divided ligaments [111]. The cited studies are small, and firm conclusions are difficult to make. However, it seems sensible to preserve the nerves, as the impact on recurrence rates has not been reproduced.

With the aim of decreased constipation, suture rectopexy and sigmoid resection have been used as standard abdominal procedures [112] or in a selective manner [113]. Some strategies to select patients for resection rectopexy based on the dominating symptoms have been attempted [113, 114]. Available data show improved constipation following resection rectopexy (Table 2). The added sigmoidectomy can be performed without major increase in morbidity [67]. In 1990, Sayfan et al. found 44% postoperative constipation after posterior mesh rectopexy compared with only 8% after resection rectopexy [115]. They concluded that a randomised trial was justified. At present, there are two similar, larger randomised studies ongoing, one in the UK and one in Sweden, where the benefit of a resection is addressed as well as a comparison between the abdominal and perineal approaches. These studies may provide enough data to outline some guidelines for operative treatment in the future. From a strict evidence-based perspective, there is still much to be studied [116].

References

1. Moschcowitz AV (1912) The pathogenesis, anatomy and cure of the prolapse of rectum. Surg Gynecol Obstet 15:7–21
2. Graham RR (1942) The operative repair of massive rectal prolapse. Ann Surg 115:1007–1012
3. Snellman B (1961) Pelvic floor repair for rectal prolapse. Dis Colon Rectum 4:199–202
4. Porter NH (1962) Collective results of operation for rectal prolapse. Proc R Soc Med 55:1087–1091
5. Kupfer CA, Goligher JC (1970) One hundred consecutive cases of complete rectal prolapse treated by operation. Br J Surg 57:481–487
6. Klaaborg KE, Qvist N, Kongborg O (1985) Rectal prolapse and anal incontinence treated with a modified Roscoe Graham operation. Dis Colon Rectum 28:582–584
7. Hughes ESR, Gleadell LW (1962) Abdominoperineal repair of complete prolapse of the rectum. Proc R Soc Med 55:1077–1080
8. Pemberton J, Stalker LK (1939) Surgical treatment of complete rectal prolapse. Ann Surg 109:799–808
9. Mortensen NJ McC, Vellacott KD, Wilson MG (1984) Lahaut's operation for rectal prolapse. Ann R Coll Surg 66:17–18
10. Muir EG (1962) The surgical treatment of rectal prolapse in the adult. Proc R Soc Med 55:105–109
11. Thauerkauf FJ, Bears OH, Hill JR (1970) Rectal prolapse: causation and surgical treatment. Ann Surg 171:819–835
12. Schlinkert RT, Beart RW, Wolf BG, Pemberton JH (1985) Anterior resection for complete rectal prolapse. Dis Colon Rectum 28:409–412
13. Brodén B, Snellman B (1968) Procidentia of the rectum studied with cineradiography: a contribution to the discussion of a causative mechanism. Dis Colon Rectum 11:330–347
14. Scaglia M, Fasth S, Hallgren T et al (1994) Abdominal rectopexy for rectal prolapse; influence of surgical technique on function outcome. Dis Colon Rectum 37:805–813
15. Portier G, Iovino F, Lazorthes F (2006) Surgery for rectal prolapse: Orr-Loygue ventral rectopexy with limited dissection prevents postoperative constipation without increasing recurrence. Dis Colon Rectum 49:1136–1140
16. Raftopoulos Y, Senagore AJ, Di Giuro G, Bergamaschi R (2005) Recurrence rates after abdominal surgery for complete rectal prolapse: a multicenter pooled analysis of 643 individual patient data. Dis Colon Rectum 48:200–1206
17. Ripstein CB (1952) Treatment of massive rectal prolapse. Am J Surg 83:68–71
18. Ripstein CB (1965) Surgical care of massive rectal prolapse. Dis Colon Rectum 8:34–38

19. Karulf RE, Madoff RD, Goldberg SM (2001) Rectal Prolapse. Current Probe Surg 38:771–832
20. Wells C (1959) New operation for rectal prolapse. Proc R Soc Med 52:602–604
21. Keighley MRB, Fielding JWL, Alexander-Williams J (1983) Results of Marlex mesh abdominal rectopexy for rectal prolapse in 100 consecutive patients. Br J Surg 70:229–232
22. Athanasiadis S, Weyand G, Heiligers J et al (1996) The risk of infection of three synthetic materials used in rectopexy with or without colonic resection for rectal prolapse. Int J Colorect Dis 11:42–44
23. Frykman HM (1955) Abdominal proctopexy and primary sigmoid resection for rectal procidentia. Am J Surg 90:780–789
24. Frykman HM, Goldberg SM (1969) The surgical treatment of rectal procidentia. Surg Gynecol Obstet 129:1225–1230
25. Orr TG (1947) A suspension operation for prolapse of the rectum. Ann Surg 126:833–840
26. Loygue J, Nordlinger B, Cunci O et al (1984) Rectopexy to the promontory for the treatment of rectal prolapse. Report of 257 cases. Dis Colon Rectum 27:356–359
27. Collopy BT, Barham KA (2002) Abdominal colporectopexy with cul-de-sac closure. Dis Colon Rectum 45:522–529
28. Berman IR (1992) Sutureless laparoscopic rectopexy for procidentia. Dis Colon Rectum 35:689–693
29. Darzy AW, Lewis C, Guillou P, Monson J (1995) Stapled laparoscopic rectopexy for rectal prolapse. Surg Endosc 9:301–303
30. D'Hoore A, Penninckx F (2006) Laparoscopic ventral recto(colpo)pexy for rectal prolapse: surgical technique and outcome in 109 patients. Surg Endosc 20:1919–1923
31. Carpelan-Holmström M, Kruuna O, Scheinin T (2006) Laparoscopic rectal prolapse surgery combined with short hospital stay in the elderly and debilitated patients, Surg Endosc 20:1353–1359
32. Purkayastha S, Tekkis P, Athanasiou T et al (2005) A comparison of open vs. laparoscopic abdominal rectopexy for full-thickness rectal prolapse: a meta analysis. Dis Colon Rectum 48:1930–1940
33. Salomon MJ, Young CJ, Eyers AA, Roberts RA (2002) Randomized clinical trial of laparoscopic versus open abdominal rectopexy for abdominal prolapse. Br J Surg 89:35–39
34. Salkeld G, Bagia M, Salomon M (2004) Economic impact of laparoscopic versus open abdominal rectopexy. Br J Surg 91:1188–1191
35. Basse L, Billesbolle P, Kehlet H (2002) Early recovery after abdominal rectopexy with multimodal rehabilitation. Dis Colon Rectum 45:195–199
36. Ejerblad S, Krause U (1988) Repair of rectal prolapse by rectosacral suture. Acta Chir Scand 154:103–105
37. Graf W, Karlbom U, Påhlman L, Nilsson S (1996) Functional results after abdominal suture rectopexy for rectal prolapse and intussusception. Eur J Surg 136:905–911
38. Graf W, Stefansson T, Arvidsson D, Påhlman L (1995) Laparoscopic suture rectopexy. Dis Colon Rectum 38:211–212
39. Lundin E, Karlbom U, Westlin JE et al (2004) Scintigraphic assessment of slow transit constipation with special reference to right or left-sided delay. Colorectal Dis 6:499–505
40. Lundin E, Karlbom U, Påhlman L, Graf W (2002) Outcome of segmental resection for slow transit constipation. Br J Surg 89:1270–1274
41. Gordon PH, Hoexter B (1978) Complications of the Ripstein procedure. Dis Colon Rectum 21:277–280
42. Morgan B (1980) The Teflon sling operation (Ripstein) for repair of complete rectal prolapse. Aust N Z J Surg 50:121–123
43. Launer DP, Fazio VW, Weakley FL, Turnbull RB et al (1982) The Ripstein procedure: a 16-year experience. Dis Colon Rectum 25:41–45
44. Holmström B, Brodén G, Dolk A (1986) Results of the Ripstein operation in the treatment of rectal prolapse and internal rectal procidentia. Dis Colon Rectum 29:845–848
45. Roberts PL, Schoetz DJ, Coller JA, Veidenheimer MC (1988) Ripstein procedure: Lahey clinic experience 1963–1985. Arch Surg 123:554–557
46. Winde G, Reers H, Nottberg H et al (1993) Clinical and functional results of abdominal rectopexy with absorbable mesh-graft for the treatment of complete rectal prolapse. Eur J Surg 159:301–305
47. Tjandra JJ, Fazio VW, Church JM et al (1993) Ripstein procedure is an effective treatment for rectal prolapse without constipation. Dis Colon Rectum 36:501–507
48. Schultz I, Mellgren A, Dolk A et al (2000) Long-term results and functional outcome after Ripstein rectopexy. Dis Colon Rectum 43:35–43
49. Penfold JCB, Hawley PR (1972) Experiences of Ivalon-sponge implant for complete rectal prolapse at St Mark's Hospital 1960–1970. Br J Surg 59:846–848
50. Naughton Morgan C, Porter NH, Kugman DJ (1972) Ivalon (polyvinyl alcohol) sponge in the repair of complete rectal prolapse. Br J Surg 59:846–848
51. Jurgeleit HC, Corman ML, Coller JA, Veidenheimer MC (1975) Procidentia of the rectum: Teflon sling repair of rectal prolapse. Lahey Clinic experience. Dis Colon Rectum 18:464–467
52. Eisenstat TE, Rubin RJ, Salvati EP (1979) Surgical treatment of complete rectal prolapse. Dis Colon Rectum 22:522–523
53. Lescher TJ, Corman ML, Coller J, Veidenheimer MC (1979) Management of late complications of Teflon sling repair for rectal prolapse. Dis Colon Rectum 23:445–467
54. Romero-Torres R (1979) Sacrofixation with Marlex mesh in massive prolapse of the rectum. Surg Gynecol Obstet 149:709–711
55. Notarus MJ (1979) A technique of abdominal repair for rectal prolapse. Proctology 1:35–37
56. Anderson JR, Kinninmonth AWG, Smith AR (1981) Polyvinyl alcohol sponge rectopexy for complete rectal prolapse. J R Coll Surg Engl 26:292:294
57. Hilsabeck JR (1981) Transabdominal posterior proctopexy using an inverted T of synthetic material. Arch Surg 116:41–44
58. Keighley MRB, Fielding JWL (1983) Management of faecal incontinence and results of surgical treatment. Br J Surg 70:463–468

59. Atkinson KG, Taylor DC (1984) Wells procedure for complete rectal prolapse: a ten years experience. Dis Colon Rectum 27:96–98
60. Anderson JR, Wilson BG, Parks TG (1984) Complete rectal prolapse: the results of Ivalon sponge rectopexy. Post Grad Med J 60:411–414
61. Vongsangnak V, Varma JS, Watters D, Smith AN (1985) Clinical manometric and surgical aspects of complete prolapse of the rectum. J R Coll Surg Edinb 30:251–254
62. Boulos PB, Stryker SJ, Nicholls RJ (1984) The long term results of polyvinyl alcohol (Ivalon) sponge for rectal prolapse I young patients. Br J Surg 71:213–214
63. Mann CV, Hoffman C (1988) Complete rectal prolapse: the anatomical and functional results of treatment by an extended abdominal rectopexy. Br J Surg 75:34–37
64. Kuijpers JHC, de Morree H (1988) Towards a selection of the most appropriate procedure in the treatment of complete rectal prolapse. Dis Colon Rectum 31:355–357
65. McCue JL, Thompson JPS (1991) Clinical and functional results of abdominal rectopexy for complete rectal prolapse. Br J Surg 78:921–923
66. Novell JR, Osborne MJ, Winslet MC, Lewis AA (1994) Prospective randomized trial of Ivalon sponge versus sutured rectopexy for full-thickness rectal prolapse. Br J Surg 81:904–906
67. Luukkonen P, Mikkonen V, Jarvinen H (1992) Abdominal rectopexy with sigmoidectomy vs. rectopexy alone for rectal prolapse: A prospective randomized study. Int J Colorectal Dis 7:219–222
68. Galili Y, Rabau M (1997) Comparison of polyglycolic acid and polypropylene mesh for rectopexy in the treatment of rectal prolapse Eur J Surg 163:445–448
69. Yakut M, Kaymakciioglu N, Simsek A et al (1998) Surgical treatment of rectal prolapse. A retrospective analysis of 94 cases. Int Surg 83:53–55
70. Aitola PT, Hiltunen KM, Matikainen MJ (1999) Functional results of operative treatment of rectal prolapse over an 11-year period: emphasis on transabdominal approach. Dis Colon Rectum 42:655–660
71. Loygue J, Huguier M, Malafosse M, Biotois H (1971) Complete prolapse of the rectum. A report of 140 cases treated by rectopexy. Br J Surg 58:847–848
72. Carter AE (1983) Rectosacral suture fixation for complete rectal prolapse in the elderly, the frail and the demented. Br J Surg 70:522–523
73. Goligher JC Prolapse of the rectum (1984). In: Goligher JC (ed) Surgery of the anus, rectum and colon, 5th edn. London Baillière Tindall, pp 267–279
74. Graham W, Clegg JF, Taylor V (1984) Complete rectal prolapse repair by a simple technique. Ann R Coll Surg Engl 66:87–89
75. Blatchford GJ, Perry RE, Thorson AG, Christensen MA (1989) Rectopexy without resection for rectal prolapse. Am J Surg 158:574–576
76. Keighley MRB Rectal prolapse. In: Keighley MRB (1999) Williams NS (eds) Surgery of the anus, rectum and colon, 2nd edn. WB Saunders, London, pp 794–842
77. Sayfan J, Koltun L, Orda L (1997) Constipation in rectal prolapse – the key to choosing the appropriate rectopexy. Techniques Coloproctol 5:38–41
78. Khanna AK, Misra MK, Kumar K (1996) Simplified sutured sacral rectopexy for complete rectal prolapse in adults. Eur J Surg 162:143–146
79. Watts JD, Rothenberger DA, Buls JG et al (1985) The management of procidentia: 30 years experience. Dis Colon Rectum 28:96–102
80. Sayfan J, Pinho M, Alexander-Williams J, Keighley MRB (1990) Sutured abdominal rectopexy with sigmoidectomy compared with Marlex rectopexy for rectal prolapse. Br J Surg 77:143–145
81. Deen KI, Grant E, Billingham C, Keighley MRB (1994) Abdominal resection rectopexy with pelvic floor repair versus perineal sigmoidectomy and pelvic floor repair for full-thickness rectal prolapse. Br J Surg 81:302–304
82. Huber FT, Stein H, Siewert JR (1995) Functional results after treatment of rectal prolapse with rectopexy and sigmoid resection. World J Surg 19:138–143
83. Douard R, Frileux P, Brunel M et al (2003) Functional results after the Orr–Loygue transabdominal rectopexy for complete rectal prolapse. Dis Colon Rectum 46:1089–1096
84. Yoshioka K, Heyen F, Keighley MRB (1989) Functional results after posterior abdominal rectopexy for rectal prolapse. Dis Colon Rectum 32:835–838
85. Madden MV, Kamm MA, Nicholls RJ et al (1992) Abdominal rectopexy for complete prolapse: prospective study evaluating changes in symptoms and anorectal function. Dis Colon Rectum 35:48–55
86. Himpens J, Cadière GB, Bryuns J, Vertruyen M (1999) Laparoscopic rectopexy according to Wells. Surg Endosc 13:139–141
87. Zittel TT, Manncke K, Haug S et al (2000) Functional results after laparoscopic rectopexy for rectal prolapse. J Gastrointest Surg 4:632–641
88. Benoist S, Taffinder N, Gould S et al (2001) Functional results two years after laparoscopic rectopexy. Am J Surg 182:168–173
89. Heah SM, Hartley JE, Hurley J et al (2000) Laparoscopic suture rectopexy without resection is effective for full-thickness prolapse. Dis Colon Rectum 43:638–643
90. Kairaluoma MV, Viljakka MT, Kellokumpu IH (2003) Open vs. laparoscopic surgery for rectal prolapse. A case controlled study assessing short-term outcome. Dis Colon Rectum 46:353–360
91. Luai L, Ashari S, Lumley JW et al (2005) Laparoscopically assisted resection rectopexy for rectal prolapse: ten years experience. Dis Colon Rectum 48:982–987
92. Kariv Y, Delaney CP, Casillas S et al (2006) Long-term outcome after laparoscopic and open surgery for rectal prolapse. Surg Endosc 20:35–42
93. D'Hoore A, Cadoni R, Penninckx F (2004) Long-term outcome of laparoscopic ventral rectopexy for total rectal prolapse. Br J Surg 91:1500–1505
94. Hiltunen KM, Matikainen M, Auvinen O, Hietanen P (1986) Clinical and manometric evaluation of anal sphincter function in patients with rectal prolapse. Am J Surg 151:489–492
95. Parks AG, Swash M, Ulrich H (1977) Sphincter denervation in anorectal incontinence and rectal prolapse. Gut 18:656–659

96. Schultz I, Mellgren A, Nilsson BY et al (1998) Preoperative electrophysiologic assessment cannot predict continence after rectopexy. Dis Colon Rectum 41:1392–1398
97. Birnbaum EH, Stamm L, Raferty JF et al (1996) Pudendal nerve motor latency influences surgical outcome in treat of rectal prolapse. Dis Colon Rectum 39:1215–1221
98. Sun WM, Read NW, Camel Donelly T et al (1989) A common pathophysiology for full-thickness rectal prolapse and solitary ulcer. Br J Surg 76:290–295
99. Farouk R, Duthie GS, MacGregor AB, Bartolo DCC (1994) Rectoanal inhibition and incontinence in patients with rectal prolapse. Br J Surg 81:743–746
100. Siproudhis L, Bellissant E, Juguet F et al (1998) Rectal adaptation to distension in patients with overt rectal prolapse. Br J Surg 85:1527–1532
101. Keighley MRB, Shouler PJ (1984) Abnormalities of colonic function in patients with rectal prolapse. Br J Surg 71:892–895
102. Brown AJ, Horgan AF, Andersson JH et al (1999) Colonic motility is abnormal before surgery for rectal prolapse. Br J Surg 86:263–266
103. Farouk R, Duthie GS, Bartolo DCC, MacGregor AB (1992) Restoration of continence following rectopexy and recovery of the internal anal sphincter electromyogram. Br J Surg 79:439–440
104. Schultz I, Mellgren A, Dolk A et al (1996) Continence is improved after the Ripstein rectopexy. Different mechanisms in rectal prolapse and rectal intussusception? Dis Colon Rectum 39:300–306
105. Sainio AP, Voutilainen PE, Husa AI (1991) Recovery of anal sphincter function following transabdominal repair of rectal prolapse: cause of improved continence, Dis Colon Rectum 34:816–821
106. Allen-Mersh TG, Turner MJ, Mann CV (1990) Effect of abdominal Ivalon sponge on bowel habit and rectal wall. Dis Colon Rectum 33:550–553
107. Felt-Bersma RJF, Sloots CEJ, Poen AC et al (2000) Rectal compliance as routine measurement. Extreme volumes have direct clinical impact and normal volumes exclude rectum as a problem. Dis Colon Rectum 43:1732–1738
108. Brown AJ, Nicol L, Anderson H et al (2005) Prospective study of the effect on colonic motility in patients with rectal prolapse. BrJ Surg 92:1417–1422
109. Pak-art R, Tansatit T, Mingmalairaks C et al (2005) The location and contents of the lateral ligaments of the rectum: A study in human soft cadavers. Dis Colon Rectum 48:1941–1944
110. Speakman CTM, Madden MV, Nicholls RJ, Kamm MA (1991) Lateral ligament division during rectopexy causes constipation but prevents recurrence. Results of a prospective randomized study. Br J Surg 78:1431–1433
111. Mollen RMHG, Kuijpers JHC, van Hoek F (2000) Effects of rectal mobilization and lateral ligament division on colonic and anorectal function, Dis Colon Rectum 43:1283–1287
112. Kim DS, Tsang CBS, Wong WD et al (1999) Complete rectal prolapse. Evolution of management and results. Dis Colon Rectum 42:460–469
113. Brown AJ, Anderson JH, McKee RF, Finlay IG (2004) Strategy for selection of type operation for rectal prolapse based on clinical criteria. Dis Colon Rectum 47:103–107
114. Madbouly KM, Senagore AJ, Delaney CP et al (2003) Clinically based management of rectal prolapse. Comparison of laparoscopic Wells procedure and laparoscopic resection with rectopexy. Surg Endosc 17:99–103
115. Sayfan J, Pinho, M, Alexander-Williams J, Keighley MR (1990) Sutured posterior abdominal rectopexy compared with Marlex rectopexy for rectal prolapse. Br J Surg 77:143–145
116. Bachoo P, Brazelli M, Grant A (2000) Surgery for complete rectal prolapse in adults. Cochrane Database Syst Rev 2:CD001758

22 The Management of Recurrent Rectal Prolapse

Robert D. Madoff, James W. Ogilvie Jr., Scott R. Steele

Introduction

The ideal surgical procedure for full-thickness rectal prolapse should be one of minimal morbidity, effective in improving symptoms, and durable over time with a low risk of recurrence. Unfortunately, as evident from the myriad number of surgical options for prolapse, it is not surprising that recurrence continues to plague the colorectal surgeon. Recurrence rates vary widely in the literature (older reports as high as 50%), and the variation is widely perceived to reflect the different technical aspects involved with each procedure [1]. Some authors suggest, however, that surgical technique does not fully account for the variation in recurrence rates, especially among abdominal approaches [2]. Instead, differences are more likely explained by nonuniform definitions of recurrent prolapse and varying lengths of follow-up [3]. Nevertheless, it is generally accepted that recurrence following an abdominal repair (0–10%) is less common than after a perineal approach (0–25%) [4–7]. Regardless of initial procedure performed, most recurrences are detected 1–3 years postoperatively, with up to one third developing within the first 7 months [8–10].

The pathophysiology of failed primary surgical repair is not entirely clear. For example, some authors have advocated that recurrence may be prevented if during abdominal rectopexy the lateral ligaments of the rectum are divided in addition to standard posterior rectal mobilization [11]. However, others report equivalent recurrence rates when the lateral ligaments are left intact [12]. Hool et al. [9] reported that a common cause of failure during anterior rectopexy with mesh (Ripstein repair) was related to technical errors associated with mesh, such as improper placement and inadequate fixation. In terms of perineal approaches, an unclear endpoint of resection (perineal rectosigmoidectomy) [13], an incomplete mucosectomy (Delorme procedure) [14], and a failure to correct concomitant pelvic floor defects [15] have all been proposed as potential harbingers of recurrence.

Higher rates of recurrence have also been associated with comorbid psychiatric illness [16], male gender [17], unsuspected constipation, or anismus [18], whereas increasing age and higher body mass index have been implicated after laparoscopic repair [19]. On the contrary, others have failed to confirm any operative or patient factors associated with recurrence [20], and often during reoperation an obvious reason for failure is never identified [9]. Demographic data from patients who have undergone a repeat operation are notably unremarkable from those who present for initial evaluation (Table 1).

Surgical Technique

Preoperative Planning

The preoperative evaluation is essential prior to any operative approach for recurrent prolapse to ensure that failure of the initial surgery was not the result of a previously missed underlying diagnosis. Planning begins with a thorough history focusing on the nature and severity of initial symptoms (ranging from incontinence to constipation), duration and alteration of symptoms after first operative repair, timing of recurrence, details of previous operative reports (in particular mesh placement or bowel resection), and exclusion of associated medical conditions that might have contributed to recurrence (diarrhea, urinary straining, infections, polyps, neoplasms, etc.). A careful assessment of existing comorbidities is not only essential to avoid perioperative car-

Table 1. Case series of reoperative recurrent rectal prolapse

Study	Year	Number	M/F	Age, mean	Initial operation, abdominal/ perineal	Time to recurrence; months, mean	Second recurrence (%)	Follow-up; months, mean
Fengler et al. [8]	1997	14	3/11	68	13/1	14	0/14 (0)	50
Hool et al. [9]	1997	24	5/19	56[a]	15/9	24[a]	4/24 (17)	81[a]
Pikarsky et al. [21]	2000	27	1/26	69	9/18	NS	4/27 (15)	24
Watts and Thompson [20]	2000	17	1/16	75 F 79 M	0/17	NS	9/17 (53)	16
Steele et al. [10]	2005	78	8/70	67	17/61	33.5	23/78 (29)	9

NS not stated
[a] Median

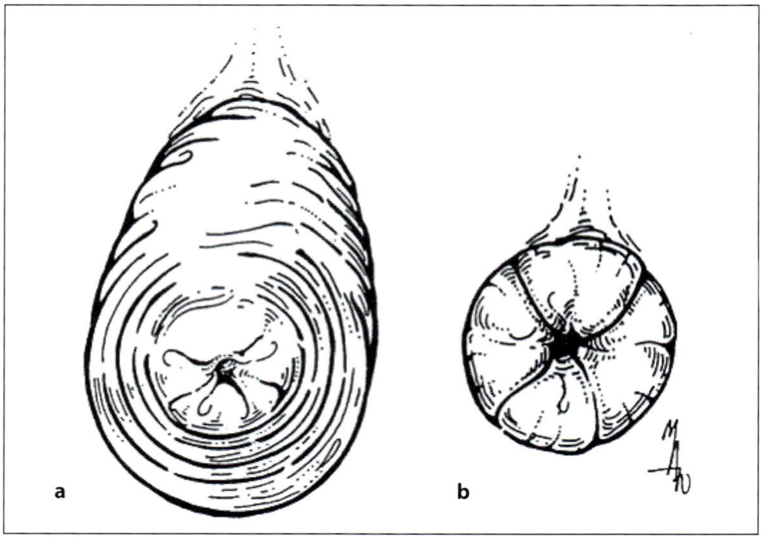

Fig. 1a, b
a Full-thickness rectal prolapse (concentric folds). **b** Partial-thickness mucosal prolapse. Reprinted from [1] with permission from Elsevier

diopulmonary complications but may potentially influence the choice of operative procedure. Physical examination should focus on differentiating full-thickness and partial-thickness mucosal prolapse (Fig. 1), the latter of which will most often not require surgical repair but can be easily controlled with dietary management and Barron rubber-band ligation. It is also important to inspect for simultaneous pelvic floor defects such as concomitant rectocele, enterocele, or pelvic floor dysfunction (i.e., paradoxical puborectalis, anismus), which may have contributed to the initial failure and may need to be addressed prior to or concomitant with any surgical repair.

If not performed previously, ancillary studies should start with endoscopic examination of the colon to exclude diverticular disease, neoplasia, or solitary rectal ulcer. Patients with a history of prior resection and symptoms of constipation should also undergo endoscopic examination to exclude an anastomotic stricture. In addition, constipated patients should undergo colonic transit studies along with anal manometry and electromyography (EMG) to assess for motility disorders, such as slow transit constipation or outlet obstruction from paradoxical puborectalis contraction [22]. Cinedefecography may prove useful in identifying internal intussusception or other pelvic floor abnormalities. For incontinent patients, there are conflicting reports whether anal manometry and pudendal nerve terminal motor latency (PNTML) are useful in predicting postoperative continence after primary prolapse repair [23–26]. In recurrent disease, the manometric findings are often similar to findings in primary disease [21], and hence these tests are not routinely performed at our institution. Endorectal ultrasound may be performed to evaluate for sphincter defects contributing to incontinence, although we recommend avoiding repair of concomitant sphincter defects in the setting of recurrent prolapse. We therefore recommend a selective approach to evaluation with anorectal physiology testing based preoperative symptoms of incontinence or constipation and the extent of testing done at the time of initial presentation.

Operative Approach

The surgical options for recurrent prolapse are the same as those employed for repair of primary disease. Successful repairs have been accomplished using almost all types of approaches [8–10, 21, 27]; however, the most commonly performed operations for recurrent prolapse are abdominal rectopexy (with or without resection) and perineal rectosigmoidectomy (Altemeier procedure). The Delorme procedure has also been employed in the reoperative setting and is one of the least invasive operations. Proponents cite its ability to avoid a full-thickness resection, especially in patients with a previous resection who may be at risk for vascular compromise. Unfortunely it has been limited by its relatively high rates of recurrence: 13–37% after primary surgery [28–30] and up to 53% after 16 months for recurrent prolapse [20].

Operative details in the setting of recurrence are similar to those for initial prolapse and are described elsewhere in detail in this book. There are, however, important caveats to remember during reoperative prolapse surgery with each approach. Given the lower recurrence rates with abdominal operations, recurrent disease should ideally be performed via an abdominal approach as long as patients are able to safely tolerate laparotomy [10]. Various forms of rectopexy with or without resection have all been accomplished in the reoperative setting, with satisfactory results.

An important consideration during resective procedures is to ensure adequate blood supply to the remaining rectum and any anastomosis present. For this reason, some authors suggest that an abdominal approach with resection should be avoided when the initial operation was an Altemeier procedure [9]. In their series of reoperative prolapse cases, Fengler et al. [8] reported on one patient who underwent anterior resection with rectopexy after an initial perineal procedure who sloughed rectal mucosa postoperatively. Although the patient remained free of recurrence, an area of ischemia was created between the two anastomoses. In the series by Steele et al. [10], two patients developed postoperative strictures, both of whom had undergone an initial perineal rectosigmoidectomy followed by rectopexy with resection. We therefore recommend that every effort be made to resect the prior anastomosis to avoid ischemic complications to the remaining bowel.

When performing sigmoid resection with an abdominal rectopexy, complications may be minimized by ensuring adequate blood supply to a new anastomosis via careful preservation of the superior rectal artery. Although there is also the potential for rectal devascularization when performing an Altemeier operation in the setting of a previous rectosigmoid resection, there are few documented complications in this scenario [21].

In terms of the technical aspects of the Altemeier procedure, inadequate rectal mobilization and resection are possible explanations for its higher recurrence rates. To circumvent such problems in the reoperative setting, care should be taken to completely mobilize everted bowel by dividing all the surrounding attachments. Unfortunately, the endpoint of dissection is not always clearly defined, and it is not uncommon to find more redundant bowel even after the presumed final attachments are divided. Interestingly, Pikarsky et al. [21] found no difference in the length of bowel resected during a second Altemeier procedure than from the primary operation. The surgeon must use experience to balance an aggressive resection and potential tension-induced anastomotic complications with that of leaving behind too much bowel and experiencing higher recurrence rates.

The final option for recurrent prolapse is the creation of a low Hartmann pouch with end sigmoid colostomy [1]. This radical approach is an important consideration for a select group of patients with gross fecal incontinence and stable comorbidities (such as certain psychiatric diseases or paraplegia) without severe underlying cardiopulmonary disease. For primary prolapse, low anterior resection is associated with significant morbidity and varying effects on incontinence [31, 32], yet the addition of end colostomy not only eliminates concern over incontinence but decreases the morbidity associated with a low pelvic anastomosis.

Personal Experience

At the University of Minnesota, we reported on the largest series to date of patients who underwent surgery for recurrent rectal prolapse [10]. From a cohort of 685 patients over a 16-year period, the recurrence rate for initial procedures was 16.7% for perineal approaches and 7.7% for abdominal approaches. We identified 70 women and 8 men with a full-thickness recurrent rectal prolapse who underwent subsequent operative repair (Fig. 2). At the discretion of the operating surgeon, 51 patients had a perineal approach (Altemeier operation) and 27 an abdominal approach (rectopexy with or without resection). At a mean follow-up of 9 months, 29% of all patients developed a second recurrence. When stratified by operative approach, we observed a significantly higher second recurrence rate in the group who underwent a perineal procedure compared with those who had an abdominal procedure (37% vs. 15%; p=0.03).

Of the four patients who developed second recurrences following an abdominal approach for initial recurrence, three had additional operations at a later date. One patient had a third abdominal rectopexy (no recurrence), one underwent perineal resection (recurrence after 25 months), and one underwent placement of an artificial bowel sphincter. Of the 19 patients who developed second recurrences after a perineal approach, 11 underwent an abdominal approach (one recurrence; 9%), and five underwent a second perineal approach (two recurrences; 40%). Combining the results of all patients who underwent a third repair, 50% (3/6) of perineal approaches recurred, whereas 8% (1/12) of abdominal approaches recurred (p=0.07). Finally, when evaluating the overall recurrence rate following any repair for recurrent prolapse (whether it be the first, second,

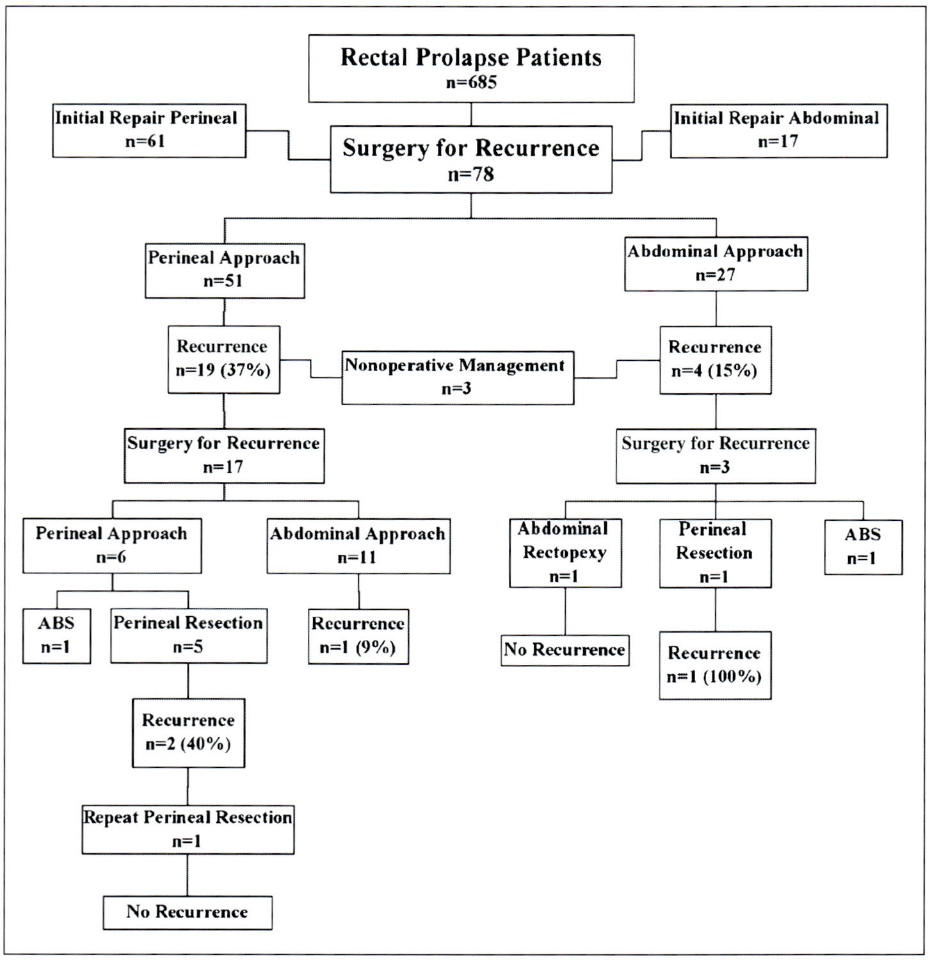

Fig. 2 Patient management and outcome following recurrent prolapse surgery. *ABS* artificial bowel sphincter. Reprinted with permission from [10]

or third repair), patients undergoing an abdominal procedure had a significantly lower recurrence (13%) compared with those undergoing a perineal repair (39%) after a mean follow-up of 10 months ($p<0.01$). Rates of major and minor postoperative complications were similar between perineal and abdominal approaches. Pelvic abscess in conjunction with anastomotic leak was the most commonly encountered major complication, occurring in 5% of all repairs.

Based on our findings, we recommend that an abdominal approach be employed for treatment of recurrent rectal prolapse if the patient's risk profile permits. Although it is unclear exactly what factors account for the increased success, we surmise that a more accurate determination of complete rectal mobilization and determination of extent of resection can be facilitated when using an abdominal approach. Nevertheless, the perineal approach has advantages for those patients with significant comorbidities, a lesser degree of prolapsed bowel, or incarcerated prolapse.

Overview of the Literature

In 1953, Sir Kenneth Starr from Sydney, Australia, first reported on a series of operative repairs for recurrent rectal prolapse. He published three cases of recurrent prolapse that were successfully treated via a combined procedure of anal encirclement with strips of fascia lata or plantaris tendon, along with rectal mobilization and sigmoidopexy [33]. In 1959, the Russian surgeon Dmitrii Chukhrienko published a series of 12 patients where T-shaped mesh bands were used to fixate the mobilized rectum to the presacral fascia in a fashion similar to the mesh methods used today. In 11 cases with recurrent or massive prolapse, the operation was deemed successful, and in one case, the same technique was applied for fixation of uterine prolapse [34].

Almost 40 years later, Fengler et al. [8] reported on a series of 14 patients over a 10-year period who were operatively managed for recurrent rectal prolapse. In 13 patients, the initial procedure was performed via a perineal approach and in one patient via an abdominal approach. The mean time to recurrence was 14 months. The authors performed a repeat perineal approach (Altemeier, Delorme, or anal encirclement) in nine patients and an abdominal approach (rectopexy with and without resection) in the remaining five. As mentioned previously, one patient developed postoperative mucosal sloughing after anterior resection with rectopexy following an initial perineal resection. There were no second recurrences after a mean follow-up of 50 months, yet three patients with preoperative fecal incontinence had no symptom resolution. The authors concluded that whereas recurrent resection is safe, any prior anastomosis should be removed to avoid ischemia to the remaining bowel segment.

That same year, Hool et al. [9] identified 24 patients over a 30-year period in whom they performed 29 operations for recurrent prolapse. There were 25 abdominal procedures (72% of which were the Ripstein procedure) and four perineal procedures. After almost 7 years of follow-up, the overall recurrence rate for all reoperations was 17%. Major postoperative complications were only seen among those who had abdominal procedures, occurring in 24% of cases (6/25). Similar to the Fengler et al. [8] series, reoperative surgery rarely altered preoperative bowel function. Incontinence improved in only three of ten patients, and new-onset constipation developed in one patient. The authors concluded that despite the success in terms of treating the recurrent prolapse by using an abdominal approach, bowel dysfunction persists in the majority of patients.

In order to compare recurrent prolapse surgery with primary repair, Pikarsky et al. [21] analyzed 27 cases of reoperative recurrent prolapse with an equal number of cases matched for age, gender, and type of repair performed. Compared with the primary repair group, recurrent cases were no different in terms of the results from anal physiologic studies (manometry, EMG, defecography) or coexistient anal pathology (i.e., paradoxical puborectalis contraction or associated sphincter defects). The authors performed a mixture of abdominal and perineal procedures, and after a mean follow-up of 2 years, recurrence rates were similar between the two groups (recurrent repair 15%, primary repair 11%). Postoperative incontinent scores and complication rates were also similar between groups. Unlike previous series, these authors did not preferentially advocate the abdominal approach given the relatively equivalent rates of re-recurrent prolapse and safety profile seen with the perineal procedures.

In 2002, Tsugawa et al. [27] demonstrated an

effective laparoscopic approach to repair recurrent prolapse in two patients who had undergone a primary perineal repair (Gant-Miwa operation). They performed sacral rectopexy using braided absorbable suture without the use of mesh or sigmoid resection. There were no complications, and patients were free of recurrence after 24 months.

Conclusion

Recurrent rectal prolapse continues to be an often-encountered but not well-delineated problem. Although it may occur at any time, most recurrences are detected within 1–3 years after the initial operation. It is often helpful to perform adjunctive tests such as anophysiologic studies, defecography, or transit studies to evaluate for factors such as straining with severe constipation or concomitant pelvic floor disorders that might have led to the recurrence. A careful review of the technical details of the prior operation is essential to aid in identifying potential intraoperative clues as to why the initial operation failed. Resection of the prior anastomosis will lessen the chances of ischemic complications such as sloughing, stricture, or leak. Unfortunately, repairing recurrent prolapse may not improve – and perhaps may worsen – any associated constipation or incontinence. Patients should therefore be counseled realistically regarding expectations for functional outcomes, and in select cases, abdominal proctectomy with end colostomy should be considered. Although perineal approaches can be safely and successfully used for recurrent prolapse, abdominal approaches are consistently associated with lower recurrence rates regardless of the number of prior failures.

References

1. Karulf RE, Madoff RD, Goldberg SM (2001) Rectal prolapse. Curr Probl Surg 38:771–832
2. Raftopoulos Y, Senagore AJ, Di Giuro G, Bergamaschi R (2005) Recurrence rates after abdominal surgery for complete rectal prolapse: a multicenter pooled analysis of 643 individual patient data. Dis Colon Rectum 48:1200–1206
3. DiGiuro G, Ignjatovic D, Brogger J, Bergamaschi R (2006) How accurate are published recurrence rates after rectal prolapse surgery? A meta-analysis of individual patient data. Am J Surg 191:773–778
4. Kim DS, Tsang CB, Wong WD et al (1999) Complete rectal prolapse: evolution of management and results. Dis Colon Rectum 42:460–466; discussion 466–469
5. Madiba TE, Baig MK, Wexner SD (2005) Surgical management of rectal prolapse. Arch Surg 140:63–73
6. Jacobs LK, Lin YJ, Orkin BA (1997) The best operation for rectal prolapse. Surg Clin North Am 77:49–70
7. Bullard Dunn K, Madoff R (2007) Rectal Prolapse. In: Wexner S, Stollman N (eds) Diseases of the colon. Informa Healthcare, New York, pp 81–97
8. Fengler SA, Pearl RK, Prasad ML et al (1997) Management of recurrent rectal prolapse. Dis Colon Rectum 40:832–834
9. Hool GR, Hull TL, Fazio VW (1997) Surgical treatment of recurrent complete rectal prolapse: a thirty-year experience. Dis Colon Rectum 40:270–272
10. Steele SR, Goetz LH, Minami S et al (2006) Management of recurrent rectal prolapse: surgical approach influences outcome. Dis Colon Rectum 49:440–445
11. Speakman CT, Madden MV, Nicholls RJ, Kamm MA (1991) Lateral ligament division during rectopexy causes constipation but prevents recurrence: results of a prospective randomized study. Br J Surg 78:1431–1433
12. Scaglia M, Fasth S, Hallgren T et al (1994) Abdominal rectopexy for rectal prolapse. Influence of surgical technique on functional outcome. Dis Colon Rectum 37:805–813
13. Williams JG, Rothenberger DA, Madoff RD, Goldberg SM (1992) Treatment of rectal prolapse in the elderly by perineal rectosigmoidectomy. Dis Colon Rectum 35:830–834
14. Oliver GC, Vachon D, Eisenstat TE et al (1994) Delorme's procedure for complete rectal prolapse in severely debilitated patients. An analysis of 41 cases. Dis Colon Rectum 37:461–467
15. Uhlig BE, Sullivan ES (1979) The modified Delorme operation: its place in surgical treatment for massive rectal prolapse. Dis Colon Rectum 22:513–521
16. Marceau C, Parc Y, Debroux E et al (2005) Complete rectal prolapse in young patients: psychiatric disease a risk factor of poor outcome. Colorectal Dis 7:360–365
17. Zbar AP, Takashima S, Hasegawa T, Kitabayashi K (2002) Perineal rectosigmoidectomy (Altemeier's procedure): a review of physiology, technique and outcome. Tech Coloproctol 6:109–116
18. Delaney CP, Senagore AJ (2005) Rectal Prolapse. In: Fazio VW, Church JM, Delaney CP (eds) Current therapy in colon and rectal surgery,2nd edn. Elsevier Mosby, Philadelphia, pp 125–134
19. Kariv Y, Delaney CP, Casillas S et al (2006) Long-term

outcome after laparoscopic and open surgery for rectal prolapse: a case-control study. Surg Endosc 20:35–42
20. Watts AM, Thompson MR (2000) Evaluation of Delorme's procedure as a treatment for full-thickness rectal prolapse. Br J Surg 87:218–222
21. Pikarsky AJ, Joo JS, Wexner SD et al (2000) Recurrent rectal prolapse: what is the next good option? Dis Colon Rectum 43:1273–1276
22. Dolk A, Broden G, Holmstrom B et al (1990) Slow transit of the colon associated with severe constipation after the Ripstein operation. A clinical and physiologic study. Dis Colon Rectum 33:786–790
23. Birnbaum EH, Stamm L, Rafferty JF et al (1996) Pudendal nerve terminal motor latency influences surgical outcome in treatment of rectal prolapse. Dis Colon Rectum 39:1215–1221
24. Glasgow SC, Birnbaum EH, Kodner IJ et al (2006) Preoperative anal manometry predicts continence after perineal proctectomy for rectal prolapse. Dis Colon Rectum 49:1052–1058
25. Johansen OB, Wexner SD, Daniel N et al (1993) Perineal rectosigmoidectomy in the elderly. Dis Colon Rectum 36:767–772
26. Schultz I, Mellgren A, Nilsson BY et al (1998) Preoperative electrophysiologic assessment cannot predict continence after rectopexy. Dis Colon Rectum 41:1392–1398
27. Tsugawa K, Sue K, Koyanagi N et al (2002) Laparoscopic rectopexy for recurrent rectal prolapse: a safe and simple procedure without a mesh prosthesis. Hepatogastroenterology 49:1549–1551
28. Agachan F, Pfeifer J, Joo JS et al (1997) Results of perineal procedures for the treatment of rectal prolapse. Am Surg 63:9–12
29. Marchal F, Bresler L, Ayav A et al (2005) Long-term results of Delorme's procedure and Orr-Loygue rectopexy to treat complete rectal prolapse. Dis Colon Rectum 48:1785–1790
30. Tsunoda A, Yasuda N, Yokoyama N et al (2003) Delorme's procedure for rectal prolapse: clinical and physiological analysis. Dis Colon Rectum 46: 1260–1265
31. Schlinkert RT, Beart RW, Jr., Wolff BG, Pemberton JH (1985) Anterior resection for complete rectal prolapse. Dis Colon Rectum 28:409–412
32. Cirocco WC, Brown AC (1993) Anterior resection for the treatment of rectal prolapse: a 20-year experience. Am Surg 59:265–269
33. Starr KW (1953) Recurrent rectal prolapse; an operative method of treatment. Med J Aust 40:190
34. Chukhrienko DP (1959) [Operative treatment of recurrent and massive forms of rectal prolapse with the use of capron material.]. Vestn Khir Im I I Grek 83:78–83

23 Surgery for Rectal Prolapse: General Criteria for the Selection of the Best Treatment

Giovanni Romano, Francesco Bianco, Luisa Caggiano

Introduction

Rectal prolapse is an intussusception of the rectum, which may be classified as mucosal, internal (occult) or complete (full thickness). Mucosal prolapse is a protrusion of the mucosa only without sliding of the muscular layer, which remains in place. Internal rectal prolapse does not come down beyond the anal canal and, frequently, is not associated with any symptoms; it is likely to be a precursor of a complete prolapse. Complete rectal prolapse is a full-thickness protrusion through the anal canal.

Until to the 1990s, there was some debate as to whether rectal prolapse is due to a sliding hernia or intussusception or a combination of both. Defecography demonstrated that rectal prolapse is due to an intussusception and that anatomical abnormalities, such as redundant rectosigmoid, weakness of pelvic and sacral attachments, loss of anorectal angle, perineal descent, diastasis of the levator and denervation of anal sphincter, are the results of the prolapse rather than its cause. This consideration constitutes the theoretical basis of the surgical management of rectal prolapse in order to achieve curative treatment. Whereas the exact pathophysiology of rectal prolapse remains unclear, several factors have been associated with its development, including constipation, female gender, pregnancies, menopausal status and previous anorectal surgical procedures. Colonic inertia, neurologic disease, psychiatric illness and obstructed defecation are frequently the causes of the initial constipation. Obstructed defecation is often a consequence of anismus and/or paradoxical nonrelaxing puborectalis syndrome. These patients experience painful and difficult evacuation, with the need for straining and digital manoeuvres. Chronic constipation and straining are supposed to be two important initial causes of the rectal protrusion. Progression of the prolapse leads to lengthening of the mesorectum and the lateral ligaments, whereas weakness of pelvic floor muscles and sphincters and pudendal neuropathy contribute to rectal descent. Consequently, rectal prolapse is frequently associated with other diseases, such as rectocele, enterocele, cystocele and uterine and vaginal prolapse. Assessment of functional disturbances of the pelvic floor and knowledge as to how they contribute to the development of rectal prolapse are essential to determine the appropriate operative approaches for long-term management of these patients.

Conservative Treatment after Surgery

Conservative management of rectal prolapse is usually unsuccessful; however, in some constipated patients, and particularly younger patients, it is advisable to restore normal bowel habit by dietary means and laxatives and educate these patients to evacuate without straining, as it is likely that some early recurrences after operation are the consequences of the repeated straining during evacuation before the rectum has been fixed to the surrounding structures by perineal fibrosis.

On the opposite end of a broad spectrum of patients with a combination of symptoms are some incontinent elderly patients who are no longer able to contract pelvic floor muscles. In these patients, pelvic floor training and biofeedback could help restore continence after the surgery, although some authors report that these means are often not useful, as patients with low basal pressure remain incontinent even after successful surgery for the prolapse and restoration of the normal anatomy [1].

Objectives of Surgical Treatment

The aim of surgical treatment should be both to correct anatomic modifications and ameliorate impaired bowel functions, as functional disturbances greatly affect the patient's social life. As demonstrated by some questionnaires, patients become afraid to engage in a normal life due to concern of a sudden prolapse descent. Frequently, elderly patients are too embarrassed to participate in routine activities because of the incontinence. They are often not correctly informed about the possibility of curative surgical treatment, and some constipated patients describe evacuation as a routinely distressing experience because of fear that the prolapse may come down and the subsequent need for complicated manipulations to replace it. Therefore, surgical treatment has a double aim: to correct anorectal and pelvic anatomy in order to control the prolapse, and to restore continence and prevent constipation.

Many surgical procedures have been developed over the years to treat full-thickness rectal prolapse, so the first problem for the surgeon is the choice of operation: which one has the higher possibility of controlling the prolapse with minimal risk of morbidity and mortality, always considering the different symptoms associated with the disease as well as the patient's age? Moreover, patient expectations of functional results should be taken in account, and they should be adequately informed about the different surgical options and their possibility to be curative.

Surgical correction of the anatomic defect does not always imply resolution or improvement in functional symptoms and, frequently, other multifactorial causes are associated to the disorder of bowel function, such as colonic inertia, as demonstrated by the experience of many authors. Patients should be made aware about the limitations of surgical procedures through written informed consent and drawings in order to avoid unpleasant disappointment of patient expectations. Because the aetiology and pathophysiology of rectal prolapse are not well understood and the causes appear to vary, it is not possible to determine a single procedure as the best surgical option for all patients. From the above-mentioned considerations, it is quite clear that there is no gold standard for treating rectal prolapse, but the choice of operation should be tailored for each patient.

Choice of Surgical Procedure

The aims of all authors in the current literature are to develop some general criteria to match specific patients to specific procedures that are most appropriate for them. Therefore, the choice of operation should be determined by different factors such as the patient's gender and age, operative risk, other associated pelvic floor defects, degree of incontinence or constipation and the surgeon's experience with different techniques. Considering such factors increases the likelihood of rectifying the greatest portion of functional and anatomical defects and reducing perioperative morbidity and postoperative recurrences. Therefore, a perineal rectosigmoidectomy, which is reported to have a recurrence rate of between 10% and 30%, may be the most appropriate choice for an elderly constipated patient with a shorter life expectancy. A younger incontinent patient, on the other had, might be better treated with an abdominal rectopexy, whereas a rectopexy with an associated colonic resection might be more appropriately proposed for a young constipated patient. Likewise, patients with small circumferential partial-thickness prolapse, less than 3 cm, might constitute a good indication for the Delorme procedure or for stapled transanal rectal resection (STARR). However, it must be noted that a further problem is the lack of long-term and homogeneous comparative follow-up, particularly for the elderly, who constitute a large part of these patients. Therefore, reported series are often incomplete, and the real incidence of recurrences and residual disorders of bowel function are not always correctly deduced.

Moreover, the surgeon must consider some technical details that are different between men and women. In most elderly women who have had a greater number of pregnancies, there is an important perineal descent, which implies a multidisciplinary treatment in association with the gynaecologist and/or urologist. These women usually have a long peritoneal pouch that extends between the rectum and the back of the vagina to the level of the pelvic floor and the anorectal junction. A deep peritoneal pouch is not always present in the men. Consequently, the presence of anatomical abnormalities of the perineum and pelvic floor, and the need of correcting these defects, may incline the surgeon towards using a perineal technique that will allow this repair. The surgeon's decision is also influenced by some favourable anatomic aspects usually existing in these patients that make rectal mobilisation easier than in patients affected by different diseases. In fact, in most cases, the large bowel has a normal aspect with a redundant sigmoid, and the rectum is extremely mobile. In a patient with an attenuated mesorectum that provides little support to the rectum, the lateral ligaments are usually floppy, with a frequent lack of the middle rectal vessel so that the retrorectal space is wide. Posterior or lateral dissection of the rectum is therefore quite easy and bloodless. Another problem to be considered is the perineal body that is frequently deficient with an atrophic pelvic floor, particularly the puborectalis sling and the rectovaginal septum.

Surgical Outcomes

For objective comparison of the outcome of different surgical procedures, a standardised classification system for rectal prolapse is needed. Some authors report the following classification system: first-degree rectal prolapse is defined by rectal intussusception above the anal canal (internal or incomplete prolapse), second-degree rectal prolapse is an intussusception of the rectal wall into the anal canal, whereas a third-degree rectal prolapse is a complete (full-thickness) rectal prolapse through the anus [2]. However, this classification system does not mention the mucosal prolapse, which is considered a different pathologic entity that requires a different surgical approach. According to these authors, the indications for surgery were third-degree rectal prolapse outlet obstruction caused by morphological changes such as sigmoidoceles with consecutive compression of the rectum during defecation combined with second- and third-degree rectal prolapse, and patients with second- and third-degree rectal prolapse combined with chronic diverticulitis of the sigmoid colon. Conversely, patients with first-degree rectal prolapse were excluded from surgery and treated conservatively with biofeedback or with other surgical procedures only in case of clinical outlet obstruction syndrome or when associated with other disorders (e.g. sigmoidocele, rectocele). When internal prolapse is an isolated finding without associated disorders, the patient does not benefit from repair and, obviously, surgery is not advised.

Surgical Procedures

More than 100 procedures have been reported for the repair of rectal prolapse, but they may be generally divided into two broad categories: abdominal and perineal. Different abdominal procedures may be performed as open or laparoscopic operations. These procedures differ due to extent of rectal mobilisation, division of lateral ligaments, anterior or posterior fixation of the rectum, fixation material used and whether or not a sigmoid resection is included in the procedure, such as in the Frykman–Goldberg procedure. Suture rectopexy is the most common procedure performed to treat rectal prolapse, with an associated resection (Frykman–Goldberg) in case of a coexisting significant constipation. The different posterior rectopexies, both with sutures or meshes, are more commonly used than anterior fixation of the rectum (Ripstein procedure) or the Ivalon sponge operation (a sponge placed posterior to the rectum to create an inflammatory reaction; Wells procedure) because of the risk related to the use of prosthetic material, including stenosis, infections and erosion. Overall, abdominal procedures yield better results and functional outcome than do perineal operations, with recurrence rates ranging from 0% to 8% [3]. These procedures allow a more complete rectal mobilisation and better fixation of the rectum to the sacrum, thus implying better prevention of recurrences.

According to the presence or not of different functional disorders such as constipation or incontinence, abdominal procedures should be selected and tailored for each patient by adding or not a sigmoid resection. Many authors consider the posterior rectopexy the procedure of choice because of its low morbidity and recurrence rate, and more than 50% of incontinent patients achieve improvement in their condition. In these incontinent patients, a bowel resection might produce reduction of the reservoir function, with a worsening of continence, so that a resection is not advisable for these patients. On the contrary, it must be noted that up to 50% of patients experience a new onset of constipation or exacerbation of their preexisting constipation [4]. Constipation is likely to be a consequence of denervation of the rectum due to division of the lateral ligaments; however, preservation of the ligaments is reported to be associated with higher recurrence rates [5].

Several prospective randomised trials demonstrated that a sigmoid resection associated with a rectopexy reduces postoperative constipation [3, 6, 7]. In these cases, continence is preserved because the rectal reservoir is maintained by limiting the resection of the large bowel to the upper part of the rectum above the peritoneal reflection. Some authors maintain that isolated resection of the colon is an effective method of permanently preventing recurrence, because reduction of bowel length definitively prevents rectal mobility. Recurrence rate after rectopexy and resection rectopexy are similar, and although resection implies more risks, such as anastomotic leakage and sepsis, the morbidity rate seems to be comparable, so that choosing this procedure should depend only on the patient's specific symptoms. Moreover, an extended resection as a subtotal colectomy with ileorectal anastomosis may be indicated in patients with rectal prolapse and constipation due to a colonic inertia.

Some disadvantages of the open abdominal procedures, such as more extensive intra-abdominal invasion with a significantly higher incidence of peritoneal adhesions, scarring and longer recovery time, may be reduced by the laparoscopic approach [2, 3, 8, 9]. Laparoscopic rectopexy with or without resection is both safe and effective. Advantages include low morbidity, improved cosmesis, rapid return of intestinal function and early discharge from hospital. The outcome in terms of recurrences, faecal continence and constipation are comparable with those obtained with open procedures. Recently, Raftopoulos et al. [10] reported that the results achieved by treating these patients with rectal mobilisation only, without fixation and/or resection, are similar to those obtained by rectopexy with or without resection.

The perineal operations include anal encirclement (the Thiersch wire procedure), mucosal sleeve resection (the Delorme procedure) and perineal rectosigmoidectomy (the Altemeier procedure). Despite the simplicity of the operation, the results are so discouraging that the anal encirclement is actually an option only for high-risk patients who cannot be selected for any other type of procedures. The Delorme procedure is a rectal mucosectomy that can be performed under regional anaesthesia with few postoperative complications, making it suitable for high-risk patients [11, 12]. This operation has been reported to resolve faecal incontinence to varying degrees and has not been found to be associated with constipation after operation, but the physiological reasons for these improved functions are not clear. Although this procedure is widely adopted to treat mucosal intussusception, most authors consider the role of the Delorme procedure still controversial when dealing with a full-thickness rectal prolapse. This is due to the higher rate of recurrences, so that it is indicated for a small protrusion of less than 3 cm, elderly or high-risk patients and as a secondary procedure for elderly or high-risk patients with recurrence who previously underwent other surgical techniques [11].

The perineal rectosigmoidectomy according to Altemeier offers a combination of repairs of anatomic alterations associated with rectal prolapse. Scarring following rectal mobilisation allows rectopexy, resection removes the redundant bowel, dissection and ligation of the enterocele allows obliteration of the hernia pouch and levatorplasty provides pelvic floor reconstruction. The advantages of the perineal procedures include reduced pain, short hospital stay, avoidance of peritoneal adhesions, lower risk of pelvic nerve injuries and the possibility of treatment with a single intervention for other diseases, such as rectocele, vaginal prolapse, haemorrhoids and sphincter defect. Therefore, the concomitant presence of these other pathologies may induce the surgeon to choose this procedure.

The recurrence rate with the perineal approach ranges between 0% and 29% and is higher than those for transabdominal techniques [3, 13, 14], although the perineal procedures can be repeated multiple times both in the same patient and in patients who previously underwent different procedures. Perineal procedures generally have a lower morbidity than abdominal procedures because they are less invasive and are therefore particularly indicated in elderly and high-risk patients. In these patients, constipation may be improved with a perineal rectosigmoidectomy, whereas compared with abdominal rectopexy, there may be a lesser improvement in continence. This is likely due to sphincter stretching and loss of the rectal reservoir after perineal rectosigmoidectomy.

A combination of various perineal procedures,

including the Delorme procedure, the Altemeier procedure and perineal rectosigmoidectomy with levatorplasty resulted in significant improvement in terms of continence and the lowest recurrence rates in these patients [15]. The incidence of rectal prolapse increases with age and is higher between 50 and 70 years, so that many of these patients are elderly and have many associated diseases. The perineal techniques, which may be considered low-risk procedures, are advantageous for these elderly patients as well as for high-risk patients and those who need combined intervention from different pelvic specialists, such as a gynaecologist or urologist. In elderly patients, who have a limited life expectancy, the higher risk of recurrence associated with perineal procedures may be considered not so significant and may be balanced by the benefit of undergoing a low-risk procedure. Moreover, the Altemeier procedure may also be indicated for patients who are suspected of having peritoneal adhesions due to previous multiple abdominal operations, as well as for young men who choose not to take the risk related to an abdominal intervention, such as impairment of sexual function.

Surgical Approaches to Prolapse Recurrence

The recurrence rate is higher with the perineal procedures than with abdominal operations, and the causes are not always identified. Although surgical procedures correct the anatomical defect, frequently, the underlying functional disorders persist and provide the basis for prolapse recurrence. It is generally supposed that early recurrences – occurring less than 2 years after operation – are related to technical factors associated with the primary procedures. The surgical approach to these recurrences remains an unresolved problem in which the optimal treatment is still debated. As mentioned earlier, the primary operation is chosen by considering many different factors. All those factors maintain their importance when choosing the technique for the second repair, but first, the second procedure to treat the recurrence has to be carefully chosen by considering the primary procedure.

The reported data demonstrate that a second, or even third, abdominal procedure, irrespective of the number of previous failures, is related to a lower re-recurrence rate than a second perineal repair (13% vs. 39% re-recurrence rates) [16]. Therefore, it has been suggested that abdominal repair of recurrent rectal prolapse should be always undertaken if the patient's risk profile allows this approach. Because of the success rate and personal experience, some authors prefer to repeat an abdominal procedure regardless of what the first operation was; however, some considerations must be noted. Whether a rectopexy without resection has been performed to initially manage a rectal prolapse, a resection as secondary procedure – either transabdominal or perineal – may be safely accomplished. On the contrary, for patients who had previously undergone a resection as primary surgery, a second resection to treat the recurrence may be dangerous due to the risk of bowel ischaemia between the two anastomoses. This may occur both in the case of an abdominal anterior resection after an Altemeier procedure or in the opposite sequence. Therefore, a repeat resectional procedure should always be avoided unless the surgeon may absolutely be sure of resecting the previous anastomoses in the second procedure. The only exception is constituted by the patients who underwent perineal rectosigmoidectomy as primary surgery; in these cases, a second Altemeier procedure can be safely repeated because, as the previous procedure is an ultralow coloanal anastomoses, it is always contained in the recurrent prolapse.

To overcome these problems, some surgeons have suggested treating rectal recurrences after primary resectional surgery with a Delorme procedure. Overall re-recurrence rate and morbidity after surgery for recurrent rectal prolapse are similar to those reported after the primary treatment and range between 10% and 20% [16–19].

References

1. Hamalainen KPJ, Raivio P, Antila S et al (1996) Biofeedback therapy in rectal prolapse patients. Dis Colon Rectum 39:262–265
2. Schiedeck THK, Shwandner O, Scheele J et al (2005) Rectal prolapse: which surgical option is appropriate? Langenbecks Arch Surg 390:8–14

3. Gourgiotis S, Baratsis S (2007) Rectal prolapse. Int J Colorectal Dis 22:231–243
4. Aitola PT, Hiltunen KM, Matikainen MJ (1999) Functional results of operative treatment of rectal prolapse over an 11-years period: emphasis on transabdominal approach. Dis Colon Rectum 42:655–660
5. Mollen RM, Kuijpers HC, van Hoek F (2000) Effects of rectal mobilization and lateral ligaments division on colonic and anorectal function. Dis Colon Rectum 43:1283–1287
6. Lukkonen P, Mikkonen U, Jarvinen H (1992) Abdominal rectopexy with sigmoidectomy vs rectopexy alone for rectal prolapse: a prospective, randomized study. Int J Colorectal Dis 7:219–222
7. McKee RF, Lauder JC, Poon FW et al (1992) A prospective randomized study of abdominal rectopexy with and without sigmoidectomy in rectal prolapse. Surg Gynecol Obstet 174:145–148
8. Lechaux D, Trebuchet G, Siproudhis L et al (2005) Laparoscopic rectopexy for full-thickness rectal prolapse. Surg Endosc 19:514–518
9. Salomon MJ, Young CJ, Eyers AA et al (2002) Randomized clinical trial of laparoscopic versus open abdominal rectopexy for rectal prolapse. Br J Surg 89:35–39
10. Raftopoulos Y, Seragore AJ, Bergamaschi R et al (2005) Recurrence rates after abdominal surgery for complete rectal prolapse: a multicenter pooled analysis of 643 individual patient data. Dis Colon Rectum 48:1200–126
11. Tsunoda A, Yasuda N, Yokoyama N et al (2003) Delorme's procedure for rectal prolapse. Dis Colon Rectum 46:1260–1265
12. Watts AM, Thompson MR (2000) Evaluation of Delorme's procedure as a treatment for full-thickness rectal prolapse. Br J Surg 87:218–222
13. Takesue Y, Yokoyama T, Murakami Y (1999) The effectiveness of perineal sigmoidectomy for the treatment of rectal prolapse. Surg Today 29:290–293
14. Johansen OB, Wexner SD, Daniel N (1993) Perineal rectosigmoidectomy in the elderly. Dis Colon Rectum 36:767–772
15. Agachan F, Reissman P, Pfeifer J et al (1997) Comparison of three perineal procedures for the treatment of rectal prolapse. South Med J 90:925–932
16. Steele SR, Goetz LH, Minami S et al (2006) Management of recurrent rectal prolapse: surgical approach influences outcome. Dis Colon Rectum 49:440–445
17. Pikarskj AJ, Joo JS, Wexner SD et al (2000) Recurrent rectal prolapse: what is the next good option? Dis Colon Rectum 43:1273–1276
18. Hool GR, Hull TL, Fazio VW (1997) Surgical treatment of recurrent complete rectal prolapse: a thirty-year experience. Dis Colon Rectum 40:270–272
19. Fengler SA, Pearl RK, Prased ML et al (1997) Management of recurrent rectal prolapse. Dis Colon Rectum 40:832–834

24 Management of Associated Pelvic Dysfunctions: External Rectal Prolapse and Faecal Incontinence

Giuseppe Dodi, Luca Amadio

Introduction

Rectal prolapse syndrome (RPS) seems to be an appropriate term for a group of diseases in which rectal prolapse is just one of the signs, usually the most evident, but not necessarily the most annoying for the patient. External rectal prolapse is in itself a circumferential, full-thickness procidentia of the rectal wall through the anal orifice, a sliding hernia that develops in patients who often have a deep pouch of Douglas [1]. RPS includes several relatively well-defined clinical conditions in which full rectal prolapse, intussusception, mucosal prolapse, haemorrhoids, genital prolapse, descending or descended perineum, solitary rectal ulcer, weak pelvic floor muscles, faecal incontinence, hypertonic and nonrelaxing sphincters, constipation, "rather odd" personality (as stated by Goligher [2]) and eating disorders are variably associated. The nosographic setting of these conditions as a *syndrome* apparently has never been described in the medical literature.

Prolapse most often appears after straining through a weakened pelvic floor. The theory that the prolapse originates from an internal intussusception before progressing to a full-thickness procidentia is not supported by the literature. Mellgren et al. [3] followed 38 patients with internal intussusception with defecography, and only one developed external rectal prolapse. These findings confirm the results of a previous study by Ihre et al. suggesting that rectal intussusception and full-thickness rectal prolapse are two different entities, and that intussusception is not a risk factor for rectal prolapse and probably not an indication for surgery [4]. The onset of rectal prolapse in most cases is gradual. The earliest symptom of external prolapse is a reducible anal procidentia associated with mucous discharge. Other symptoms are unsatisfactory defecation with different types of stool retention (constipation with feeling of incomplete evacuation, tenesmus, need for straining, etc.) and some degree of anal or faecal incontinence.

The reported rate of faecal incontinence associated with full-thickness rectal prolapse is approximately 50–75% in most series, where incontinence appears as a late symptom. One theory is based on the stretching of sphincter muscles and pudendal nerves, causing progressive loss of control. Incontinence, however, may be observed in patients with intussusception. Patients with rectal prolapse have a significantly increased anal sphincter asymmetry index at rest, the other manometric parameters being normal, without other anal sphincter defects. Rectal prolapse or rectoanal intussusception probably increases the anal asymmetry index in the same proportions as anal sphincter defects. These data may be important in explaining why with rectal prolapse we can observe anal incontinence and why prolapse treatment may also improve incontinence.

Several hypotheses have been suggested to explain why rectal prolapse can be associated with decreased resting anal pressure: associated pudendal neuropathy, functional inhibition of the internal anal sphincter mechanical activity, associated sphincter defects [5–7]. Anal sphincter distortion induced by the prolapse may also be responsible for decreased contractile activity (functional inhibition) [8]. Whether prolonged rectal prolapse causes the sphincter defect or abnormal sphincteric relaxation at baseline contributes to the subsequent development of prolapse is unclear and subject to debate. Similarly, the relative pathogenic contribution of pudendal nerve injury is uncertain. Nevertheless, surgical correction of procidentia is reported to produce improvement in both resting and squeeze pressures over time, particularly in patients with normal pudendal nerve terminal motor latency (PNTML) testing [9].

In some patients with rectal prolapse, endoanal ultrasound showed a typical aspect with an asymmetric anal sphincter and heterogeneous thickening of the anal submucosa internal hyperechoic layer. Woods et al. [10] reported that 71% of patients with rectal prolapse and incontinence had an abnormal anal sphincter complex on endoanal ultrasound. In 19% of the patients, there was a defect isolated to the internal anal sphincter, in 14% the defects were limited to the external anal sphincter and in 38% they were present in both structures. Probably, anal sphincter tears contribute to faecal incontinence after surgical correction of prolapse [8, 10].

In patients with full-thickness rectal prolapse, reduction of external anal sphincter pressure is probably also due to pudendal neuropathy. Parks et al. [11] in histologic specimens demonstrated denervation of the external anal sphincter muscle in patients with faecal incontinence and full external prolapse, suggesting it was the result of pudendal neuropathy, a consequence of rectal descent produced by continuous straining at defecation. Electromyographic studies supported this suggestion, showing an increased fibre density in the puborectalis and external sphincter of incontinent patients compared with normal controls, and in patients with rectal prolapse but who where completely continent. Similarly, PNTML was significantly increased in incontinent patients with rectal prolapse [6, 12]. Postoperative manometry showed a significant improvement in maximum resting and squeeze pressures and a significant decrease of the volume at which rectal sensation was first perceived.

It should be kept in mind that, as with constipation, it is quite difficult to define faecal incontinence and measure its severity. For this reason, quality of life is now considered the more useful pretreatment and outcome severity measure in the most recent literature.

Many operations have been described for full-thickness rectal prolapse. The approach can be abdominal or perineal. The choice is based on many factors, including the presence of faecal incontinence or simply to evaluate the risk of developing this dysfunction in the future or in relation to the appearance of RPS or to the surgical procedure itself.

Abdominal rectopexy has become the most commonly performed operation [13, 14]. Rectal mobilisation and fixation both appear to have an effect on colonic and anorectal motility, and several authors have reported an increase in the incidence of constipation, whereas faecal incontinence improves presumably due to the restored anatomy of the anal canal [15], as happens with perineal procedures.

Authors' Personal Experience

Between 1990 and 2006, 92 patients with full external rectal prolapse were operated by one surgeon (GD) with the following procedures (Table 1): modified Orr–Loygue and Wells rectopexy, Delorme procedure with and without sphincteroplasty, Altemeier procedure, artificial bowel sphincter implant in incontinent patients with lax sphincters, Thiersch encirclement, Saraffof anoplasty (in patients with residual mucosal ectropion after Whitehead haemorrhoidectomy performed in cases of unrecognised rectal prolapse), electrostimulated graciloplasty, and anterior rectal resection with coloanal anastomosis (in a patient with severe bleeding after dehiscence of a Delorme procedure).

Of 32 incontinent patients, 13 underwent an Orr–Loygue, six a Wells procedure, two a colporectosacropexy for associated genital prolapse and 11 a Delorme rectal placation. After a mean follow-up of 50 months, an acceptable faecal continence was restored in all but seven patients (21%): two after Orr–Loygue rectopexy and five after the Delorme procedure. Four preoperatively continent patients, followed up for more than

Table 1. Rectal prolapse surgery: the authors' experience (1990–2006)

Procedure	Number
Orr–Loygue modified rectopexy	43
Wells rectopexy	4
Delorme mucosectomy and rectal plication	22
with levatorplasty	3
Altemeier rectal prolapse resection	6
Artificial bowel sphincter	5
Thiersch anal encirclement	5
Saraffof procedure	2
Electrostimulated graciloplasty	1
Rectal anterior resection	1
Total	92

Table 2. Outcome in constipation (*C*) and incontinence (*IA*) (mean follow-up 50 months)

Preoperative symptoms [*n* (%) patients]		Postoperative symptoms (*n* patients)	
IA (-) C (-)	29 (31%)	IA (-) C (-)	21
		IA (+) C (-)	2
		IA (-) C (+)	6
		IA (+) C (+)	0
IA (+) C (-)	11 (12%)	IA (-) C (-)	6
		IA (+) C (-)	2
		IA (-) C (+)	3
		IA (+) C (+)	0
IA (-) C (+)	31 (34%)	IA (-) C (-)	24
		IA (+) C (-)	1
		IA (-) C (+)	5
		IA (+) C (+)	1
IA (+) C (+)	21 (23%)	IA (-) C (-)	12
		IA (+) C (-)	4
		IA (-) C (+)	4
		IA (+) C (+)	1
Total	92 (100%)	Total	92

(+), present; (–), absent

8 years, developed mild anal incontinence after perineal surgery.

Fifty-two patients complained of some degree of preoperative constipation, being associated to anal incontinence in 21. After surgery only 11 were still more or less severely constipated. Among 40 patients not constipated preoperatively, following abdominal rectopexy, nine were affected by annoying stool retention (Table 2).

Overview of the Literature

Patients with rectal prolapse often complain of other pelvic floor dysfunctions and require an accurate peroperative and multidisciplinary evaluation. A routine screening evaluation of the colon with endoscopy or barium enema is recommended to exclude coexisting conditions such as cancer or inflammatory bowel disease (IBD). Specific tests include (cystocolpo) defecography, solid sphere test [16], electromyography, anorectal manometry, colon transit study and transanal ultrasound.

Despite recovery of anal sphincteric tone after prolapse repair, faecal incontinence persists in at least one third of cases regardless of the surgical approach (Table 3). The persisting incontinence may be due to sphincter dilatation by the prolapse or to pudendal neuropathy caused by chronic traction of the nerves. Some authors have attempted to correlate postoperative outcome with preoperative physiologic testing (anal manometry and PNTML) to predict which patients are more likely to experience improved continence. This would allow selection of the best surgical option and provide comprehensive preoperative counselling. Patients with the most severe physiologic derangements generally have little or no improvement in incontinence after surgery. Glasgow et al. [9] demonstrated that preoperative squeeze pres-

Table 3. Cure of faecal incontinence after rectal prolapse surgery. Review of the literature

Reference	No. patients	Type of surgery	Continence status	
Brown et al. 2004 [17]	102	Perineal (Altemeier/Delorme)	Continent	53%
	41	Abdominal	Continent	41%
Portier et al. 2006 [18]	73	Orr–Loygue	Continent	62.5%
			Improved	29.2%
Lechaux et al. 2004 [19]	48	Rectopexy (laparoscopic)	Continent	31%
Tsunoda et al. 2003 [20]	31	Delorme	Continent	30%
Marchal et al. 2005 [21]	49	Orr–Loygue rectopexy	Continent	73%
	60	Delorme	Continent	42%
Schultz et al. 2000 [22]	69	Ripstein rectopexy	Continent	43%
Aitola et al. 1999 [23]	96	Posterior rectopexy	Continent	26%
			Improved	42%
Zittel et al. 2000 [24]	29	Rectopexy (laparoscopic)	Improved	76%
Benoist et al. 2001 [25]	48	Rectopexy (laparoscopic)	Continent	30%
			Improved	60%
Pescatori et al. 1998 [26]	33	Delorme	Continent	30%
Kohler and Athanasiadis 2001 [27]	16	Altemeier + posterior levator plasty	Continent	84%
Kim et al. 1999 [28]	183	Altemeier	Continent	55%
	176	Abdominal rectopexy	Continent	53%
Dodi G, Amadio L 2007 (present report)	32	Orr–Loygue, Wells rectopexy	Continent	85%
		Delorme	Continent	55%

sure >60 mmHg is associated with significantly lower incidence of postoperative faecal incontinence, with a postproctectomy continence rate of 84.6%. Only 36% of preoperatively incontinent patients with maximal squeeze pressures <60 mmHg became continent after surgery. Maximum squeeze pressure >60 mmHg seemed therefore to be a predictive parameter of improved functional outcome after perineal proctectomy. According to Williams et al. [7], a resting pressure <10 mmHg predicts incontinence after surgery. Other authors found no correlation between resting pressure, unilateral or bilateral PNTML abnormality and postoperative faecal incontinence [29, 30].

Continence improves after all surgical procedures for treatment of rectal prolapse, the best results being observed after abdominal surgery [17]. Ripstein rectopexy incontinence improves in 3–40% of cases [22, 31], and the success of the Orr–Loygue procedure for continence dysfunction is a total cure in 62–73% of cases, an improvement in 29% and a complete failure in 8–22% [18, 21]. Deen et al. [32] compared perineal rectosigmoidectomy with abdominal resection rectopexy associated with pelvic floor repair and showed that perineal surgery has a greater risk of faecal incontinence (odds ratio 8.07). Other studies prove that rectopexy with sigmoid resection in incontinent patients is associated with an increased risk of postoperative continence dysfunction [17, 33]. Rectal mobilisation with division of lateral ligaments guarantees a minor risk of prolapse recurrence but has no influence on faecal continence [34].

Continence improvement after perineal procedure occurs in 43% of patients, with a significant reduction of incontinence scores [21, 32–35]. In 1997, Agachan et al. [36] compared rectal plication and perineal rectosigmoidectomy with or without levatorplasty. Postoperative scores improved after all procedures, with the best results after perineal rectosigmoidectomy associated with levatorplasty [36]. Pescatori et al. [26] found continence improvement in 30% of Delorme procedures with sphincteroplasty. Kohler and Athanasiadis associated posterior levatorplasty with abdominal or perineal procedures, with significant improvement of continence (84% of with posterior levatorplasty vs. 67% without; $p < 0.05$) [27].

Management of persistent postoperative incontinence remains a difficult problem to treat. Conservative therapy includes dietary regimes, antidiarrhoeal medications and rehabilitation. A surgical option is represented by postanal repair. Setti Carraro and Nicholls found modest improvement in seven of nine patients: two became continent to solid and liquid stools and five to solid stool only [37]. Sacral nerve stimulation (SNS) is an alternative treatment for idiopathic incontinence. Three studies deal with SNS after surgical correction of rectal prolapse. There was a reduction in monthly faecal incontinence episodes, an improvement in urgency and a better ability to defer defecation, but the small number of patients is the limitation of these works. Multicentric studies are necessary to confirm these results [38–40].

In an Italian multicentric study, 11 patients with rectal prolapse and incontinence were treated with an artificial bowel sphincter (ABS). In six the prolapse had been treated before prosthesis implantation, and five underwent ABS implantation without prolapse treatment. Five had the device removed for infection or erosion and displacement into the rectum. Obstructed defecation was a frequent problem that led several patients to deactivate the system. Manometric findings of low anal canal resting pressure suggest that the ABS may function as a passive obstacle to the passage of faeces in the long term rather than as a dynamic sphincter [41].

Anal encirclement for prolapse is a safe procedure useful for patients unfit for more extensive surgery, but overall results are poor and include associated faecal incontinence that improves only in 27% of patients [42].

Conclusion

Many surgical techniques have been described for treating rectal prolapse. The high number of different procedures indicates that none are entirely satisfactory. The different techniques, abdominal or perineal, guarantee similar results overall on faecal incontinence, and the surgeon can basically choose the operation, evaluating the performance status of the patient. Abdominal surgery, however, appears to be mandatory for low-risk patients because of a better postoperative outcome (continence, recurrence).

Anal continence is based on several factors: internal and external anal sphincter and anal canal integrity in their anatomy and nervous supply, anal canal and rectum sensitivity, rectal compliance, peristalsis and patient mental function and mobility. In the different forms of RPS, damage of the above factors is variously associated, and this should be considered when evaluating the results obtained with the different operations.

For anal incontinence, the outcome, especially after a long follow-up, must be viewed considering the specific RPS evolution in each patient as a sort of personal biological history of the disease. Surgery takes place, early or late, in a specific moment of the progressive worsening of some factors of anal continence and pelvic floor stability only. We must therefore take into a serious consideration patient age and general health as defined by his or her physical and mental conditions. The item "G" (general factors) is an important part of the IPGH (incontinence, pelvic floor and prolapse, general factors, handicap) classification system, but it is seldom considered in the scientific reports [43–45].

Anal incontinence is a complex dysfunction with multiple causes, and in RPS, it may be difficult to understand if it is due only to anatomical defect (full rectal eversion, abnormal sphincter dilatation, etc.) or to a functional lesion (abnormal rectal sensitivity, loss of rectal reservoir function, etc.). This can explain why in some cases treating only the prolapse may not be sufficient to cure all symptoms of RPS. Furthermore, evaluation of faecal incontinence severity is such a difficult problem that quality of life seems to be the most acceptable measurement. Only the recent literature, however, is updated on this matter.

References

1. Moschcowitz AW (1912) The pathogenesis, anatomy and cure of prolapse of the rectum. Surg Gynecol Obstet 15:7–21
2. Goligher JC (1975) Surgery of the anus rectum and colon, 3rd end. Baillière Tindall, London
3. Mellgren A, Schultz I, Johansonn C, Dolk A (1997) Internal rectal intussusception seldom develops intc total rectal prolapse. Dis Colon Rectum 40:817–820
4. Ihre T, Seligson U (1975) Intussusception of the rectum-internal procidentia: treatment and result in 90 patients. Dis Colon Rectum 18:391–396
5. Shafik A (1997) Role of pudendal canal syndrome in the etiology of faecal incontinence in rectal prolapse. Digestion 58:489–493
6. Snooks SJ, Henry MM, Swash M (1985) Anorectal incontinence and rectal prolapse: differential assessment of the innervation to puborectalis and external anal sphincter muscles. Gut 26:470–476
7. Williams JG, Wong WD, Jensen L et al (1998) Incontinence and rectal prolapse: a prospective manometric study. Dis Colon Rectum 41:1392–1398
8. Damon H, Henry L, Roman S et al (2003) Influence of rectal prolapse on asymmetry of the anal sphinctere in patients with anal incontinence. BMC Gastroenterol 3:23
9. Glasgow SC, Birnbaum EH, Kodner I et al (2006) Preoperative anal manometry predicts continence after perineal proctectomy for rectal prolapse. Dis Colon Rectum 49:1052–1058
10. Woods R, Voyvodic F, Scholoithe AC et al (2002) Anal sphincter tears in patients with rectal prolapse and incontinence. Colorectal Dis 5:544–548
11. Parks AG, Swash M, Urich H (1977) Sphincter denervation in anorectal incontinence and rectal prolapse 18:656–665
12. Neill ME, Parks AG, Swash M (1981) Physiological studies of the anal sphincter musculature in fecal incontinence and rectal prolapse. Br J Surg 68(8): 531–536
13. Karulf RE, Madoff RD, Goldberg SM (2001) Rectal prolapse. Curr Probl Surg 38(10):771–832
14. Madiba TE, Baig MK, Wexner SD (2005) Surgical management of rectal prolapse. Arch Surg 140:63–23
15. Mollen RM, Kuijpers HC, van Hoek F (2000) Effects of rectal mobilization and lateral ligaments division on colonic and anorectal function. Dis Colon Rectum 43:1283–1287
16. Cavallari F, Dodi G (2004) Test della sfera solida: validazione metodologica e dati preliminari nella stipsi da anismo. Pelvi-Perineologia 23:132–135
17. Brown AJ, Anderson JH, McKee RF, Finlay IG (2004) Strategy for selection of type of operation for rectal prolapse based on clinical criteria. Dis Colon Rectum 47:103–107
18. Portier G, Iovino F, Lezorthes F (2006) Surgery for rectal prolapse: Orr–Loygue ventral rectopexy with limited dissection prevents postoperative induced constipation without increasing recurrence. Dis Colon Rectum 49:1136–1140
19. Lechaux D, Trebuchet G, Siproudhis L, Campion JP (2005) Laparoscopic rectopexy for full-thickness rectal prolapse. A single-institution retrospective study evaluating surgical outcome. Surg Endosc 19:514–518
20. Tsunoda A, Yasuda N, Yokoyama N et al (2003) Delorme's procedure for rectal prolapse. Clinical and physiological analysis. Dis Colon Rectum 46:1260–1265
21. Marchal F, Bresler L, Ayav A et al (2005) Long-term results of Delorme's procedure and Orr–Loygue rectopexy to treat complete rectal prolapse. Dis Colon

Rectum 48:1785–1790
22. Schultz I, Mellgren A, Dolk A et al (2000) Long-term results and functional outcome after Ripstein rectopexy. Dis Colon Rectum 43:35–43
23. Aitola PT, Hiltunen KM, Matikainen MJ (1999) Functional results of operative treatment of rectal prolapse over an 11-year period. Emphasis on transabdominal approach. Dis Colon Rectum 42:655–660
24. Zittel TT, Maniche K, Haug S et al (2000) Functional results after laparoscopic rectopexy for rectal prolapse. J Gastrointest Surg 4:632–641
25. Benoist S, Taffinder N Gouls S et al (2001) Functional results two years after laparoscopic rectopexy. Am J Surg 182:168–173
26. Pescatori M, Interisano A, Stolfi VM, Zoffoli M (1998) Delorme's operation and sphincteroplasty for rectal prolapse and fecal incontinence. Int J Colorectal Dis 13:223–227
27. Kohler A, Athanasiadis S (2001) The value of posterior levator repair in the treatment of anorectal incontinence due to rectal prolapse – a clinical and manometric study. Langenbeck's Arch Surg 386:188–192
28. Kim DS, Tsang CB, Wong WD et al (1999) Complete rectal prolapse: evolution of management and results. Dis Colon Rectum 42:460–469
29. Johansen OB, Wexner SD, Daniel N et al (1993) Perineal rectosigmoidectomy in the elderly. Dis Colon Rectum 36:767–772
30. Sainio AP, Vou tilainen PE, Husa AI (1991) Recovery of anal sphincter function following transabdominal repair of rectal prolapse: cause of improved continence? Dis Colon Rectum 34:816–821
31. Roberts PL, Schoetz DJ, Coller JA et al (1988) Ripstein procedure: Lahey Clinic experience: 1963–1985. Arch Surg 123:554–557
32. Deen KI, Grant E, Billingham C, Keighley MR (1994) Abdominal resection rectopexy with pelvic floor repair versus perineal rectosigmoidectomy and pelvic floor repair for full-thickness rectal prolapse. Br J Surg 81(2):302–304
33. Madoff RD, Williams JG, Wong WD et al (1992) Long-term functional results of colon resection and rectopexy for overt rectal prolapse. Am J Gastroenterol 87:1001–1004
34. Speakman CTM, Madden MV, Nicholls RJ, Kamm MA (1992) Lateral ligament division during rectopexy causes constipation but prevents recurrence of prolapse. Br J Surg 79(5):465
35. Boccasanta P, Venturi M, Barbieri S, Roviaro G (2006) Impact of new technologies on the clinical and functional outcome of Altemeier's procedure: a randomized, controlled trial. Dis Colon Rectum 49:652–660
36. Agachan F, Reissman P, Pfeifer J et al (1997) Comparison of three perineal procedure for the treatment of rectal prolapse. South Med J 90(9):925–932
37. Setti Carraro P, Nicholls RJ (1994) Postanal repair for faecal incontinence persisting after rectopexy.Br J Surg 81(2):305–307
38. Matzel KE, Stadelmaier U, Hohenfellner M, Hohenberger W (2001) Chronic sacral spinal nerve stimulation for faecal incontinence: long-term results with foramen and cuff electrodes. Dis Colon Rectum 44:59–66
39. Kenefick NJ, Vaizey CJ, Cohen RG et al (2002) Medium term results of sacral nerve stimulation for faecal incontinence. Br J Surg 89:896–901
40. Jarrett MED, Matzel KE, Stosser M (2005) Sacral nerve stimulation for faecal incontinence following surgery for rectal prolapse repair: a multicenter study. Dis Colon rectum 48:1243–1248
41. Altomare DF, Dodi G, La Torre F et al (2001) Multicentre retrospective analysis of the outcome of artificial anal sphincter implantation for severe faecal incontinence. Br J Surg 88(11):1481–1486
42. Sanio AP, Halme LE, Husa AI (1991) Anal encirclement with polypropylene mesh for rectal prolapse and incontinence. Dis Colon Rectum 34(19):905–908
43. Artibani W, Benvenuti F, Di Benedetto P et al (1996) Staging of female urinary incontinence and pelvic floor disorders. Proposal of IPGH system. Urodinamica, Neurology, Urodynamics & Continence 6(1):1–5
44. Dodi G, Lucio P, Spella M et al (2006) La raccolta dati nel paziente pelvi-perineologico. Pelvi-Perineologia 25:19–27
45. Farnsworth B, Dodi G (2007) Short-IPGH system for assessment of pelvic floor disease. Pelviperineology 26(2):73–77

25 Management of Associated Pelvic Dysfunctions: External Rectal Prolapse and Genital Prolapse

Mauro Cervigni, Franca Natale, Anna Padoa

Introduction

Genital prolapse, or pelvic organ prolapse (POP), is an emerging problem among women over the age of 65 and is a common disorder in Western countries [1]. Besides age, well-established risk factors include race, genetic predisposition, pregnancy, parity, obstetric trauma, menopause and previous gynaecological surgery. Among these variables, Caucasian women have a higher odds ratio (1.0) than do African Americans (0.6) [2].

Considering the different vaginal segments involved in the development of POP, a study of 27,000 American women determined that the anterior vaginal wall and the bladder in particular represented the site most frequently affected (34% of the group) compared with the posterior and apical segments (rectocele 19% and uterine prolapse 14%, respectively) [2]. The incidence of rectal prolapse (RP) in the general population is unknown, although it is less common than genital prolapse. Women are more commonly affected, representing 80–90% of RP patients [3].

In the literature, very few series have reported upon combined simultaneous treatment of RP and POP (Fig. 1). In 1968, Amico and Marino described women with prolapse of the vagina and rectal procidentia, claiming that this was the second such case published since 1920 [4]. Tancer et al. [5], in 1987, found it remarkable that the world gynaecological literature of the preceding 50 years provided almost no evidence that POP and RP can be concurrent.

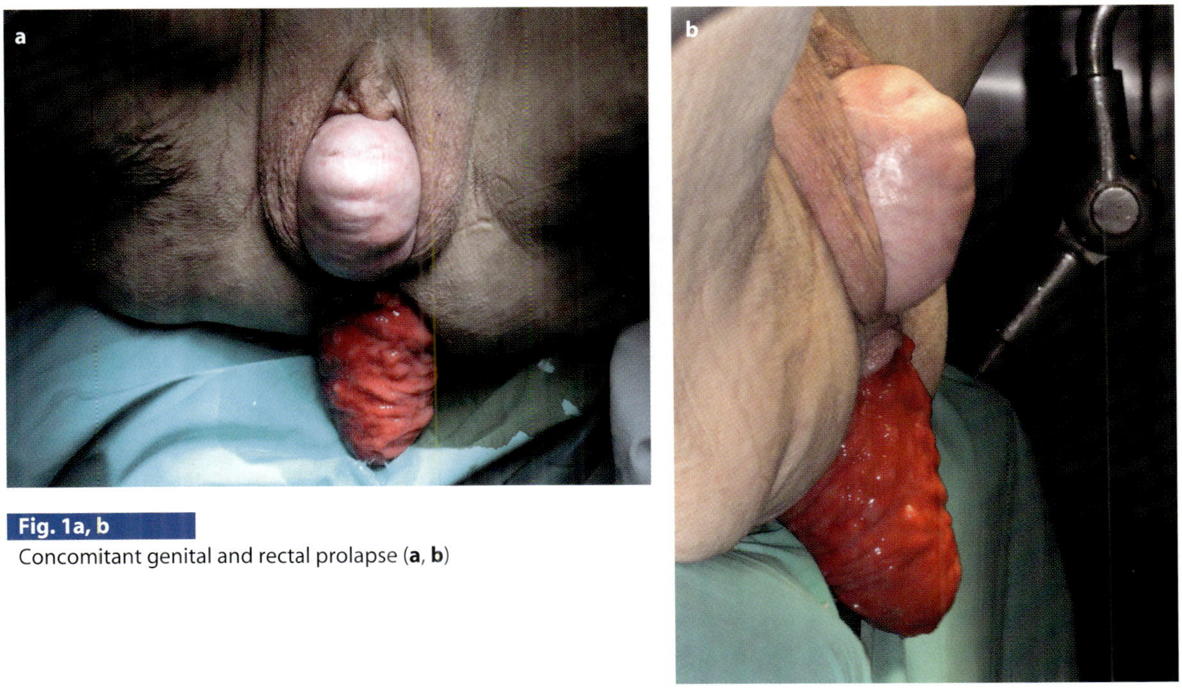

Fig. 1a, b
Concomitant genital and rectal prolapse (**a**, **b**)

Pathophysiology, Epidemiology and Predisposing Factors

An association between rectal and genital prolapse is biologically plausible, as both conditions involve laxity of pelvic organ supportive tissues. Some of the risk factors presumably predisposing for RP, such as chronic straining at defecation, previous pelvic surgery, elevated intra-abdominal pressure and increasing age, are often associated with POP as well [6, 7]. Concomitant pelvic floor disorders have been reported in 8–27% of patients with RP [8, 9]. Current knowledge on the relationship between rectal and genital prolapse is mostly limited to anecdotal reports and case series [4]. Epidemiologic studies agree that pregnancy and delivery are important risk factors for POP [10]. Evidence demonstrates that direct tissue trauma at delivery may have a harmful effect on pelvic floor innervation [11]. Similarly, parity and vaginal delivery have been associated with an increased risk of RP [12], although a high percentage of patients with this disorder were found to be nulliparous by some authors [13, 14]. Associated medical conditions may contribute to the development of POP, particularly those involving chronically increased intra-abdominal pressure or connective tissue defects. Psychiatric disorders were noted in 52% of patients by Altemeier et al. [15] and in a sizeable percentage Goligher's series [16]; he found uterine prolapse to be commonly coincident with RP.

Clinical Findings

Genital Prolapse

POP is defined as the descent of either the anterior, posterior or apical segment of the vagina beyond the introitus. POP symptoms are often vague, which makes it difficult to correlate specific symptoms with the prolapse site or severity. POP symptoms may include a sensation of pelvic pressure or vaginal "heaviness", recurrent irritative bladder symptoms, voiding difficulties, incontinence or defecatory difficulty. Other symptoms such as low back or pelvic pain may or may not be related to POP.

Physical examination is essential in the assessment of all women with POP. The patient should be examined in the lithotomy position, and the anterior, superior and posterior vaginal segments should be evaluated. Several systems for the description and classification of POP have been developed. The Baden and Walker classification, or "half-way system", has been used within this scope [17]. Nowadays, the method of choice is the "POP-Q system", recommended by the International Continence Society in 1996 [18].

As regards ancillary testing, imaging with traditional X-ray (cystourethrography and defecography) or magnetic resonance imaging (MRI) could help the clinician obtain a more detailed morphological visualisation of pelvic organs. Conventional urodynamic studies are an essential tool for the evaluation of bladder-function alterations in the presence of POP, such as stress urinary incontinence (SUI), detrusor overactivity and/or bladder outlet obstruction.

Rectal Prolapse

RP is defined as a protrusion of all layers of the rectum through the anal orifice. Patients usually complain of a protrusion at the anal area, a feeling of incomplete evacuation after bowel movements and sometimes of stool incontinence. Early in the disease course, the protrusion may be present only when the patient is straining during evacuation or lifting heavy objects; with disease progression, however, prolapse occurs with standing or walking. Attempts by the patients to reduce the prolapse manually become increasingly ineffective until finally the rectum protrudes constantly. At this point, a continuous mucoid discharge and frequent bleeding from irritation of the mucosa are present.

Examination of the patient with suspect RP should begin with the patient sitting on a toilet and straining. In order to define RP, the rectal surface is usually oedematous and hyperaemic, and superficial ulceration may be present. Both walls of the bowel can be palpated in the prolapsed segment; thickening is more likely to be prominent anteriorly. Excoriation of perineal skin resulting from faecal soiling and mucous discharge is common. Neill and colleagues showed that in two thirds of patients, sphincter function was similar to patients with faecal incontinence [19]. Anal manometry and electrophysiologic testing evaluate anorectal and sphincteric function. Manometry may diagnose internal and external sphincter weakness, identifying reduced resting and squeeze pressure as well as reduced sphincter length. Pudendal nerve motor conduction studies can show prolonged latencies when a neuropathy is present [20].

Some patients with RP complain of constipation, which may be associated with prolonged colonic transit time. Flexible sigmoidoscopy should be carried out to exclude a solitary rectal ulcer, rectal polyp, tumour or mucosal disease. Defecating proctography is not routinely required if a full-thickness RP is evident clinically, although it may be useful in order to predict the chances of return of continence.

Surgical Techniques

Pelvic Organ Prolapse Repair

Traditional pelvic reconstructive surgery restores the position of the pelvic organs using autologous tissue. Numerous surgical procedures have been proposed in the past century to correct all types of anterior vaginal wall defects (central, paravaginal, combined) with either an abdominal or vaginal approach. Despite improved understanding of pelvic anatomy and organ function and the advancement of surgical techniques, the long-term success rate is still variable. The different surgical procedures for anterior vaginal prolapse report a recurrence rate of 3–20% [21, 22] after single anterior colporrhaphy (AC); 22–92% [23, 24] if the AC is combined with other procedures (sacrospinous ligament suspension); 2–59% [25, 26] after four-corner suspension; 5–50% [27, 28] after vaginal paravaginal repair. The reasons for such a discrepancy are several: poor patient selection; suboptimal surgical technique; inappropriate choice of suture material; persistence of predisposing risk factors for prolapse (constipation, chronic lung disease) [29]. Moreover, Farrel et al. [30] doubted the very existence of the pubocervical fascia used during AC. During surgical procedures for the correction of anterior defect, they observed that the so-called fascia is adequately identified only 58% of the time and therefore concluded this finding called into question techniques relying on isolated fascia for the repair of anterior and posterior defects.

Due to these findings and the high recurrence rate with traditional techniques for POP repair, prosthetic surgery has gained increased popularity in recent years. The goal of prosthetic surgery is to replace the damaged visceral fascia, to restore cohesion between visceral and parietal fascia and to rebuild the hammock connected to the arcus tendineus fascia pelvis (ATFP), thus respecting the bladder neck and stabilising the bladder hammock, the apex of the vagina and the rectovaginal septum. Initial experience utilised an overlaid synthetic mesh reinforcing a traditional AC [31]. Later, the concept of transvaginal suspension of pelvic floor defects was introduced with the four-corner suspension [7]. An evolution of this technique included a prosthetic reinforcement of the central segment utilising mesh applied with a double-needle suspension [32].

The new "tension-free" concept acquired by general surgeons in treating abdominal hernia and the advancement in the treatment of female SUI achieved with tension-free vaginal tape (TVT) were applied in POP repair. A new proposal utilising a Prolene mesh positioned below the bladder tension free, i.e. without any fixation, was developed [33]. Since then, other authors have proposed various transvaginal tension-free mesh repairs [34–36].

In 2001, a new approach utilising the transobturator route, based on the same tension-free principles as TVT, was proposed for the treatment of SUI [37]. The excellent preliminary results incited the development of a wider concept of transperineal pelvic floor repair [38–40]. Much research is underway in order to determine the efficacy and safety of this promising new technique, and more studies on large groups of patients, with medium- to long-term follow-up, are required to encourage the spread of such an approach. A brief schematic summary of the commercially available kits follows.

Prolift

Material:	Prolene soft (Gynemesh)
System delivery:	one reusable long, curved needle
Anchoring system:	low-tension (friction) – Velcro effect
Tension free:	in the vesicovaginal space; Retzius space; paravesical space; ischiorectal fossa

Arms: anteriorly; two superficial and two deeper-positioned apical and distal at the ATFP posteriorly; two deeper-positioned at the transsacrospinous ligament (Figs. 2 and 3)

Perigee

Material: polypropylene

System delivery: four disposable needles connected with a special connector

Anchoring system: low tension (friction) – Velcro effect

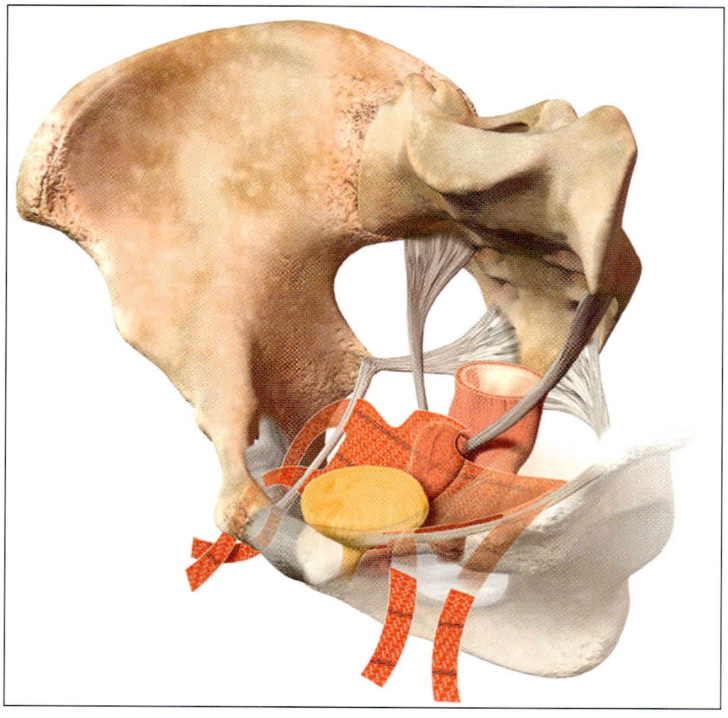

Fig. 2

Final position of Prolift total vaginal mesh in the pelvis. ETHICON, Inc. Reproduced with permission

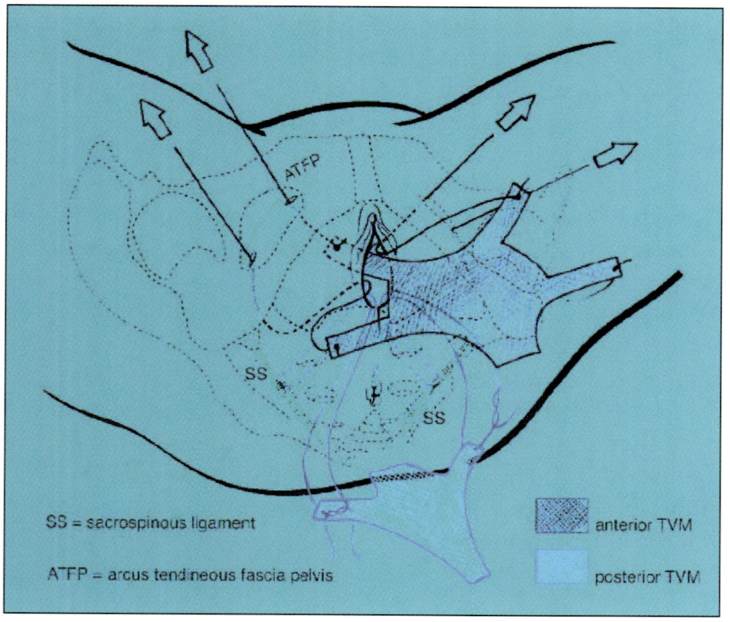

Fig. 3

Female pelvis showing correct positioning of the anterior and posterior transvaginal mesh segments. ETHICON, Inc. Reproduced with permission

Tension free: in the vesicovaginal space; Retzius space; paravesical space

Arms: two superficial and two deeper positioned apical and distal at the ATFP (Figs. 4 and 5)

Apogee

Material: polypropylene

System delivery: two disposable needles connected with a special connector

Anchoring system: low tension (friction) – Velcro effect

Tension free: in the pararectal space; ischiorectal fossa

Arms: two deeper, transfixing the sacrospinous ligament (Fig. 6)

Avaulta

Material: polypropylene covered by collagen in the central part

System delivery: one reusable curved needle

Anchoring system: low tension (friction) – Velcro effect

Tension free: in the vesicovaginal space; Retzius space; paravesical space; pararectal space

Arms: two superficial and two deeper positioned apical and distal at the ATFP; two deeper positioned at the trans-sacrospinous ligaments, two superficial at the transperineal membrane (Figs. 7 and 8)

Table 1 shows the preliminary results of the use of transperineal mesh.

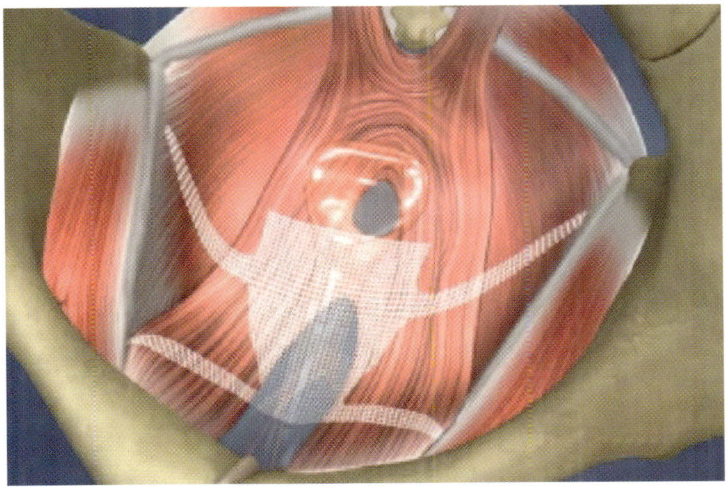

Fig. 4
Final position of the Perigee mesh in the pelvis. Perigee (Transobturator Anterior Prolapse Repair System). Courtesy of American Medical Systems, Inc., Minnetonka, Minnesota. www.AmericanMedicalSystems.com

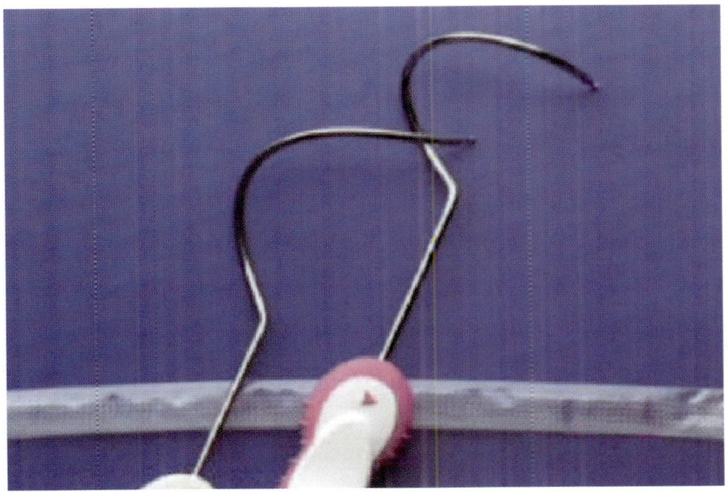

Fig. 5
Perigee needles. Perigee (Transobturator Anterior Prolapse Repair System). Courtesy of American Medical Systems, Inc., Minnetonka, Minnesota. www.AmericanMedicalSystems.com

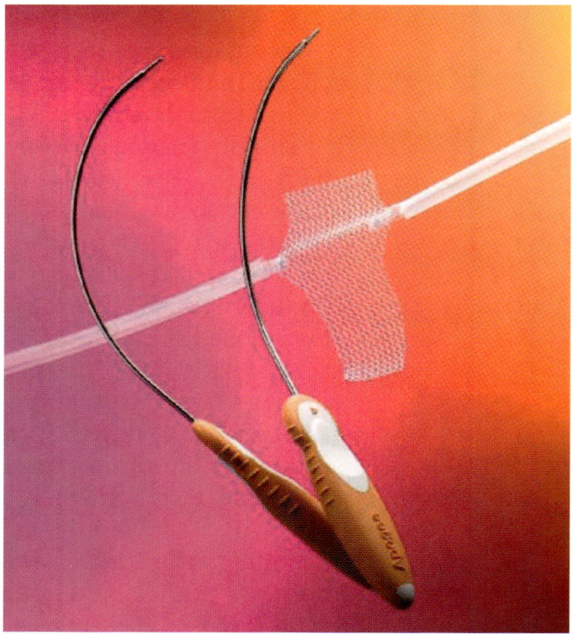

Fig. 6
Apogee needles and mesh. Apogee (Vaginal Vault Prolapse Repair Suystem). Courtesy of American Medical Systems, Inc., Minnetonka, Minnesota. www.AmericanMedicalSystems.com

Surgical Treatment of Rectal Prolapse

More than 100 different operative procedures have been described for RP. The aim of treatment is to correct the prolapse and restore continence while preventing constipation or impaired evacuation. The different procedures for RP repair are classified as transabdominal or perineal approaches. Perineal repairs are less invasive and cause less morbidity. They are preferred for frail, elderly patients, but some authors favour perineal repairs for younger, healthy patients as well. The perineal route carries a risk of infection and possible complications related to the wound's suture line. Abdominal approaches are favoured by other authors due to a higher success rate compared with perineal procedures. However, the abdominal approach has potentially severe complications, such as anastomotic leak, abdominal sepsis, stricture and adhesions, and it usually requires general anaesthesia. The introduction of laparoscopy in the past decade added a new dimension to RP surgery and is very promising, as it reduces postoperative recovery time following abdominal repairs.

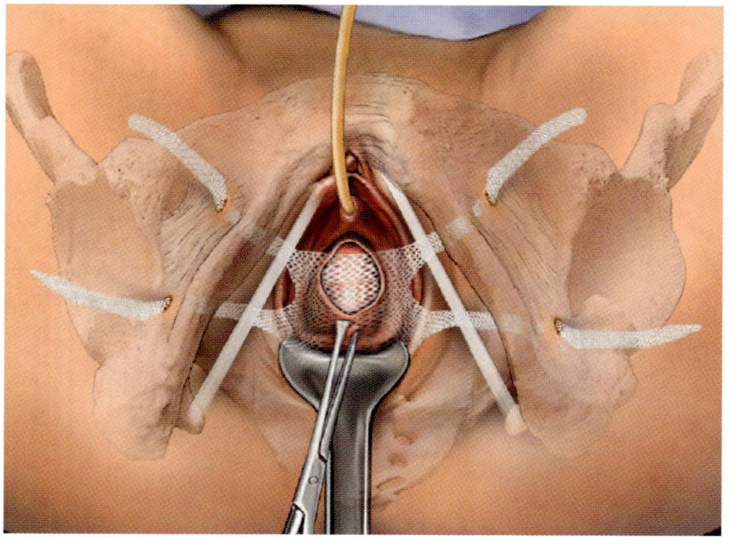

Fig. 7
Final position of the anterior Avaulta mesh in the anterior vaginal wall. Figure from www.bardurological.com

Table 1. Outcome following pelvic organ prolapse surgery with mesh

Author	Mesh	Patients	follow-up	Cure rate	Sequelae
De Tayrac et al. 2002 [41]	Gynemesh	48	18 months	97.9%	8.3% erosion
Von Theobald and Labbe 2003 [42]	Prolene mesh; Posterior IVS[a]	92			3 erosions; 1 haematoma
Yan et al. 2004 [43]	Synthetic	30	6.7 months	97%	7% erosion; 14% dyspareunia
Bader et al. 2004 [44]	Gynemesh	40	16.4 months	95%	2 erosions

[a] Posterior intravaginal slingplasty

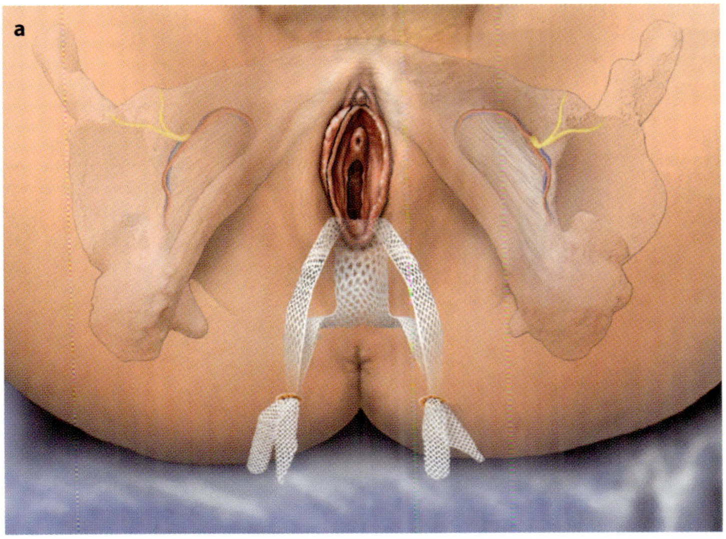

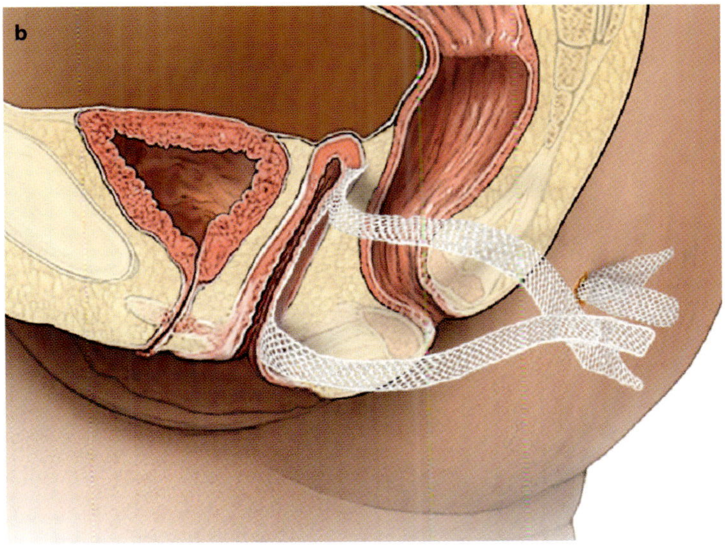

Fig. 8a,b
Final position of the posterior Avaulta mesh in the posterior vaginal wall. Figures from www.bardurological.com (**a**, **b**)

Authors' Experience in the Management of POP and RP

From 1997 through 2006, six women were referred to our centre with total genital descensus (≥2 according to the "half-way" system) and RP (>10 cm). Ages ranged from 67 to 91 (mean 74.2) years; parity ranged from two to five (median two). All patients were postmenopausal. All had a long history of POP symptoms and moderate to severe constipation, associated with faecal incontinence in one patient. Preoperative evaluation included questionnaires, voiding diaries, physical examination, urodynamics, cystoscopy, defecography and anal manometry. Patients with associated faecal incontinence treated recently also underwent endoanal ultrasound and pudendal nerve terminal motor latency.

Vaginal hysterectomy was performed in four patients. A prosthetic anterior repair utilising a polypropylene mesh (Marlex) applied tension free was carried out in all cases. Four patients were treated with a sacrospinous ligament suspension (bilateral in one case) for prolapse of the vaginal apex. In two cases, an intravaginal slingplasty (posterior IVS, or infracoccygeal sacropexy) was carried out (Figs. 9 and 10). A midline prerectal fascia plication was performed in all women. All patients underwent a Delorme procedure. No continence procedure (either faecal or urinary) was performed.

No intraoperative complications were ob-

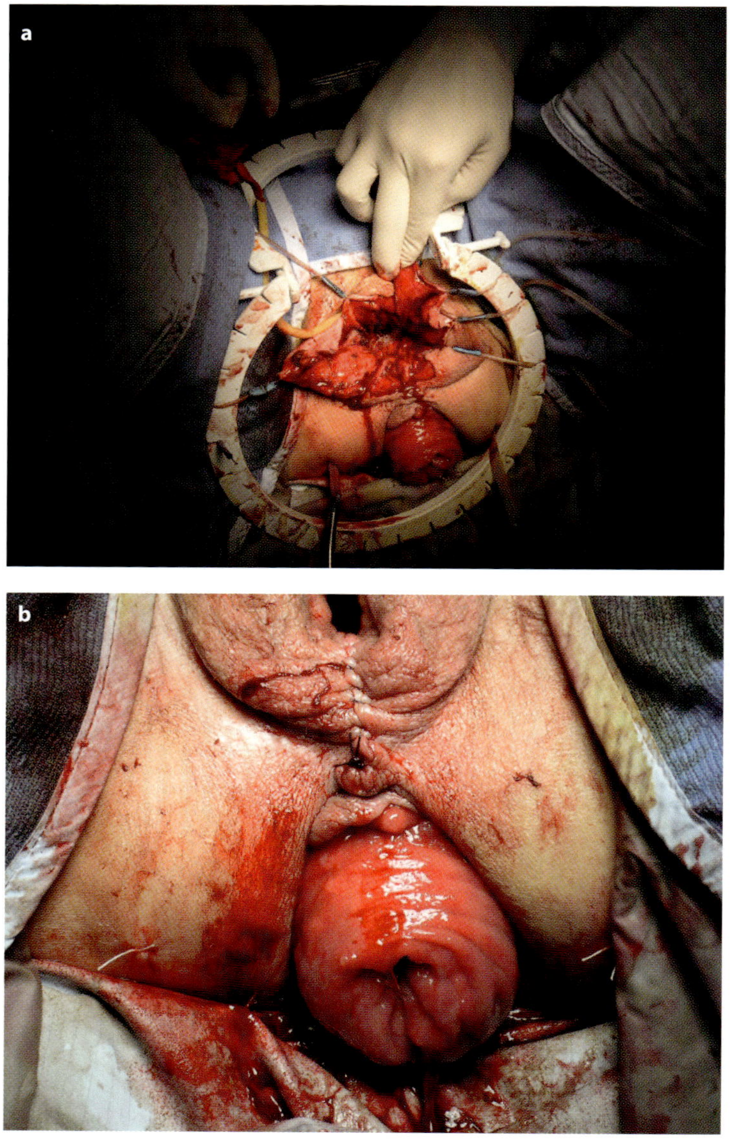

Fig. 9a,b
Pelvic organ prolapse repair with posterior intravaginal slingplasty in a patient with concomitant rectal prolapse (**a**, **b**)

served. Postoperatively, there were two pelvic hematomas, which were subsequently treated conservatively; one vaginal-vault abscess, which resolved after drainage; and one case of pelvic pain, with spontaneous resolution 2 months after surgery. With a mean follow-up of 2 years, anatomical correction of POP was achieved, as shown in Table 2.

No de novo SUI occurred; however, two patients developed de novo urge urinary incontinence. Anatomical correction of RP was achieved in four out of six patients; four women referred de novo faecal incontinence, and only two complained of persistent constipation.

Table 2. Pre- and postoperative vaginal profile

	Preoperative	Postoperative
Cystocele ≥2°	6	4
Vaginal vault ≥2°	6	6
Posterior colpocele ≥2°	6	5

Treatment of Combined RP and GP

Although there is a trend toward a more comprehensive and holistic approach to pelvic floor disorders, their management continues to suffer from compartmentalisation among medical sub-

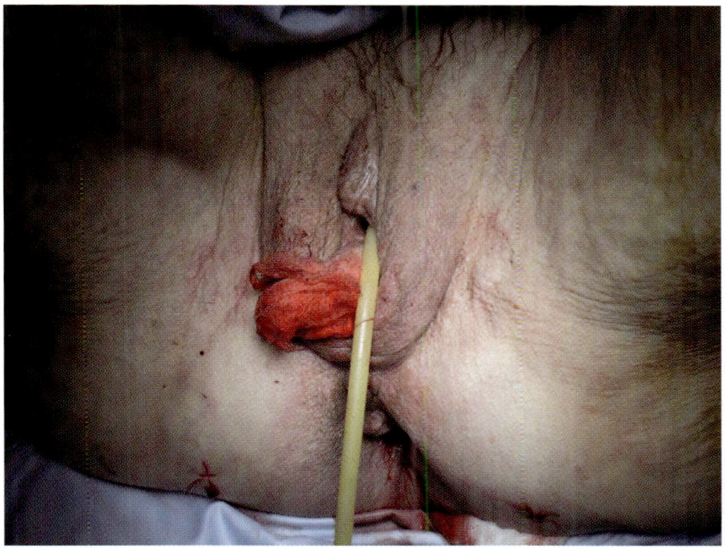

Fig. 10
Final anatomical result following rectal prolapse repair with the Delorme procedure

specialties [45], and RP and POP are often treated at separate surgical sessions. Literature regarding the combined surgical treatment of POP and RP is scarce and contains mainly case reports and a few small series of patients. In 1993, Barham and Collopy reported their experience with 24 posthysterectomy patients with combined vault prolapse and RP [46]. The operative procedure consisted of a Wells-type rectopexy modification in which the sling was extended to anchor the vaginal vault after abdominal correction of the enterocele. With a mean 15.6 months of follow-up, they reported good symptomatic relief with minimal morbidity. That same year, another group reported treatment of six patients with POP and RP by uterine fixation to the promontory and rectopexy using the Orr–Loygue technique [47]. With a 20-month follow-up, there were no recurrences in their small series. In 2000, Dekel et al. [48] presented their prospective assessment of ten patients treated with vaginal hysterectomy and AC with plication sutures combined with the Altemeier procedure for RP. At the 3-year follow-up, there were no recurrences of either rectal or vault prolapse. Three women complained of gas incontinence at 18–24 months following surgery. Ayav et al. [49] reported in 2005 on eight patients with combined prolapse treated with colpohysteropexy associated with mesh or sutured rectopexy and sigmoid resection. With a follow-up of 7 months, no prolapse recurrences were observed. Three of six patients remained constipated postoperatively; one patient had new-onset constipation postoperatively. None of the patients became faecally incontinent.

In light of these data, it is difficult to draw conclusions regarding the preferred approach for this synchronous condition. In our opinion, a multidisciplinary approach should be adopted for patient evaluation, and we also believe that combined surgery for POP and RP should be recommended in such patients. In the literature we reviewed on combined surgery for POP and RP, the main route for RP repair was abdominal. In our experience, the transperineal approach may be a safe and more effective alternative and has the following advantages:

1. It should cause less postoperative morbidity [50] and a shorter postoperative course.
2. It can be done using regional anaesthesia, which is less dangerous than general anaesthesia in elderly patients [51].
3. The proximity of the defect enables the use of the lithotomy position for both procedures, allowing better access and shorter operative time.

Clinical studies on larger groups of patients with POP and RP are required in order to achieve a clear conclusion on the best therapeutic option.

References

1. Azpuru CE (1974) Total rectal prolapse and total genital prolapse: a series of 17 cases. Dis Colon Rectum 17:528–531
2. Hendrix SL (2002) Urinary incontinence and menopause: an evidence-based treatment approach. Dis Mon 48:622
3. Jacobs KL, Lin YJ, Orkin BA (1997) The best operation for rectal prolapse. Surg Clin North Am 77:49–70
4. Amico JC, Marino AW Jr (1968) Prolapse of the vagina in association with rectal procidentia. Dis Colon Rectum 11(2):115–119
5. Tancer ML, Fleischer M, Berkowitz BJ (1987) Simultaneous colpo-recto-sacropexy. Obstet Gynecol 70(6):951–954
6. Rinne KM, Kirkinen PP (1999) What predisposes young women to genital prolapse. Eur J Obstet Gynecol Reprod Biol 84:23–25
7. Swift SE, Pound T, Dias JK (2001) Case-control study of etiologic factors in the development of severe pelvic organ prolapse. Int Urogynecol J Pelvic Floor Dysfunct 12:187–192
8. Kupfer CA, Goligher JC (1970) One hundred consecutive cases of complete prolapse of the rectum treated by operation. Br J Surg 57:482–487
9. Peters WA 3rd, Smith MR, Drescher CW (2001) Rectal prolapse in women with other defects of pelvic floor support. Am J Obstet Gynecol 184:1488–1494
10. MacLennan AH, Taylor AW, Wilson DH, Wilson D (2000) The prevalence of pelvic floor disorders and their relationship to gender, age, parity and mode of delivery.Br J Obstet Gynaecol 107:1460–1470
11. Snooke SJ, Swash M, Henry MM, Serchell M (1985) Risk factors in childbirth causing damage to the pelvic floor innervation. Br J Surg 72:S15–17
12. Altman D, Zetterstrom J, Schultz I et al (2005) Pelvic organ prolapse and urinary incontinence in women with surgically managed rectal prolapse: a population-based case-control study. Dis Colon Rectum 49:28–35
13. Ryan P (1980) Observations upon the etiology and treatment of complete rectal prolapse. ANZ J Surg 50:109–115
14. Watts JD, Rothemberger DA, Bulls JG et al (1985) The management of procidentia. 30 years' experience. Dic Colon Rectum 28:96–102
15. Altemeier WA, Culbertson WR, Schowegerdt C, Hunt J (1970) Nineteen years' experience with the one-stage perineal repair of rectal prolapse. Ann Surg 173(6):993–1006
16. Goligher J (1984) The skeptical chirurgeon. Ann R Coll Surg Engl 66(3):207–210
17. Baden WF, Walker T (1972) Genesis of the vaginal profile: a correlated classification of vaginal relaxation. Clin Obstet Gynecol 15(4):1048–1054
18. Bump RC, Mattiasson A, Bo K et al (1996) The standardization of terminology of female pelvic organ prolapse and pelvic floor dysfunction. Am J Obstet Gynecol 175 (1):10–17
19. Neill ME, Parks AG, Swash M (1981) Physiological studies of the anal sphincter musculature in faecal incontinence and rectal prolapse. Br J Surg 68(8):531–536
20. Osterberg A, Graf W, Edebol Eeg-Olofsson K et al (2000) Results of neurophysiologic evaluation in fecal incontinence. Dis Colon Rectum 43(9):1256–1261
21. Porges RF, Smilen SW (1994) Long-term analysis of the surgical management of pelvic support defect. Am J Obstet Gynecol 171:1518–1528
22. Macer GA (1978) Transabdominal repair of cystocele, a 20 years experience, compared with the traditional vaginal approach. Am J Obstet Gynecol 131:203–207
23. Morley GW, DeLancey JOL (1988) Sacrospinous ligament fixation for eversion of the vagina. Am J Obstet Gynecol 158:872–881
24. Holley RL, Varner RE, Gleason et al (1995): recurrent pelvic support defects after sacrospinous ligament fixation for vaginal vault prolapse. J Amer Coll Surg 180:444–448
25. Raz S, Klutke CG, Golomb J (1989) Four-corner bladder and urethral suspension for moderate cystocele. J Urol 142(3):712–715
26. Miyazaki FS, Miyazaki DW (1994) Raz four-corner suspension for severe cystocele: Poor results. Int Urol J 5:94–97
27. Richardson AC, EdmondsPB, Williams NL (1981) Treatment of stress urinary incontinence due to paravaginal defect. Obstet Gynecol 57(3):357–362
28. Benson JT (1992) Female pelvic floor disorders. WW Norton, New York, pp 280–294
29. Birch C (2005) The use of prosthetics in pelvic reconstructive surgery. Best Practice and Research Clin Obstet Gynaecol 19(1):979–991
30. Farrell SA, Dempsey T, Geldenhuys L (2001) Histologic examination of "fascia" used in colporrhaphy. Obstet Gynecol 98:794–798
31. Flood CG, Drutz HP, Waja L (1988) Anterior colporrhaphy reinforced with Marlex mesh for the treatment of systoles. Int Urogynecol J Pelvic Floor Dysfunct 9(4):200–204
32. Migliari R, Usai E (1999) Treatment results using a mixed fiber mesh in patients with grade IV cystocele. J Urol 161(4):1255–1258
33. Cervigni M, Natale F, Conti Puorger C et al (1998) Cistopessi con protesi "tension-free": esperienze preliminari. Acta Urol Ital XII(Suppl):120–121
34. De Tayrac R, Fernandez H (2002) Surgical repair of cystocele with mesh by the vaginal route. Am J Obstet Gynecol 186(4):852–853
35. Bader G, Fauconnier A, Roger N (2004) Cystocele repair by vaginal approach with a tension-free trasversal polypropylene mesh. Technique and results. Gynecol Obstet Fertil 32(4):280–284
36. Husaunndee M, Rousseau E, Deleflie M et al (2003) Surgical treatment of genital prolapse with a new lateral prosthetic hysteropexia technique combining vaginal and laparoscopic methods. J Gynecol Obstet Biol Reprod (Paris) 32(4):314–320
37. Delorme E (2001) Transobturator urethral suspension: mini invasive procedure in the treatment of stress urinary incontinence in women. Prog Urol 11(6):1306–1313
38. Deval B, Ferchaux J, Berry R et al (2006) Objective and subjective cure rates after trans-obturator tape (Obtape) treatment of female urinary incontinence. Eur

Urol 49(2):373–377
39. Wang AC, Lin YH, Tseng LH et al (2005) Prospective randomized comparison of transobturator suburethral sling (Monarc) vs. suprapubic arc (Sparc) sling procedures for female urodynamic stress incontinence. Int Urogynecol J Pelvic Floor Dynsfunct 3:1–5
40. Davila GW, Johnson JD, Serels S (2005) Multicenter experience with the Monarc transobturator sling system to treat stress urinary incontinence. Int Urogynecol J Pelvic Floor Dysfunct 29:1–6
41. De Tayrac R, Gervaise A, Fernandez H (2002) Cure de cystocèle voie basse par protese sous-vesicale libre. J Gynecol Obstet Biol Reprod 31:597–599
42. Von Theobald P, Labbè E (2003) La triple opèration pèrinèale avec prothèse. J Gynecol Obstet Biol Reprod 32:562–570
43. Yan A, Anne M, Karine A et al (2004) Cystocele repair by a synthetic vaginal mesh secured anteriorly through the obturator foramen. Eur J Obstet Gynecol Reprod Biol 115 (1):90–94
44. Bader G, Fauconnier A, Roger N (2004) Cystocele repair by vaginal approach with a tension-free transversal polypropylene mesh. Technique and results. Gynecol Obstet Fertil 32:280–284
45. Nichols DH (1972) Types of enterocele and principles underlying choice of operation for repair. Obstet Gynecol 40:257–263
46. Barham K, Collopy BT (1993) Posthysterectomy rectal and vaginal prolapse, a common overlooked problem. Aust NZJ Obstet Gynaecol 33(3):300–303
47. Zhioua F, Ferckiou M, Pira JM et al (1993) Uterine fixation to the promontory and the Orr–Loygue operation in associated genital and rectal prolapse. Rev Fr Gynecol Obstet 88(4):277–281
48. Dekel A, Rabinerson D, Rafael ZB, Kaplan B at al (2000) Concurrent genital and rectal prolapse: two pathologies – one joint operation. BJOG 107(1): 125–129
49. Ayav A, Bresler L, Brunaud L et al (2005) Surgical management of combined rectal and genital prolapse in young patients: transabdominal approach. Int J Colorectal Dis 20(2):173–179
50. Meeks JR, Harris RL (1997) Surgical approach to hysterectomy: abdominal, laparoscopic-assisted or vaginal. Clin Obstet Gynecol 40:886–894
51. Ueo H, Takeuchi H, Aringa S et al (1994) The feasibility of epidural anaesthesia without endotracheal intubation for abdominal surgery on patients over 80 years of age. Int Surg 79:158–162

26 Management Guidelines for Full-thickness Rectal Prolapse

Andrew P. Zbar, Hung Nguyen

Introduction

Given the profusion of surgical approaches in rectal prolapse, despite their history, there is currently no agreed-upon management strategy for this condition [1]. This situation, coupled with the unknown demographics of isolated full-thickness rectal prolapse or that combined with genital prolapse [2, 3], has been one of the stimulants for the ongoing PROSPER (PROlapse Surgery: PErineal or Rectopexy) trial being conducted in the UK. The trial, designed to recruit and randomise 1,000 patients, commenced in 2004 and separated short-term perioperative results and functional outcomes by comparing two main abdominal operations, abdominal rectopexy and resection rectopexy, with two principal perineal procedures, the Delorme mucosectomy and the Altemeier perineal rectosigmoidectomy. The prospective collection of this data will create the largest available randomised trial for surgical treatment of rectal prolapse in the adult. It will assess basic demography, risk factors, standardised defecatory function and quality of life. It was also felt the trial should at least provide raw postoperative morbidity and mortality data along with recurrence rates for the procedures, with some insight into the correlative physiologic derangements before and after surgery [4, 5]. The interpretation of this data is, however, likely to be comparatively difficult. There will be selective manometric, transit, and sphincteric morphologic information available, along with the less widespread expertise with the Altemeier procedure in the UK [6–8], inherent difficulties in functional equation of resectional with nonresectional procedures and a limited capacity for true case randomisation given the available patient cohort and its expected comorbidities [9].

Physiologic and Morphologic Preoperative Assessment Recommendations

There are no hard and fast recommendations concerning preoperative evaluation of patients presenting with rectal prolapse. Much of the management of children presenting with prolapse is conservative, and there is considerable benefit in determining broad colorectal transit in these patients where there is an underlying chronic constipation background [10]. There is also some evidence for basic pelvic ultrasonography in suspected cases of megarectum [11] combined with anal endosonography where the constitutive thickness of the internal anal sphincter correlates with rectal size and duration and severity of constipation symptoms [12]. In adult rectal prolapse, objective manometric and/or morphologic sphincter assessment is controversial but may serve as a medicolegally useful baseline in patients in whom there is substantial faecal incontinence and where, in particular, a perineal rectosigmoidectomy is contemplated [13, 14]. It is the authors' impression that preoperative absence of a significant rectoanal inhibitory reflex may be associated with poor functional outcome where a coloanal anastomosis is performed [15, 16]. However, this, too is unclear, as in cases where others have found similar disease-specific disturbances in rectoanal inhibition [17] but where there is little available evidence that preoperative manometry influences direct restorative proctectomy [18] or neorectal reservoir reconstruction [19]. These effects have not been age dependent, given the usually elderly cohort of patients undergoing perineal surgery for prolapse [20, 21]. It would seem logical to assess sphincter morphology before surgery in patients undergoing perineal surgery, partly as a continence predictor and possibly for prediction of recurrence where a case can be made in selected patients for concomitant sphincteroplasty or levatorplasty at the time of prolapse repair [22].

Managing Rectal Prolapse in Children

Most management in children is conservative, as rectal prolapse is commonly self-limiting. Nonoperative therapy may consist of intermittent laxative use with injection sclerotherapy, or occasional banding for circumferential mucosal cases. In children under 5 years of age, submucosal hypertonic saline has been advocated [23], whereas conventional injectable agents are used in older patients, with a comparatively low reinjection rate [24]. Prolonged follow-up of cases so treated shows this approach to be generally safe, with about a 10% recurrence rate over 2 years [25]. Decisions to operate on children for rectal prolapse are based on patient age and recurrence following conservative therapy, along with persistent, troublesome symptomatology, such as perineal pain, recurrent bleeding and perianal excoriation or the need for repeated manual prolapse reduction [26]. Recently, stapled prolapsectomy has been described for intractable cases [27].

Rectal Prolapse Recommendations in the Adult

Choosing the surgical approach in full-thickness adult rectal prolapse is dependent upon many factors, including patient age, attendant comorbidity, presence or absence of significant constipation (and sigmoid redundancy), admission of faecal incontinence, associated genital descensus, gender, body habitus and the surgeon's procedural familiarity and expertise. In general, coloproctologists will have their stock abdominal and perineal approaches, which may be modified in accordance with presentation, including some form of abdominal rectopexy in relatively fit patients and a perineal approach for those with worse performance status. Of the abdominal approaches, it would appear that mesh utilisation has disappeared in favour of a suture rectopexy [28, 29] and that that process is better performed to the lumbosacral disc by rectosacropexy rather than with presacral fixation [30, 31] – a lesson relearned since its original exposition by Cutait [32]. There is little difference between either the laparoscopic or the open approach, dependent upon surgical expertise [33–35]. Technical aspects of carrying the procedure to the territory of the lateral ligaments are probably moot [36, 37]: adequate dissection posteriorly to the levator plate and limitation of the anterior dissection through the fascia of Denonvilliers is adequate [38], with the impression that the laparoscopic suture rectopexy in male patients is superior given the 3-fold higher recurrence rate in men compared with women when open abdominal rectopexy is employed [39].

The choice for sigmoidectomy still seems to be based on a somewhat subjective assessment of the severity of attendant constipation and impression on contrast enema, computed tomography, colonoscopy or at surgery regarding the presence of sigmoid redundancy [40, 41]. It is recognised that in these circumstances, rectopexy alone can be associated with a high incidence of severe postoperative constipation. In patients without contraindication and with acceptable performance status and in the absence of prospective randomised data, this approach (as initially advocated by Frykman and Goldberg) appears today to act as the gold standard whether performed open or laparoscopically assisted [42–44].

For frailer patients with attendant comorbidity or chronic brain syndrome, in particular where there is substantial reproducible prolapse, a perineal approach has been favoured, with the main choices being between a Delorme-style mucosectomy or a formal resection and coloanal anastomosis. It is the authors' view that the very redundant prolapse lends itself to a perineal rectosigmoidectomy (and coincident sigmoidectomy), which is favoured when there is no substantial history of incontinence that will be aggravated by prolonged intraoperative endoanal distraction. This approach might be supported by the finding of disrupted sphincters on endosonography or manometric evidence of internal anal sphincter nonfunction. Utilisation of the harmonic scalpel and stapled coloanal anastomosis appears to reduce operative time and blood loss during perineal rectosigmoidectomy, although there is no demonstrable benefit on manometric variables or reported postoperative continence [45]. Both mucosal and full-thickness prolapse lend themselves well to a Delorme approach, which has very little attendant morbidity but is associated with a moderate short-term recurrence rate [46, 47]. In general, we do not favour the combined use of a transperineal levatorplasty with either procedure at the time of the first perineal operation for rectal prolapse, as correction of the full-thickness prolapse results in improvement in continence function in about two thirds of cases [48, 49].

Managing Recurrent Rectal Prolapse

Reported recurrence rates vary widely, and this is partly indicative of what by definition represents a recurrence where mild mucosal prolapse can be a relatively common finding after perineal mucosectomy [50] and where there is variable length and accuracy of follow-up. In nonrandomised analyses, there is general acceptance that full-thickness recurrence is less common following abdominal procedures, although most recurrences with both abdominal and perineal approaches tend to occur within the first year after surgery [51, 52]. Patient demographics such as age and gender provide little information concerning recurrence, although there is acceptance that actuarial recurrence rates exceed reported recurrence rates [53].

The purported causes for recurrence after abdominal and perineal approaches are speculative and are discussed in more detail elsewhere in this book. If preoperative formal anorectal assessment in primary cases is controversial, there is little data to support its use in recurrence, although it is advised to exclude organic colorectal pathology by colonoscopy and to perform broad-transit analysis in these patients. A trend in patients with prior perineal surgery in cases deemed fit enough for an abdominal approach is to perform an abdominal rectopexy, with the caveat of resecting an anastomosis if the prior procedure was an Altemeier operation. This is because nonresectional approaches appear to be associated with moderately high recurrence rates [54]. Moreover, failure to resect the previous anastomosis has been associated with significant morbidity from colorectal ischaemia. The impression is that provided the patient is fit for abdominal surgery, even a multiple repeat abdominal procedure is associated with a lower overall recurrence rate than secondary perineal surgery [52].

It has also been argued that repeat Delorme mucosectomy is technically more challenging [55], although this has not been the authors' experience. Patients should be warned, however, that recurrence after repeat perineal surgery is moderately high (up to 50%) on relatively short-term follow-up [56]. Here an alternative to consider is the Altemeier procedure in selected cases after a failed Delorme operation (an approach also advocated after an initial failed Altemeier resection in which anastomotic resection is part of the coloanal procedure). However, this can be moderately challenging, as considerable adherence may be encountered, which prevents adequate mobilisation and repeat tension-free anastomosis [57]. Data pertaining to functional outcome after reoperative surgery is lacking (both in terms of evacuatory dysfunction and faecal incontinence), and the occasional patient may be encountered who requires an abdominal proctectomy and end colostomy. Functional evacuatory results in some young patients undergoing reoperative prolapse surgery should be guarded, particularly where there is a significant psychiatric history [58].

Summary

It would seem logical in adults to morphologically assess sphincter integrity if presentation is with full-thickness rectal prolapse and faecal incontinence. If patients are deemed sufficiently fit, abdominal sacrorectopexy (either open or laparoscopic) is the procedure of choice, with resection rectopexy being reserved for patients with significant constipation, demonstrated delayed colonic transit and operative sigmoidorectal redundancy. Perineal procedures are reserved for frailer cases with significant comorbidity, and for males, where a Delorme mucosectomy is used for moderate prolapse and an Altemeier rectosigmoidectomy is utilised for extensive prolapse. The latter procedure is not employed when there is associated faecal incontinence, particularly when there is demonstrable sphincter disruption and internal anal sphincter dysfunction. In the absence of prospective controlled randomised studies, this decision is subjectively based on the length of the prolapse, although there is no real difference in resected bowel or mucosal lengths between the perineal operations. There is little data to support sphincteroplasty and/or levatorplasty at the time of the primary surgery. It is anticipated that earlier recurrence (however that is defined) is more common after a perineal procedure and that a secondary operation is selectively abdominal (with repeat anastomotic resection if that has previously been performed) when the patient's performance status permits, or by repeat mucosectomy in frailer cases. In the absence of an available evidence base, an algorithm for primary and recurrent full-thickness rectal prolapse in the adult is proffered in Figs. 1 and 2.

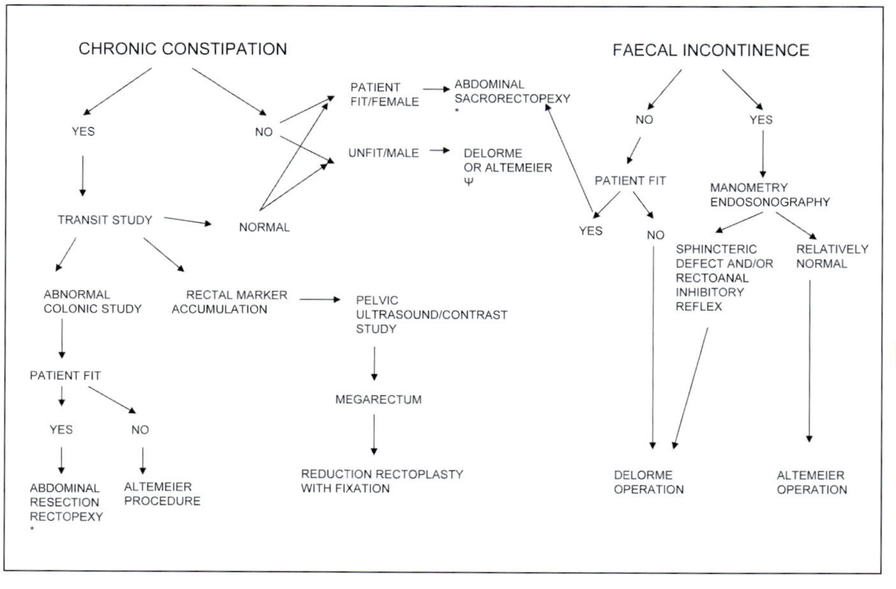

Fig. 1 Primary management algorithm for full-thickness rectal prolapse in the adult. * Procedure may be performed open or laparoscopically. ψ Either procedure may be primarily performed depending upon prolapse extent

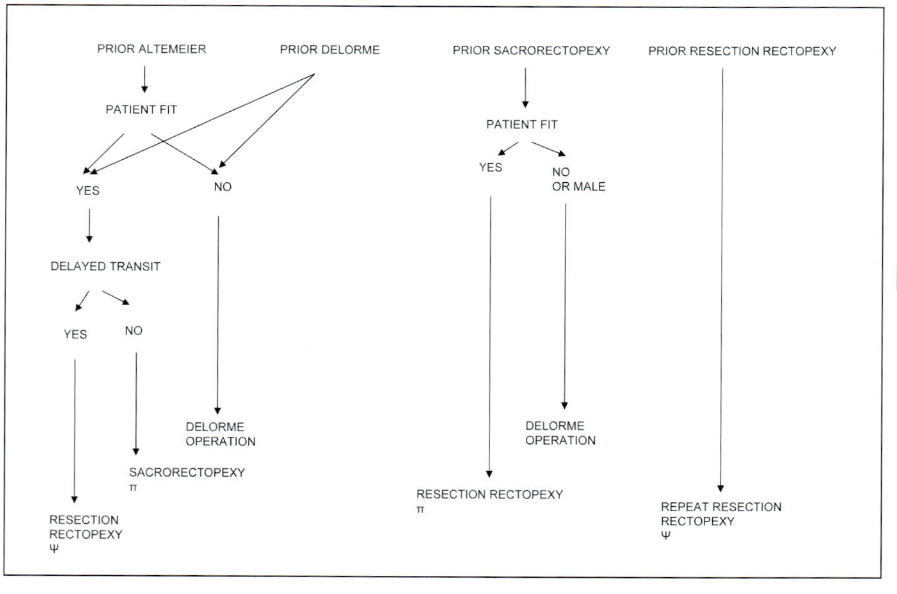

Fig. 2 Management algorithm for full-thickness rectal prolapse recurrence in the adult. Prior to treatment, colonoscopy and transit studies routinely performed. ψ Procedure should include repeat resection of the primary anastomosis. Π Procedure may be performed open or laparoscopically

References

1. Bachoo P, Brazelli M, Grant A (2000) Surgery for complete rectal prolapse in adults. Cochrane Database Syst Rev 2:CD001758
2. Kriplani A, Banerjee N, Kriplani AK et al (1998) Uterovaginal prolapse associated with rectal prolapse. Aust N Z J Obstet Gynaecol 38:325–326
3. Dekel A, Rabinerson D, Rafael ZB et al (2000) Concurrent genital and rectal prolapse: two pathologies – one joint operation. BJOG 107:125–129
4. Gray R, Jan S, Hills RK et al (2003) PROSPER: Association of Coloproctology of Great Britain & Ireland randomized trial of rectal prolapse surgery. Colorectal Dis 5 (Suppl 1):A 131
5. Jan S, Gross L, Senapati A et al (2005) Persistent benefits in bowel function and quality of life following rectal prolapse surgery – the ACPGBI PROSPER Trial. Colorectal Dis 7 (Suppl 1):A 234
6. Zbar AP, Takashima S, Hasegawa T, Kitabayashi K (2002) Perineal rectosigmoidectomy (Altemeier's procedure): a review of physiology, technique and outcome. Techn Coloproctol 6:109–116
7. Carditello A, Milone A, Stilo F et al (2003) Surgical treatment of rectal prolapse with transanal resection according to Altemeier. Experience and results. Chir Ital 55:687–692
8. Sailer M, Bonicke L, Petersen S (2007) Surgical options in the treatment of rectal prolapse: indications, techniques and results. Zentralb Chirurg 132:350–359
9. Phillips RKS (2004) Rectal prolapse – update on the PROSPER trial. Royal Australasian College of Surgeons Annual Scientific Congress: CR 33
10. Brown AJ, Nicol L, Anderson JH et al (2005) Prospective study of the effect on colonic motility in patients with rectal prolapse. Br J Surg 92:1417–1422
11. Singh SJ, Gibbons NJ, Vincent MV et al (2005) Use of pelvic ultrasound in the diagnosis of megarectum in children with constipation. J Pediatr Surg 40:1941–1945
12. Keshtgar AS, Ward HC, Clayden GS, Sanei A (2004) Thickening of the internal anal sphincter in idiopathic constipation in children. Pediatr Surg Int 20:817–823
13. Zbar AP (2005) The role of functional evaluation before anorectal surgery. Societa Italiana di Chirurgia ColoRettale 9:74–83
14. Glasgow SC, Birnbaum EH, Kodner IJ et al (2006) Preoperative anal manometry predicts continence after perineal proctectomy for rectal prolapse. Dis Colon Rectum 49:1052–1058
15. Zbar AP, Aslam M, Gold DM et al (1998) Parameters of the rectoanal inhibitory reflex in patients with idiopathic fecal incontinence and chronic constipation. Dis Colon Rectum 41:200–208
16. Zbar AP, Aslam M, Hider A et al (1998) Comparison of vector volume manometry with conventional manometry in anorectal dysfunction. Techn Coloproctol 2:84–90
17. Kaur G, Gardiner A, Duthie GS (2002) Rectoanal reflex parameters in incontinence and constipation. Dis Colon Rectum 45:928–933
18. Teleky B, Jech B, Karner-Hanusch J et al (2006) Straight and colonic J-pouch reconstruction after low anterior resection. Arch Chir Iugosl 53:109–112
19. Ho YH, Tan M, Seow-Choen F (1996) Prospective randomized controlled study of clinical function after low anterior resection: comparison of straight and colonic J pouch anastomosis. Br J Surg 83:978–980
20. Johansen OB, Wexner SD, Daniel N et al (1993) Perineal rectosigmoidectomy in the elderly. Dis Colon Rectum 36:767–772
21. Habr-Gama A, Jacob CE, Jorge JM et al (2006) Rectal procidentia treatment by perineal rectosigmoidectomy combined with levator ani repair. Hepatogastroenterology 53:213–217
22. Chun SW, Pikarsky AJ, You SY et al (2004) Perineal rectosigmoidectomy for rectal prolapse: role of levatorplasty. Techn Coloproctol 8:3–9
23. Shah A, Parikh D, Jawaheer G, Gornall P (2005) Persistent rectal prolapse in children: sclerotherapy and surgical management. Pediatr Surg Int 21:270–273
24. Sasaki Y, Iwai N, Kimura O, Hibi M (2004) The treatment of rectal prolapse in children with phenol in almond oil. Eur J Pediatr Surg 14:414–417
25. Fahmy MA, Ezzelarab S (2004) Outcome of submucosal injection of different sclerosing materials for rectal prolapse in children. Pediatr Surg Int 20:353–356
26. Antao B, Bradley V, Roberts JP, Shawis R (2005) Management of rectal prolapse in children. Dis Colon Rectum 48:1620–1625
27. Lee JI, Vogel AM, Suchar AM et al (2006) Sequential linear stapling technique for perineal resection of intractable pediatric rectal prolapse. Am Surg 72:1212–1215
28. Detry RJ, Vanheuverzwijn R, Mahieu P, Kestens PJ (1984) The use of prosthetic materials in rectopexies. Int Surg 69:301–304
29. Gourgiotis S, Baratsis S (2007) Rectal prolapse. Int J Colorect Dis 22:231–243
30. Loygue J, Nordlinger B, Malafosse M et al (1984) Rectopexy to the promontory for the treatment of rectal prolapse: report of 257 cases. Dis Colon Rectum 27:356–359
31. Khanna AK, Misra MK, Kumar K (1996) Simplified sutured sacral rectopexy for complete rectal prolapse in adults. Eur J Surg 162:143–146
32. Cutait D (1959) Sacro-promontory fixation of the rectum for complete rectal prolapse. Proc R Soc Med 52 (Suppl):105
33. Heah SM, Hartley J, Hurley J et al (2000) Laparoscopic suture rectopexy without resection is effective treatment for full-thickness rectal prolapse. Dis Colon Rectum 43:638–643
34. Solomon MJ, Young CJ, Eyers AA, Roberts RA (2002) Randomized clinical trial of laparoscopic versus open abdominal rectopexy for rectal prolapse. Br J Surg 89:35–39
35. Purkayastha S, Tekkis P, Athanasiou T et al (2005) A comparison of open vs. laparoscopic abdominal rectopexy for full-thickness rectal prolapse: a meta-analysis. Dis Colon Rectum 48:1930–1934

36. Speakman CT, Madden MV, Nicholls RJ, Kamm MA (1991) Lateral ligament division during rectopexy causes constipation but prevents recurrence: results of a prospective randomized study. Br J Surg 78:1431–1433
37. Mollen RM, Kuijpers HC, van Hoek F (2000) Effects of rectal mobilization and lateral ligaments division on colonic and anorectal function. Dis Colon Rectum 43:1283–1287
38. Nelson R, Spitz J, Pearl RK, Abcarian H (2001) What role does full rectal mobilization alone play in the treatment of rectal prolapse? Techn Coloproctol 5:33–35
39. Roberts PL, Schoetz DJ, Coller JA, Veidenheimer MC (1988) Ripstein procedure: Lahey Clinic experience 1963–1985. Arch Surg 123:554–557
40. Lukkonen P, Mikkonen U, Järvinen H (1992) Abdominal rectopexy with sigmoidectomy vs rectopexy alone for rectal prolapse: a prospective, randomised study. Int J Colorect Dis 7:219–222
41. McKee RF, Lauder JC, Poon FW et al (1992) A prospective randomised study of abdominal rectopexy with and without sigmoidectomy in rectal prolapse. Surg Gynecol Obstet 174:145–148
42. Frykman HM, Goldberg SM (1969) The surgical management of rectal procidentia. Surg Gynecol Obstet 129:1225–1230
43. Stevenson AR, Stitz RW, Lumley JW (1998) Laparoscopic-assisted resection-rectopexy for rectal prolapse: early and medium follow-up. Dis Colon Rectum 41:46–54
44. Carpelan-Holmström M, Kruna O, Scheinin T (2006) Laparoscopic rectal prolapse surgery combined with short hospital stay is safe in elderly and debilitated patients. Surg Endosc 20:1353–1359
45. Boccasanta P, Venturi M, Barbieri S, Roviaro G (2006) Impact of new technologies on the clinical and functional outcome of Altemeier's procedure: a randomized, controlled trial. Dis Colon Rectum 49:652–660
46. Agachan F, Reissman P, Pfeifer J et al (1997) Comparison of three perineal procedures for the treatment of rectal prolapse. South Med J 90:925–932
47. Pascual Montero JA, Martinez Puente MC, Pascual I et al (2006) Complete rectal prolapse clinical and functional outcome with Delorme's procedure. Rev Esp Enferm Dig 98:837–843
48. Pescatori M, Interisano A, Stolfi VM, Zoffoli M (1998) Delorme's operation and sphincteroplasty for rectal prolapse and faecal incontinence. Int J Colorect Dis 13:223–227
49. Serventi A, Sallustio P, Lobascio P, Binda GA (2005) Role of levatorplasty in total rectal prolapse treatment using a perineal approach. II. Joint Meeting ECCP/EACP SICCR Congress. Bologna A:155–157
50. DiGiuro G, Ignatovic D, Brogger J, Bergamaschi R: Rectal Prolapse Recurrence Study Group (2006) How accurate are published recurrence rates after rectal prolapse surgery? A meta-analysis of individual patient data. Am J Surg 191:773–778
51. Hool GR, Hull TL, Fazio VW (1997) Surgical treatment of recurrent complete rectal prolapse: a thirty-year experience. Dis Colon Rectum 40:270–272
52. Steele SR, Goetz LH, Minami S et al. (2006) Management of recurrent rectal prolapse: surgical approach influences outcome. Dis Colon Rectum 49:440–445
53. Raftopoulos Y, Senagore AG, DiGiuro G, Bergamaschi R: Rectal Prolapse Recurrence Study Group (2005) Recurrence rates after abdominal surgery for complete rectal prolapse: a multicenter pooled analysis of 643 individual patient data. Dis Colon Rectum 48:1200–1206
54. Fengler SA, Pearl RK, Prasad ML et al (1997) Management of recurrent rectal prolapse. Dis Colon Rectum 40:832–834
55. Nicholls RJ (2005) Combined ECCP/EACP Meeting Bologna Italy
56. Watts AM, Thompson MR (2000) Evaluation of Delorme's procedure as a treatment for full-thickness rectal prolapse. Br J Surg 87:218–222
57. Pikarsky AJ, Joo JS, Wexner SD et al (2000) Recurrent rectal prolapse: what is the next good option? Dis Colon Rectum 43:1273–1276
58. Marceau C, Parc Y, Debroux E et al (2005) Complete rectal prolapse in young patients: psychiatric disease a risk factor of poor outcome. Colorectal Dis 7:360–365

Subject Index

L

M

O

P

R

Printed in October 2007